LOCATING HEALTH: HISTORICAL AND ANTHROPOLOGICAL INVESTIGATIONS OF HEALTH AND PLACE

STUDIES FOR THE SOCIETY FOR THE SOCIAL HISTORY OF MEDICINE

Series Editors: David Cantor
                  Keir Waddington

TITLES IN THIS SERIES

1 Meat, Medicine and Human Health in the Twentieth Century
David Cantor, Christian Bonah and Matthias Dörries (eds)

FORTHCOMING TITLES

Medicine in the Remote and Rural North, 1800–2000
J. T. H. Connor and Stephan Curtis (eds)

www.pickeringchatto.com/sshm

LOCATING HEALTH: HISTORICAL AND ANTHROPOLOGICAL INVESTIGATIONS OF HEALTH AND PLACE

EDITED BY

Erika Dyck and Christopher Fletcher

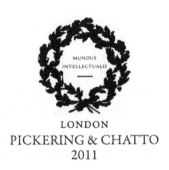

LONDON
PICKERING & CHATTO
2011

Published by Pickering & Chatto (Publishers) Limited
21 Bloomsbury Way, London WC1A 2TH

2252 Ridge Road, Brookfield, Vermont 05036-9704, USA

www.pickeringchatto.com

BRITISH LIBRARY CATALOGUING IN PUBLICATION DATA

Locating health: historical and anthropological investigations of place and
health. – (Studies for the Society for the Social History of Medicine)
1. Public health – Anthropological aspects. 2. Medical geography.
I. Series II. Dyck, Erika. III. Fletcher, Christopher.
306.4'61-dc22

ISBN-13: 9781848931497
e: 9781848931503

This publication is printed on acid-free paper that conforms to the American
National Standard for the Permanence of Paper for Printed Library Materials.

Typeset by Pickering & Chatto (Publishers) Limited
Printed in the United Kingdom at MPG Books Group, Bodmin and King's Lynn

CONTENTS

LIST OF TABLES

LIST OF CONTRIBUTORS

Hugo De Burgos is an assistant professor at the University of British Columbia Okanagan, was born and raised in El Salvador. He earned his BA at the McGill University; his M.A. from the University of Toronto; and his PhD degree at the University of Alberta. He has published three books of anthropology and history focusing on three colonial cities in El Salvador in a collection titled *City and Memory*, as well as several medical anthropology articles.

Erika Dyck is an associate professor and a Tier 2 Canada Research Chair in the History of Medicine in the Department of History at the University of Saskatchewan. From 2005–8 she was the Co-Director of the History of Medicine Program at the University of Alberta. She is the author of *Psychedelic Psychiatry* and is currently working on a history of eugenics in western Canada as well as a collaborating with a number of Canadian scholars, practitioners and former patients on the history of deinstitutionalization.

Alvin Finkel is a professor of history at Athabasca University in Athabasca, Alberta. His major areas of research are social policy history and labour history. His latest book is *Social Policy and Practice in Canada: A History* (Waterloo, Ont.: Wilfrid Laurier Press, 2006).

Christopher Fletcher is an associate professor in the Department of Anthropology at the University of Alberta. He received a PhD from l'Université de Montréal in 2002. His research interests include health and healing in northern Canadian Aboriginal communities, 'equivocal illnesses', the imbrications of place and culture, visual and sensory culture generally.

Maureen Lux teaches Canadian history at Brock University and is the author of *Medicine that Walks: Disease, Medicine and Canadian Plains Native People, 1880–1940*. She is currently researching the Canadian government's 'Indian Hospitals' established in the twentieth century.

Stephen E. Mawdsley is a PhD candidate at the University of Cambridge, United Kingdom. He has published on the history of poliomyelitis and the politics of immunization in twentieth-century America.

Sasha Mullally is assistant professor of History at the University of New Brunswick, where she teaches courses in Atlantic Canadian History, Women's History and the Social History of Medicine. Her article is taken from her forthcoming book *Unpacking the Black Bag: Country Doctor Stories from Canada and the United States, 1900–1950* (Toronto: University of Toronto Press).

Liza Piper teaches Environmental and Canadian history in the Department of History and Classics at the University of Alberta. Her research examines the rise of industrial resource economies across the subarctic, and the history of disease and climate in changing human relations to the natural world in the Northwest. Her book, *The Industrial Transformation of Subarctic Canada* was published with UBC Press in 2009 and won the Canadian Historical Association's 2010 Clio Book Prize for Northern history.

Jonathan Reinarz is Director of the History of Medicine Unit at the University of Birmingham Medical School. His research addresses the history of medical institutions, including specialist hospitals and provincial medical schools, from the 18th to the 20th centuries. His recent publications include *Healthcare in Birmingham: the Birmingham Teaching Hospitals, 1779–1939* (Woodbridge: Boydell Press, 2009) and *Permeable Walls: institutional visiting in historical perspective* (Amsterdam: Rodopi, 2009).

Mathew Smith is a Wellcome Trust research fellow at the University of Exeter's Centre for Medical History where he is studying the history of food allergy. His PhD, on the history of the Feingold diet and hyperactivity, will be published by Rutgers University Press in 2011. He is past winner of the Roy Porter Prize and the Pressman-Burroughs Wellcome Career Development Award. His essay in this volume is based on one that was awarded the 2007 Cadogan Prize by the British Society for the History of Paediatrics and Child Health.

Susan L. Smith is a professor of history at the University of Alberta in Canada. She is the author of *Sick and Tired of Being Sick and Tired: Black Women's Health Activism in America, 1890–1950* (Philadelphia, PA: University of Pennsylvania Press, 1995) and *Japanese American Midwives: Culture, Community and Health Politics, 1880-1950* (Chicago, IL: University of Illinois Press, 2005). She is currently conducting research on the human and environmental health consequences of military medical experimentation with mustard gas during World War 2 in the US and Canada.

Helen Vallianatos is an assistant professor in the Department of Anthropology, University of Alberta. Her current research interests include understanding migration experiences, and concepts of health and the body, through food memories, beliefs and practices. Recent publications include H. Vallianatos, *Poor and Pregnant in New*

Delhi, India (International Institute for Qualitative Methodology Series, Walnut Creek, CA: Left Coast Press, 2007), and H. Vallianatos and K. Raine, 'Consuming Food, Constructing Identities: A Symbolic Analysis of Diet among Arabic and South Asian Immigrant Women', *Food, Culture and Society*, 11 (2008), pp. 355–73.

Marko Živković studied clinical psychology and Japanese in his native Belgrade and social-cultural anthropology at the University of Chicago. He taught at Reed College in Portland, Oregon and is currently teaching anthropology at the University of Alberta in Edmonton. His main work is on the social life of stories and the national imaginary in Serbia, while he still maintains his old interests in the cross-cultural uses of imagery in healing and in Japanese intellectual history. He has lately ventured into anthropology of art and is particularly interested in exploring artistic practice as research and research as artistic practice.

ACKNOWLEDGEMENTS AND PREFACE

We are grateful to everyone who has helped this collaborative project come to fruition, it has been a long journey. The inspiration for this collection initially grew out of an interdisciplinary conference held in Edmonton, Alberta in October 2007. That conference, 'Putting Region in its Place' evolved out of a series of conversations, initially among a group of Canadian historians of medicine who had grown impatient with how scholars in that field were largely ignoring considerations of place and region in their studies. Chief among the original voices in these discussions were Chris Dooley and Kristin Burnett, who would later participate as key conference organizers. Our concerns originated from a tendency that we identified then as graduate students to undertheorize the use of 'region' or 'place' in historical analyses of human experiences. Regional analyses, within histories of medicine and health at least, seemed to suggest something parochial, local and perhaps even uncritical. As our own studies progressed, we became increasingly dissatisfied with this perspective and decided to look beyond our disciplinary and national borders for guidance.

Chris Fletcher broadened our thinking on this subject, especially by bringing an enthusiastic dose of ethnography and indigenous studies to these discussions. It became clear that medical anthropologists and medical historians shared certain subjective interests, but our methods for collecting and interpreting evidence differed, challenging us to think carefully about the edges of our own crafts. Over many lunches and countless coffees it became obvious to both of us that the more we came to appreciate the other's discipline, the more we were forced to define our own.

By 2006 the idea of organizing an interdisciplinary conference around the themes of health and place gained traction and we (Chris, Kristin, Chris and Erika) began searching for others who shared our sympathies for spatial analyses of health studies. The University of Alberta was a fertile environment for such collaborative pursuits. It isn't really clear why this western Canadian university attracts, or indeed stimulates, a higher number of researchers who are concerned with the role of 'place' in their work, though perhaps it is the institution's relatively northern, western and somewhat isolated environment that fosters a place consciousness. Perhaps too it is the relative newness of the city in vast space.

The original plan expanded from a historical pursuit to one that embraced other disciplinary perspectives. Shannon Stunden Bower and Nairne Cameron, both with geography backgrounds, pushed us in new directions as we entertained layers of urbanism, environmentalism and natural versus constructed concepts. Rob Shields, a sociologist with training in architecture and a theoretician of space, reminded us of ways to capture ideas about the utility of space by looking at its embodiment in architecture, without losing sight of the importance of human experience and sensory investigation within different environments. Our medical colleagues reminded us that regional concerns from their perspective introduced an entirely different set of connotations. Region, to the Canadian physician, connoted a particular distribution of health services, the political management of those services, and the competition that existed between urban and rural locations for access to health resources. In the medical and nursing faculties, colleagues bristled at the thought of tackling an issue as politically charged as 'region' and its connection to health; for them this word contained the trappings of the labour disputes, resource shortages, financial pressures and (un) coordinated services that fell within the jurisdiction of the regionalized health boards. In spite of the differences in vocabulary, it became abundantly clear that health and place existed in an abstract yet fragile relationship.

By 2007 our idea had grown from a few grumblings about the lack of regionally conscientious scholarship in medical history, to a more sophisticated articulation as to how health and medicine have been shaped by and experienced through local or spatial realities. The overwhelming response to the call for papers indicated that several others had been considering some of the same thematic intersections. Jonathan Reinarz in Birmingham welcomed the chance to bring a group of scholars from the United Kingdom to begin weaving together some of the historiographical territory that spanned the Atlantic. A number of students, researchers and administrators joined us from across North America, and whose research areas spilled into several different geographical regions and political jurisdictions from Nicaragua to Serbia, and from black women's health clinics in the United States to evaluating the environmental health of the Canadian North. Nearly 100 participants from two continents attended a three-day meeting. A number of strong themes emerged at that gathering, such as the ways in which place becomes shorthand for memory, nostalgia, culture and even sovereignty. Others engaged the subtle intersections between notions of health, authority, ethnicity and authenticity. This concept was perhaps best displayed in papers that explored Aboriginal health in North and Latin America. These authors examined colonial peoples both as bodies that had been acted upon by medicines authorized elsewhere as part of a colonial project, as well as individuals whose legitimacy as healers derived from a physical and spiritual connection with the local flora and fauna. This second category invoked discussions of memory, evidence and authority in ways that strengthened the value of interdisciplinary engagement.

The resulting collection is not merely a reconstruction of the papers presented at the conference, but rather a careful selection of studies that explored intersections of health and place along innovative lines.

We would like to draw special attention to the many people who helped put this collection together. We are grateful to the conference organizers: Pamela Brett-MacLean, Kristin Burnett, Nairne Cameron, Chris Dooley and Shannon Stunden-Bower. The exceptional talents and energies of the undergraduate and graduate students helped tremendously: Aaron Denham, Pieter de Vos, Matthew Eisler, Patrick Farrell, Nicole Freydberg, Meghan Horn, Roberta Lexier, Frances Reilly, Kaila Simoneau and Katherine Zwicker. We also received funding from the Social Sciences and Humanities Research Council, the Alberta Heritage Foundation for Medical Research, the Faculties of Medicine & Dentistry and Arts at the University of Alberta. At the University of Saskatchewan graduate students Amy Samson and Marc Macdonald chased up references and assisted with the copyediting process, while Caitlin Alton contributed to the editing and layout at the University of Alberta. Lastly, we are grateful to all of the authors who participated in this volume and to everyone who contributed to our ongoing discussions about the importance of considering place in our historical and anthropological analyses of health and medicine.

INTRODUCTION: HEALTHSCAPES: HEALTH AND PLACE AMONG AND BETWEEN DISCIPLINES

Erika Dyck and Christopher Fletcher

The essays in this book are concerned with the dynamic relationship between health and place. In presenting this collection we explore a selection of historical and cultural instances in which the multiple meanings of health and place intersect. Some of these are rooted in materialist or physical interpretations; others preface the role of sentiment and affect in place attachment and illness experience; and others still delve into ontological and subjective engagements that help us to understand how health and place connect with aspects of identity, authenticity and sovereignty.

These concepts acquire texture through their material presence; for example, the observable symptoms of disease, the institutions of medical practice, or the political or geographical boundaries that delineate a place. In terms of experience, behaviour is conditioned through health and illness and is further mediated by social context, local practices and resources. These concepts are also applied more abstractly; place becomes a plastic and ephemeral ingredient in the formulation of memory, in attitudes that culminate in response to historical injustices, or where health is interpreted through beliefs and practices that are profoundly shaped by ethno-cultural identities. Moving from a materialist analysis to a more abstract conceptualization destabilizes our understandings of health, place, and the interactions between the two, but also enriches our appreciation of how people respond to illness in rooted and constructive ways.

As we began assembling this collection it became clear that the terms health and place held different meanings across the disciplines. The subtle differences in substantive meanings escalated as we tried to reach consensus on the kinds of interpretive strategies necessary for developing more coherent definitions and analytical frameworks. At that point the methodological and conceptual gulf characterizing our respective disciplines emerged more clearly and encouraged us to rethink. Just as it was difficult to find common language through which historians and anthropologists discussed the role of place in health, it became clear that the conceptual worlds we occupied had also introduced different variables for defining these terms. For example, as we move from materialist analyses into the realm of interpreting cultural experiences we shift into different methodological territory and the historians' craft is sometimes stretched. Here especially, historians draw benefits from interdisciplinary dialogue with medical anthropologists, whose discipline offers a fundamentally different approach to interpreting culture. Where historians cherish a degree of distance from their subjects that time provides, anthropologists embrace a more intimate relationship with their subjects through close interaction in the present and, by default, in situ.

This book privileges historical and anthropological approaches to studying health and medicine. Both disciplines are in the midst of a renewal of theoretical and methodological frameworks for critically analyzing the role of location, place, or space in their work. For anthropologists fieldwork has always been paramount in methods grounded in participant observation. Historians often anchor their studies in locales, but temporal contexts frequently serve as the primary guide for evaluating subjects. Merely adding location to these disciplines introduces new risks. Simply borrowing terminology or approaches from geographers, for example, potentially threatens the integrity of extant disciplines, rendering them undisciplined. The challenge, therefore, and one that we attempt to address in this volume, is to develop fruitful interdisciplinary dialogue that respects the integrity of respective disciplines but also adds a level of methodological complexity that enhances rather than dilutes each craft.

Health: Construct and Experience

Health is formed, nurtured, lived and denied in places. Throughout the world people seek out places that provide the material conditions that foster physical health and that also offer spiritual, psychological, and existential solace. At the same time, the human condition in its physical and existential dimensions is profoundly shaped by health and disease. But, meanings ascribed to healthiness and unhealthiness are individualized and engender different socio-cultural responses. Medical anthropologist Allan Young has described a kind of language used for this scenario: disease is a biological entity knowable through science and acted upon by medicine, illness is the subjective experience of affliction by disease, and sickness is the social context of disease and illness.[1] An illness experience is closely tied to the physical and social ecology in which it occurs and, in turn, it accrues social meanings, which are read into the body of the afflicted. The presence of disease has a disturbing tendency to heighten the latent social divisions among and between peoples.[2] Disease may fracture the social body as it challenges the individual. Health and place are therefore profoundly linked constructs embedded in social practice with material repercussions.

Places are constructed in the literal sense of being built, organized and occupied in ways that affect health. Where one lives, with whom, and with access to what resources, influences health outcomes. The physical designs of cities, access to potable water, health services, food, and amenities contribute to, or detract from, individual, familial and social wellbeing. Places are also constructed in a figurative sense; they are produced through imagination, pieced together out of experiences, mythologized through historical discourse and through the metonymic roots of human heritage and lineage. Their meanings are manipulated and incorporated into social, political and identity formation processes. These kinds of attachments to place engender sentiments of social and political identity with significant implications for health in a juridical and emotional sense. The qualities of place are woven into notions of health in ways that localize health, disease and medicine, while often simultaneously leaving intact powerful renderings of scientific knowledge that relies upon a more universal discourse.

This conceptualization of the health-place dynamic forces us to confront the potential contradiction between individualized health experiences and the external characterization of health and disease categories. The former are highly subjective positions that draw on physical states of wellbeing, inter-subjective reflections on health and illness, social status and cultural dispositions. The latter emerge out of myriad factors tied to political, economic and scientific perspectives that collectively define access to resources. Such resources include adequate food supplies, medical services, housing and living conditions, economic opportunities, and legal recourse for negotiating rights within a defined juridical setting. These duplicitous conceptualizations of health thus have broad implications. Individuals are subsumed into social, political and economic circumstances, which are in turn historically situated and culturally constructed. Health, as a concept, therefore becomes both an experience and a commodity at the heart of which lays a fundamental contradiction that undermines our ability to casually apply the terms health and place with any expectation of a universal understanding.

The experience of illness is a challenge to individual autonomy and integrity. In its confrontation with normative bodily conditions, illness lends itself to unique insights onto the self and the world. Through sickness individuals and groups may examine their situation vis-á-vis others. Bodily experience can contribute to the realization of a critical social perspective on the production of disease and health disparities within society. In this sense, illness and sickness may illuminate the conditions under which disparities among and between peoples and places is produced and maintained. Thus, individual states of suffering extend outwards into social spaces affording unique perspectives on the otherwise taken-for-granted conditions in which people live. Health disparities are epiphenomena of other inequities and serve to orient attention to what may be diffuse, historically embedded discrepancies. Health disparities are embodied histories.[3] The distribution of health and illness within regional, national and global scales draws attention to the rooting of historical phenomena in the bodies and lives of people. Examples are found close at hand; regions in which the young leave for better fortunes elsewhere have the particular health profiles of an aged population; tuberculosis is nearly eradicated in southern Canada yet still widespread in the North; life expectancy among poor populations is less than the wealthy almost everywhere. And so it goes.

One poignant illustration of this kind of interaction emerges out of the apparent relationship among poverty, mental illness and homelessness. The occupation of what we might consider minimal spaces by the poor, mentally ill and destitute draws our attention to the rootedness of spatial notions in characterizing the health of communities and households through social statistics. The 'vacant' lot is 'home' to the homeless. Where a census tract consists of individual or collective dwelling – households – many lives are lived in impermanent spaces, rolled out at night, hostels and work camps, semi-serviced squatters settlements and so on. Locating health among the myriad of bodies that flow through these spaces speaks to coincident shaping of personhood, health and place.[4] As this example suggests, larger scales of political spatial reasoning may subsume specific places.

The relationship between health and place is recursive and inter-animating. We see evidence of this in how particular forms of experience gather elements of space together to form connotations of landscape/places/meanings. A simple example is seen in the individual and collective representations through which people are incorporated into a given locality and how that locality then serves to shape their identity. The analogy of spatial processes to embodiment has been made such that '... as places gather bodies in their midst in deeply enculturated ways, so cultures conjoin bodies in concrete circumstances of emplacement.'[5] Thus, building knowledge of the self that constitutes an experiential certainty of sensation and awareness is much like the process of coming to see and feel a place as familiar. Discursive, ritual and symbolic constructions serve to historicize a given people's place in the landscape and frame them within a moral economy of the human place in the world.[6] Just as the rhetoric of healthfulness may underpin place ideologies; affliction uproots one from the everyday of place-based experience. Thus, in conventional language, healing can be understood as a 'journey' or 'voyage' from illness to health. It is a cultural and physical act of re-placement, a process of finding new ground on which to stand.

Disciplinary Views

Health adds depth and texture to our understanding of the human condition, in a manner that demands an application of a variety of intellectual tools. Fresh attention to experience and authenticity amid trends of globalization draws us toward the local as a space of home, comfort and familiar while still distinct from the experiences in other regions. While the temporal dimension of health is an aspect that historians sometimes take for granted, anthropologists have argued that history itself is a cultural phenomenon.[7]

The language of health and place is thereby challenged and enriched by engaging in an interdisciplinary conversation that illustrates both the limits and the elasticity of these approaches. Place is tantalizingly present in *and* absent from both anthropology and history. Gradually this situation is changing, in part, as a result of increased interdisciplinary dialogue. The influence of geographers, in particular, has drawn attention to a need to consider place as it affects a number of developments, including scientific knowledge production, health practices, disease transmission, as well as their historical interpretations.[8]

Historical analyses provide scholars with an opportunity to examine snapshots, or developments frozen in time, ripe for sustained contextual analysis. Histories of epidemics, medical professionalization, medical theories or illness narratives have captured historical attention and allowed scholars to critically analyze and contextualize such developments through a long lens. Time or temporality in part defines the historians' approach but this feature is also subsumed into the analysis, enabling historians to evaluate change over time. Historical reflection thus relies on a degree of distancing between the observer and the observed.

In histories of health and medicine the temporal context is established at the historian's discretion, and often provides parameters for determining which contextual items are important for the analysis. Recent scholarship has identified a spatial turn in historical writing, suggesting that much like analytical categories of race, gender, and class, place too demands consideration within historical methodology.[9] However, this spatial turn often operates at odds with attempts at identifying universalizing trends, or ways of understanding knowledge production, discipline, and identity formation. Nonetheless, as scholars in this volume show, place – whether understood geographically, spatially, psychologically, environmentally, or experientially – often interrupts the historical narrative and therefore demands more sustained consideration as a methodological device.

Historical scholarship, whether part of the history of science and medicine or social history of health, has struggled to interpret the role of place in its analyses. Historiographically, we have often favoured methodological approaches that allow us to broaden our studies, whether they involve top-down or bottom-up examinations; place has often slipped off the analytical radar in an effort to minimize the risk of producing a parochial study with seemingly limited value. Nonetheless, recent political, economic and academic focus on the environment has given rise to new scholarship that considers nature, environment, and geography as an actor as opposed to an object. Some of those studies even go as far as to suggest a level of geo-determinism, which gives priority to the environment over human actions. Social and cultural historians and anthropologists may be reluctant to embrace this trend wholeheartedly, but have begun to acknowledge a more complicated set of interactions between humans and nature that condition culture.

This trend encourages linkages with geographers so that scholars might examine more closely how place interacts with people, bodies, and ideas. As David Livingstone has shown in a study of place and science, this intersection, and sometimes collision, locates or situates ideas that are often connected to a pursuit of universality.[10] Health emerges as a fruitful area for investigation as it allows interrogation at the level of bodies and experiences, areas that are shaped by culture, environment, and time. Yet attempts to locate these experiences often sit at odds with contemporaneous approaches, which seek to classify or diagnose illnesses in a manner that erodes the significance of place. In spite of the tensions that exist within this model, it serves to deepen our understanding of science studies, medical theory and ultimately illness experiences when we consider how local conditions mediate those developments. Adding place to the methodological framework, therefore, allows scholars to anchor their studies in lived experiences; it bridges theoretical perspectives with materialist investigations to produce studies that are cognizant of the way that broader, more fluid and historically-contingent concepts, such as nationalism, authenticity, discipline and authority condition individual experiences.

By contrast, anthropology tends to destabilize the notion of fixed categories, whether that pertains to moments frozen in time, or diagnostic labels. Time, region, illness, and health are all rendered contingent. It is common to situate all meaning as constructed, publicly available, and interpretable by the astute observer. Cultural meaning is omnipresent yet it remains contingent, indeterminate and flexible. In this view, meanings acquire social lives, suggesting that they are shared amongst people, but that they also shift over time and between places. The meanings, however, are never fixed; they evolve. Part of that evolution relies upon repetition whereby meanings gain traction but are also subject to being reformulated, fractured and merged like blobs of mercury skittering across a table.

For a long time, anthropology conflated place as synonymous with culture or incorporated it into scholarship as a formulaic 'context' segment without sufficient theoretical or ethnographic interrogation, when it was considered at all. In recent years this approach has shifted under the influence of some particularly insightful scholarship about place and culture generally. For instance, Feld and Basso's collection of *Senses of Place* struck a cord with its nuanced ethnography of human-place relations and the challenge it posed to scholars to think with places rather than about them. For these authors, human communities are intrinsically situated, and they acknowledge the power of place in the material, cultural, cognitive and affective lives of people everywhere.

Building in this tradition, several prominent critical medical anthropologists have focused on describing the social and cultural organization of power, which includes wealth and access to resources in the naturalization of the unhealthy conditions of so many of the poor and disenfranchised.[11] That work pushes the boundaries of health conceptualizations beyond the characterization of disease and its distribution into the social and political organization of inequity and social suffering. In this view it is simply not enough to examine disease as a biological entity with spatial dimensions. Rather it is incumbent that we consider the local environment along geographical and cultural axes and recognize its formative influence in understanding healthiness and unhealthiness.

Ontology: Health and Place

Culturally shaped notions of the 'self' are critical to understanding the diversity of ways in which people organize their relations to place, and in how they conceptualize and experience health. Subjectivity, the experience of selfhood, is a form of existential truth that defies the constructed nature of social life offering genuine knowledge instead. Changes in one's life circumstances are mitigated in the first instance by subjective interpretations, which support or challenge an individual's ontological security.[12] Cross-culturally a common subjective expression involves a deep symbolic, metaphorical and experiential association between the body, bodily states and the landscape. The profoundly entrenched conviction that one is part of a place and *vice versa* is especially explicit when people draw their livelihoods directly from the land, such as among farmers, horticulturalists, gatherers, hunters, or pastoralists. And yet as some scholars have pointed out, the kind of subjectivity that is rooted in a place is historically reminiscent of 'a unique kind of human autonomy that seems to have all but disappeared in the 'modern', industrialized world.'[13] The association between place and autonomy has been theoretically conceptualized as a remnant of a bygone era, an artifact of a pre-industrial period. In contrast, the modern form of self emerges out of Enlightenment philosophy as an autonomous, discrete, self-interested and economically rational one. This conceptualization in turn engenders new systems of social and economic organization, and produces new forms of knowledge on which self and society are reproduced.

The paradigmatic shift signaled by the Enlightenment and later established during the Industrial Revolution created fundamental changes in the way that science and technology acquired authority over the human condition. This slow transition has had profound implications for human autonomy and thus the significance of individual identities, experiences and places. In a sense, this Enlightenment-based conceptualization of the self shook the individual free from place. Within this framework western/industrial society became detached from place while, somewhat ironically, laying the conditions for an unprecedented phase of territorial and imperial expansion. Perhaps within this tradition we might also find the preconditions for globalization.

This model suggests that as individuals lose autonomy, they also lose a sense of place. Moreover they are subsumed into a larger collective before re-emerging as atomized parts of a new rational order that equates bodies with commodities, machines, tools, or more generally, components of an organized system, whether that is a system of medicine, justice, government, industry or production. Science, medicine and technology flourish in this setting and acquire heightened levels of authority and rationality while eroding place-based knowledge and human autonomy. Measures of health too are subject to this kind of atomization. Disease classifications, laboratory science, and medico-scientific knowledge derive out of a desire to produce rational, placeless or universal, results. Health or disease acquires status as an entity, removed from bodies and thus places. This interpretive approach has had considerable currency in post-modern and post-structuralist scholarship and yet, as this collection indicates, there is growing resistance to the implications created by linking human agency or autonomy with place. A more careful articulation of how place and experience co-mingle to produce agency is part of what this volume addresses.

Themes and Chapters

The places covered in this collection range geographically, from India to Nicaragua, to the United States, Serbia, the British Midlands, northern and western Canada. While the jurisdictions change, the articles highlight the importance of interrogating the nexus at which health and place interact to enrich our understanding of the social history of health and illness.

The collection begins with Helen Vallianatos' anthropological study of maternal health among poor women in India. These women negotiated changing health policies while the state entered a phase of national debt repayment at the end of the 20th century that resulted in dramatic changes to funds available for public health. By carefully teasing out strands of class or caste and gender and situating them within a particular community context, Vallianatos shows how identification with a specific place, along familial and geographical lines, fundamentally affected a woman's role in the community.

Jonathan Reinarz then offers an intriguing historical analysis situated at a contested intersection of the fields of science, medicine, geography and history. By knitting together these various disciplinary threads, Reinarz identifies a yet irreconcilable tension between place and organized medicine. Medicine, he demonstrates, has increasingly embraced science as a legitimizing feature of its practice, but scientific inquiry routinely measures its progress through the discovery of universal principles, or absolutes. As a result, science in effect erases place in a pursuit of generalizations. Having identified a countercurrent, Reinarz examines a community's resistance to this modernizing impulse. Sasha Mullally takes this discussion of modernity to a different place: the backwoods of Maine, where she examines the biography of a peripatetic doctor figure. In particular she illustrates how images of the region condition the doctor's experiences, memories, and finally his celebrity status within the community. Ultimately, however, the rural physician, untainted by accoutrements of modern medicine, emerges as a somewhat static feature of the environment itself, embodying the stereotypes of the region: rustic, simple, and rugged.

The next three authors provide an historical analysis of the health-place relationship with contributions that look carefully at how state policies influence actions, which in turn feed into ideological commitments to health and medical systems, along the axes of both research and delivery. Health becomes a concept through which success or progress is evaluated within a sovereign state; belonging to a nation, volunteering on behalf of national progress, or submitting a body for an ideological cause, each of these actions become expressions of a political identity which is understood through health. In these articles the temporal context of the Cold War emphasizes the ideological consequences of accepting a western view of health and, subsequently, progress. Children's bodies en masse, as Mathew Smith tells us, become contested sites for measuring American progress as their science skills are compared with Soviet results. The offshoot of this kind of brain race contributes to the pathologization of children's attention and activity into a medicalized disorder in need of psychiatric intervention. Health, in this context, becomes the embodiment of sovereign ideological values, while place expands to connote sentiments of nationalism, progress and superior values. Identification with place, in this case the United States, becomes a shorthand expression for a particular kind of health that is evaluated and maintained through adherence to a particular ideology. This kind of discursive relationship between ideology and place influences health care systems as well as medical experiments, as Finkel then Smith and Mawdsley elaborate.

Geography, environment or nature itself, operates as a force bringing health and disease. Moreover, belief or faith in the power of the environment to transmit disease, or conversely to offer cure, depends on identification with particular belief systems. In short, ethnic identity and aboriginality are examined in the next two essays as concepts that flow from attitudes towards health, disease, and healing. Belief in healing approaches forms part of an ideological position that feeds into conceptualizations of identity and ethnic authenticity. Bringing health and environment into sharp focus, Hugo De Burgos provides a nuanced examination of the delicate and dialectic relationship that exists between identity and territory, which then produces a culturally contingent understanding of illness and healing. In this way, De Burgos complicates the idea that place is a bordered, sovereign entity by questioning the authenticity of ethnic identity and by inter-rogating the notion of legitimately belonging to a particular place. Maureen Lux's article further explores these themes concerning the meanings of health that are associated with particular environments, but does so by concentrating on how western scientific medicine viewed particular environments as healthy for specific bodies. While De Burgos examines a Veracruceños approach to dis-ease construction and its treatment, Lux demonstrates how western medicine also incorporated aspects of this approach, and indeed used it as an extension of colonial practices of racial segregation and institutionalization in Canada.

The final two chapters explore health and environment, taking methodo-logical cues from environmental studies and geography and applying them to history and anthropology respectively. Liza Piper's essay examines the interplay of geography and disease in the Canadian north and uses case studies of cancer and tuberculosis to show how over time these diseases came to be understood as products of the environment, and their treatments were increasingly mediated by geography. External factors profoundly shaped the health dynamics in the nineteenth-century north through international traffic, travel, resource develop-ment and its associated environmental contamination and government policy. Indeed health services in the Canadian north reflected a lack of coordination and permanence that seemed to typify attitudes towards the northern commu-nities – resource towns home to transient populations of mixed descent – a place where the geographical environment dominated the flow of both parasites and hosts while minimizing efforts to create institutionalized health centres. Marko Zivkovic continues in this vein by examining the inter-relationships between environment and health in post-Milošević Serbia, but in contrast with Piper, Zivkovic examines places where the natural environment is coopted as a power-ful symbol of ethnic health and identity. Zivkovic examines 'places of power', which operate as symbolic tokens of identity along ideological, ethnic and healthful lines. The places, some of which convey an image of health shrines, also contain the trappings of a particular kind of Serbian identity, one that is a product of a specific time, place and 'ethno-eco' identity.

Collectively we hope that the papers in this volume will bring new perspec-tives to discussions on the recursive relationship between health and place, build opportunities for novel interdisciplinary dialogue and introduce methodologi-cal and conceptual avenues for future developments in this field. By locating our studies we aim to bring complexity to an understanding of historical and current cultural interactions. The essays in this volume provide new models for exploring the dynamic relationships between health and place as lived phenomena in ways that move beyond the use of static categorical terms.

1 PLACING MATERNAL HEALTH IN INDIA

Helen Vallianatos

When I began my work in India, I was struck by the incongruence between stereotypes of oppressed women and what seems like a powerful position attributed to them through the iconography of Hindu culture. Social statistics such as maternal mortality and morbidity rates, women's poor literacy and educational status, and the striking numbers of missing women observable in sex ratios[1] all point to women's inferior social position while the Hindu pantheon and the manifestation of these goddesses in living women (e.g. Indira Gandhi was often depicted as Durga) spoke to their esteem and power. These two images of women, as otherworldly and subjugated, point to the need for research on the women's social condition that considers their status within a cultural tradition of gender and the social-structural conditions in which lives are lived. The timing of my research, in 1999 and again in 2001, corresponded with significant political and economic changes as India embraced neoliberal economic policies, opening her markets to the world. I emphasize that knowledge of maternal health, or any health issue, requires an understanding of the local sociocultural milieu, in order to grasp how social structures shape 'local biologies'.[2] In other words, the biology of pregnancy and maternal health is not disconnected from the place where women's everyday life is performed, a place which also encompasses past life histories of individuals, communities, and the nation-state. Emplacing maternal health then requires deconstructing the spatiotemporality of place.[3] I do this here through examining how multiple forms of power are made sensible and contested, are emplaced and embodied. Because the body is critical to emplacement,[4] and how a lived body interacts with place is variable and subjective,[5] my analysis examines how healthy subjectivities are simultaneously shaped by adjustments and contestations towards structural power relations.

In this chapter I examine the health experiences of poor, pregnant women who lived in one particular *jhuggi-jhopri* community (squatter settlement) in New Delhi. I relate how women's food acquisition, preparation and consumption strategies during pregnancy, and in turn their health and well-being, is influenced by place – by their positionings in physical and social spaces at a specific time. Social spaces of gender, age and social status (class/caste) produce and reproduce inequities. Individuals are not merely passive receptacles inhabiting social spaces, but respond and resist in myriad ways, and in the process create unique places. Time here is situated both at a macro-level, historically situating global and national policies and programmes that affect the health of populations, as well as a micro-level, in consideration of women's reproductive histories and lived experiences. I begin by summarizing political-economic health and food systems in order to examine the factors affecting local health and foodways, and in turn how women's individual experiences of wellness is shaped by such macro-level conditions and their social status. I then narrow my focus to family structures, to examine how interpersonal relationships and familial spaces construct gendered healthscapes. Thus, through my examination of 'geopolitics of the body',[6] of the way political-economic and intrafamilial power relations and social inequities shape bodies and places,[7] I portray how individual women daily navigate food and health challenges while simultaneously embodying histories of places.

This paper presents a rethinking of the role of place in understanding maternal health. I had previously examined multiparous pregnant women's food-consumption practices, of how they navigated cultural food norms in light of their prior reproductive experiences, and the consequences on their nutritional and health status.[8] Here, I consider how maternal health is shaped by place, of how the broader political-economic environment interacts with local family contexts in formation of gendered (un)healthy bodies.

Methods and Context

Research in *jhuggi-jhopri* communities is fraught with any number of difficulties. Each *jhuggi-jhopri* community has unique demographic and cultural milieus. In this particular *jhuggi-jhopri* community, residents were predominantly scheduled caste Hindus, with a significant minority of Muslims who clustered within a particular spot of the settlement, and a few Christians sparsely distributed. Although most participants had resided in Delhi for approximately fourteen years, they traced their origins to northern Indian states, predominantly from Uttar Pradesh and Rajasthan. This is unlike other *jhuggi-jhopri* settlements, that may consist primarily of migrants from South India, or Nepal. Family connections were thus forged across spaces, as *jhuggi-jhopri* residents still had kinship ties to their natal and affinal villages. The joint or extended family is the ideal family structure in India. This household would include the father and mother, their sons, daughters-in-law and their children, and unmarried daughters. Ideally, resources are obtained and shared in an equitable manner. Yet, tensions may arise around dissatisfaction with the hierarchical everyday family relations and practices. Family hierarchies are based on age and gender. Consequently, to understand how maternal health is influenced by the domestic spaces they inhabit, I also interviewed men and elder women.

Interviews were conducted with forty husbands, spouses recruited from the 154 women participants. In addition, three focus group discussions, each with five to seven mothers-in-law, were also completed. Interviews were conducted in Hindi, with the aid of a research assistant – a man for the husband interviews and a woman for the mother-in-law interviews. Interviews with the husbands were conducted in their homes, while mother-in-law focus group interviews were conducted in 'community centers' to accommodate the group. Both Muslim and Hindu family members participated; almost a quarter (23 per cent) of the husbands who were interviewed were Muslim while a third of the mothers-in-law (one focus group) were Muslim. Two-thirds of the husbands lived in a nuclear household. The husband sample mirrored the basic demographic characteristics of the woman participants. Focus group discussions with mothers-in-law were conducted according to area of residence (block), and one focus group was conducted in the block where most Muslims lived.

Political-Economic Spaces

In 2001, 13.8 million people lived in the national capital territory of Delhi.[9] An astonishing number – more than 45 per cent – lived in *jhuggi-jhopri* communities or other unauthorized and unplanned settlements.[10] In the particular squatter settlement where I worked, 50,000 people lived within four square kilometres. Resources and sanitation were inadequate. Untreated sewage and other garbage accumulated in open spaces contaminating the water where livestock slacked their thirst and, during the monsoon floods, where children played to escape the heat. These conditions enabled the spread of infectious diseases, including cholera. Drinking water was available at block hand pumps; however few blocks had working pumps. Furthermore, water was available only twice a day due to the times when electricity was available for pumping water. The result was long lines at working water pumps, as women and often children waited in queues to fill multiple containers. The daily organization of time was heavily structured around the sources of water and served to emphasize the precarity of life in the *jhuggi-jhopri*. In the summer, when water and electric shortages were particularly problematic, the Government of Delhi sent water trucks to provide residents with water. Within the settlement, there was the odd food store, as well as a meat market within the Muslim block. Just outside this squatter settlement, both food and health resources were available. There was a small produce market, consisting of about ten vendors, in addition to the roving produce vendors. Government stores providing dairy and staple grains (the latter called 'fair price shops', described in more detail below) were also within a couple of blocks. Both voluntary non-governmental and private health care clinics were located on the outskirts of the community. Dispensaries, or pharmacies, providing both allopathic and Ayurvedic medicines were within walking distance. Furthermore, unauthorized health practitioners (i.e. those without recognized qualifications) were practising both within and outside this community. Thus in this particular *jhuggi-jhopri* settlement, there was a relative plurality of resources. Arguably the most restricted access was for water. A variety of food and healthcare options existed, although access was of course limited according to financial means.

Those living in the marginal poverty of the ad-hoc social and economic space of the *jhuggi-jhopri* are particularly vulnerable to challenges arising from changes in the political-economic socioscape. One of the major impacts on the provision of government social services has been the implementation of structural adjustment programs (SAPs), which began in India in 1991, with further economic liberalization ensuing in 2001. India's debt burden in 2001 accounted for 20 per cent of the gross national product.[11] Countries that borrow money from international lending agencies, like the International Monetary Fund (IMF) and World Bank divest themselves of power over macroeconomic policy and are required to follow specific loan conditions, designed to ensure a return on the investment for the lenders. These conditions include tightening of government budgets (with resulting cuts in social services), exchange rate adjustment, deregulation, privatization, and an increased shift towards an export-oriented economy. Such economic policies can have severe consequences for the poor. The negative consequences of such policies from the perspective of those living at or near poverty has been documented not only in South Asia, but throughout the world.[12] Here, I summarize[13] how healthcare and food security affected the lives of individuals in one locale. I hope to contribute to a person- and family-centred understanding of the global and local dialectic of poverty, policy and agency.

The foundation for health services in independent India was based on the Bhore Committee's (1946) report, which recommended universal health coverage, provision of healthcare to rural areas through primary care centres, outlined plans for dealing with diseases and population growth, and inclusion of non-biomedical practitioners in the health system.[14] A number of committees were formed thereafter, including the Jain Committee (1966), the Kartar Singh Committee (1974), the Srivastava Committee (1975), and the ICMR-ICSSR Joint Panel (1980), but all emphasized the importance of universal health coverage.[15] The core of such a health system was primary health centres, imagined not only as a means of provisioning health services to the masses, but simultaneously gathering information on local needs and issues that would in inform future national health policies and programmes.

This feedback system of incorporating local voices in national policies is not isolated from the influence and agendas imposed by SAPs and donor agencies. Even before implementation of SAPS, neoliberal international development policies of the 1980s shaped healthcare in India through changes in funding donor agencies and their priorities. The major funding sources for health programmes became the World Bank and the Asian Development Bank, as opposed to country- or religious-based aid organizations.[16] This shift in funders resulted in changes in health policies and priorities, including alterations in which diseases get funding, as well as reallocation of funds from services and infrastructure towards training, supplies and research.[17] In light of these changes in funding and priorities, it has been argued that health sector reforms 'have become instruments to promote markets rather than a means to improve the health sector and ultimately, health'.[18]

Following implementation of SAPs conditions in 1991, the Government of India diminished its grants to state governments for the health sector by 6.7 per cent and by 2001, national government expenditure on public health services accounted for only 0.6 per cent of the gross domestic product.[19] The arguable outcome is heavy reliance on the private and voluntary sectors – and this has substantial ramifications for families living at or near the poverty line, such as inequitable access to care (e.g. many private facilities congregate in spaces serving wealthier clientele while voluntary facilities are dependent on potentially insecure donor funds). The push towards increased reliance on voluntary and non-governmental organizations has also been supported by the World Bank.[20] It was estimated that approximately 7,000 voluntary organizations provide health services in India.[21] State governments that are financially unable to continue, let alone improve public health services, hand over responsibility for healthcare to non-governmental organizations (NGOs). Government control remains in that grants are provided to the organizations for their expenses and user fees may be fixed at state government levels in order to (attempt to) ensure universal access.[22]

A key aspect to SAPs is the emphasis on exports in order to earn money to repay loans and for many countries including India, there is pressure to reallocate agricultural lands to produce commodities for export. Concurrently, hunger and malnutrition continue to be problematic.[23] The Public Distribution System (PDS) is the Government of India's primary means of providing food security. The PDS supplies wheat, rice, sugar, edible oils and kerosene at subsidized rates to consumers via 'fair price shops'. Because of the recognition that those in need were not obtaining access to foods through the PDS, it was revamped in 1997 to target the 'poorest of the poor'. The central government allocates food staples to state governments according to a formula enumerating the number of families living below the poverty line (BPL), plus each state's average need in the past ten years for families living above the poverty line (APL). Families who were BPL received 10 kg per month of wheat and/or rice at a highly subsidized rate.

While this description suggests substantial assistance for the poor, the reality was less auspicious. Since the introduction of the TPDS in 1997 until 2001, the Delhi government had not used any of its allotment from the federal government for BPL families.[24] Fair price shops charged higher prices than those fixed by the Government, so in Delhi, in contrast to the national PDS subsidized prices for rice and wheat of Rs. 6.1 and 4.65 per kg, average prices for these two staple foods were Rs. 10 and 9 per kg respectively.[25] Furthermore, the allocation of 10 kg per BPL family was irrespective of family size – and larger families are more often poorer than families smaller in size.[26] In fact, it is argued that the PDS throughout India has been weakened in the 1990s in large part due to implementation of liberalization policies. Evidence for this is the decrease in tons of food grains distributed (the highest distribution was in 1991), and the reduced price differential for grains between fair price shops and open markets.[27]

The Government of India is responsible to the people of India but must also balance this against its obligations of loan repayments. To provide more social assistance would cost money, and governments are required to slash expenditures. To make loan repayments, exports must be increased, which in turn means substitution of domestic food crops for export cash crops. This negatively impacts people, especially the poor, who have limited funds to purchase foods and who had relied on foods that were locally cultivated.

With this general overview of the global and national structural conditions facing India in mind I will turn to the squatter settlement in New Delhi where I undertook fieldwork to examine how access to food and health manifested in this place.

Emplacing Maternal Health I: Social Class Shaping Meanings/ Experiences of Place

Living conditions in squatter settlements are difficult. In addition to the unsanitary and crowded living conditions, funds are always limited, exacerbating nutritional stress and relatively frequent illness episodes. The public, private and voluntary sectors each provide for some healthcare services amongst the poor in Delhi to varying degrees of success. The number of institutions providing medical care in Delhi has consistently grown, to a total of 1596 in the beginning of 2002, with the vast majority (91.6 per cent) of health services provided through the private and voluntary sectors.[28]

The predominant role that the private and voluntary sectors play in healthcare delivery in Delhi exemplifies the effects of liberalization policies outlined in the previous section. Where I worked, all study participants utilized local private or non-governmental health services. Government-provided services in the immediate locality were rare, comprised only of the occasional maternal and child health clinics, immunization programmes, or technicians monitoring water quality (e.g. for malarial parasites). The main government public hospital was approximately eight kilometres away, necessitating a trip by bus or autorickshaw.

The cost of healthcare was a common concern. Residents complained about the minimal cost differences between seeing medical practitioners at voluntary versus private clinics. Private health care was available for as little as Rs10 or 20 more than the cost for access to one of the NGO clinics serving the *jhuggi-jhopri* community. Many community members seemed to have very different perceptions of the appropriate cost of healthcare to NGO expectations. NGO administrators had developed a payment scheme, which to them was a reasonable amount to charge for care, and that would make healthcare provisioning sustainable. The fact that the cost of care at this facility was a very common complaint raised by various community members suggests that an incongruity exists between at least some members of the community and the NGO officials on perceptions of affordable services.

Complaints about the cost of care in the voluntary versus the private sectors expressed more than concerns over costs of healthcare. They also situated perceptions of difference about the quality of care inherent to the two systems. I heard many people of different walks of life articulate that better healthcare is provided by private practitioners (a perception that has been reported for other places in India).[29] Any service or programme that is geared towards the poor was commonly viewed as inferior. What was commonly perceived to be lower quality of care provided at government-funded institutions was carried over to assumptions of health services at voluntary clinics.[30] Consequently, if people paid money for healthcare, they might as well have gone to a private doctor. This assumption is linked to broader issues of social hierarchies, where social position (class and caste) shapes access to resources and meanings of health-provisioning places.

The government hospital was commonly considered by all social strata to be a dirty, unkempt place, with overworked and insensitive medical personnel, which provided indifferent and inferior care. I was often told of the fear women had of having to go to the hospital to give birth. On top of the stress of travelling to a hospital because of an emergency (otherwise childbirth would have proceeded at home), women feared being turned away because of lack of facilities (especially beds – there were 198 beds in the obstetrics ward), the difficulty and expense of having to provide their own supplies (e.g. blood), and the treatment they would receive at the hands of medical personnel. Economic liberalization policies dictate a decrease in government expenditures, and infrastructure has suffered with shortages in supplies, facilities, and staff in public hospitals.[31] The public health socioscape is shaped by macrolevel policies that in turn construct the public's imaginings and experiences of publicly funded health care.

Just as health spaces were shaped by political-economic socioscapes, so too were local foodscapes. Recall that the implementation of the PDS, providing food assistance, had been problematic. To improve the system, the Government of Delhi issued a call for applications for ration cards for BPL families in 2001. Eligible beneficiaries would then receive new ration cards, but at a cost of Rs10 per card.[32] I heard a number of complaints about the hassles of getting these new ration cards. The actual cost of the new cards was four times higher, because residents had to incur extra costs for acquiring the form and identification photographs, having the form filled out (since the vast majority had limited literacy), and postage stamps. More information was required from applicants for these new cards, and if this was not provided, the card was not issued.[33] Furthermore, only those who owned their hut were eligible to apply for the new card; those who rented their home were ineligible for the service. The kinship dynamics of the extended family also impacted on access to the cards. In extended families which had divided and the elder parental generation retained control of the card, the younger segment of the family lost access to subsidized staple foods. Arguably those who needed it most were not able to access the government's scheme to provide food assistance. The eligibility rules for card ownership suggest the cards functioned as a place-making tool; a way of connecting with and demarcating where one belonged. Not having a card not only affected access to food assistance but also place identification questioning the non-card holders belongingness to the *jhuggi-jhopri,* in a political sense. Without this card, one's 'citizenship' was unproven. This in turn had wide-ranging effects on the resources and services available to families including education (to register children, one had to show their ration card) as well as subsidized food.

Owning a ration card would seem desirable for the food assistance it is intended to provide but this was not necessarily the case. The prices between the fair price shops and the open market were similar and the local fair price shop charged more than the government values.[34] Thus, the degree of economic assistance in this locale was minimal. Furthermore, people frequently preferred to purchase foods at the open market, just as they would try to utilize private healthcare when possible. Just as public health care was viewed to be of poor quality, so to were the subsidized foods available to those living in poverty. The PDS foods, particularly rice, were viewed as 'dirty,' not fit for human consumption. Similarly, in the local produce markets, different qualities were available, with the lower quality produce being anywhere between Rs2 to 10/kg cheaper.[35] Dirty or not the discourse on food and healthcare services point to a stigmatization of these services in line with the marginal position of the residents of the *jhuggi-jhopri.* This demonstrates that national and state government policies were variably implemented, constructing local healthscapes and foodscapes that mirrored structural power relations.

Thus, the health and food options available to women and their families of this squatter settlement were shaped by global and national forces that played out in a spatiotemporally specific manner, evident in the place-specific quality and cost of healthcare and food. How people interpreted and coped with these healthscapes and foodscapes, how they embodied experiences of place, is the focus of the following section.

Emplacing Maternal Health II: Gender & Age Dynamics in Domestic Spaces

Everyday experiences of womanhood are emplaced not only within a political-economic context, but also within domestic spaces. The family provides a key social site for situating self and connecting with others. Extended families – the ideal family structure – are constructed on age and gender hierarchies. The youngest daughter-in-law is in a tenuous position within the family, especially before motherhood and the birth of sons. A woman's position rises not only with the birth of sons, but as she ages, and she too becomes a mother-in-law, making decisions on household allocation of resources, and influencing family dynamics. Thus, men hold higher status than women and older women dominate younger women. Evidence of women's status within the family is seen through both food and health practices.[36] While they occupy a subordinate position, young women are not entirely powerless, for their position is affected by their education and their abilities to contribute to family status and well-being, as well as idiosyncratic interpersonal relations. This general description of gender and age hierarchies veils the range of women's lived experiences, of how domestic spaces are negotiated and experienced by 'bodies-in-place'.[37] Gender and age-based family hierarchies are not immutable, but rather materialize in place. A place-centred analysis of family power dynamics reveals the variable nature of intrafamilial relations.[38] I now consider how women negotiate and resist power relations within their local domestic spaces. To understand how interpersonal positionings within domestic spaces influence women's health during pregnancy, I examine how knowledge on maternal health was constructed by family members, and how in turn this might affect resource distribution within households. By examining husbands' and mother-in-laws' voices, in addition to experiences of motherhood shared by women, a more contextualized understanding of women's 'local biologies,' of body and health practices in specific places are explored.

In the study community only about a third of study participants lived in the traditional extended family structure. This is not surprising, because despite the idealized extended family structure, in reality most Indians live in a nuclear family structure, particularly those living in poverty and in urban spaces.[39] How then is the local biology of maternal health shaped by unequal power relations? To examine this issue, I discuss reproductive decision-making and dynamics of food consumption within the household, followed by a brief overview of maternal health.

Both men and women shared their desire to have male and female children. Having at least one son was certainly important, as has been well documented in previous studies in other locales.[40] There were families, both Hindu and Muslim, who continued to have children in order to have a boy. But having a girl is also important, as a Hindu man with four children remarked, 'I wanted a girl, but had three boys. Now, I have a girl, and that is enough.' Thus, having children of both genders is valued. It is more problematic when there are many girl children, as the economic cost of dowries becomes a concern for both Hindu and Muslim families.

While everyone desired children of both genders, the decision-making around reproduction was not equitable. Husbands' desires predominated, and husbands took responsibility for family size, by either admitting that they kept having children to meet desired gender distribution and deciding when to stop, or that it was their 'mistake' in having larger than desired families, which they ascribed to a lack of knowledge about family planning methods. Women's bodies, then, were not their own, for they represented the means of propagation for the husband's family. Women's desires and reproductive capacities could be subsumed by the family to meet the family's needs – as defined by the head of the family (usually husband or father-in-law). For instance, one thirty-two year old woman, pregnant for the seventh time (but who had only three living children; two girls and a boy), was essentially forced to carry through with her seventh pregnancy because her in-laws desired a second grandson. Having only one grandson was considered to be too risky. This woman's lack of control over her own body (and of the concurrent stresses associated with yet another mouth to feed), was expressed through her subjective experience of her pregnant body. She had described her lack of well-being, and her concerns for the future, through her body: 'lots of discomfort, weakness, more discomfort in this pregnancy. I'm angry about this pregnancy, the stress of having this child, [of the] greater responsibilities and financial stress.' But a husband's family size desires could also be subordinated to his parents' concerns, as in the case just described, where the woman's husband also did not wish to have yet another child, but ceded to his parents' wishes.

Because women's reproductive capacities are frequently placed in the family's interests, I was interested to see how their food and health practices were (or were not) controlled by higher-status family members as well. A number of studies in India have documented food proscriptions during pregnancy.[41] These food proscriptions are believed to affect the well-being of both fetus and mother, and breaking these taboos could have dire health consequences, including miscarriage. But how were such proscriptions interpreted by family members who could influence or shape women's food consumption?

Only 10 per cent of the men indicated that pregnant women did not need to eat differently. The vast majority (77 per cent) of men described the appropriate pregnancy diet as 'green vegetables, fruits, milk and *dāl* (lentils).' These foods were commonly seen as health-promoting, good sources of protein and vitamins, and would 'make blood.' Anemia was commonly described as weakness by women and so it is not surprising that husbands were interested in health promoting foods that would strengthen and increase the blood of the mother, and in turn support the health of the fetus. More interesting is that a few men (eight, or 20 per cent) recommended eating meat, while only one man indicated that a pregnant woman should not eat meat. This is fascinating because meat is considered to be a 'hot' food, and such foods are proscribed during pregnancy.[42] Mothers-in-law unanimously considered 'hot' foods items to be avoided during pregnancy, as this was a cause of miscarriage. However, mothers-in-law recognized that food consumption would also be affected by season, so in the winter, 'warm' foods would be acceptable. When compared to their husbands female elders had a more nuanced and deeper understanding of humoral categories and relations to food proscriptions. In my previous work on local food constructions, I found that while women were aware of humoral food categorizations, and that one should avoid 'hot' foods during pregnancy, there was little agreement on categorization of foods within this system.[43] Thus, it appears that it is through elders, particularly mothers-in-law, that such knowledge is propagated within the family. I also observed this to be the case, as demonstrated when a pregnant daughter-in-law would be stopped by her mother-in-law from partaking of a food item categorized as 'hot', such as papaya, that others were sharing – and from my perspective the daughter-in-law appeared willing to consume some of this fruit had she not been stopped. Thus, I suggest that with so many women living in nuclear family structures in this squatter settlement, away from the everyday dietary oversight of their mother-in-laws, they had greater freedom to interpret dietary prescriptions and proscriptions.[44] This is supported by my earlier work, which showed that women's food consumption during pregnancy did involve experimentation and decisions based on their embodied reproductive histories.[45] Furthermore, living in an urban area provided opportunities to gather and exchange knowledge from a diverse array of sources, including neighbors, television, and community health workers. For example, through discussion with neighbors, one would hear how other women behaved, what other women ate in other parts of India, and some women would use this as a justification for their own eating practices, for 'if it did not harm those women, how then could it be bad for me?' Thus, the family emplacement of these particular pregnant women provided a discrete context for management of their own food practices and pregnant subjectivities.

Even though husbands seemed to have little awareness of 'hot' food proscriptions, they did have well established ideas of what constituted good foods for pregnancy: vegetables, fruits, milk and lentils. Although most husbands (~55 per cent) stated that these were their own ideas, and that they had not ever learned anything about dietetics during pregnancy, a significant percentage (30 per cent) acknowledged their elders as their sources of information. This again points to the importance of intergenerational communication in the joint household in transmitting cultural information including folk dietetics. With nuclear households common amongst the urban poor, the knowledge networks between generations of the family are at least partly curtailed. For husbands in a nuclear family, their status as head of the family (rather than their father), gives them a position of authority, even on food consumption patterns. A number of men (42 per cent) indicated that their wives eat according to their own ideas, for her welfare and the health of the baby, as shown in the words of these husbands:

> Yes, she does eat the food I think she should eat; if she doesn't eat this way she won't live long. [father of two children, living in a nuclear Muslim family]
>
> She should take light food like khichiri,[46] moong dāl[47] and green vegetables. She shouldn't eat spicy foods; such hard food can be harmful to the child. [father of two children, living in a nuclear Muslim family]
>
> She should eat green vegetables, milk, fruits – coconut milk mostly. By eating all of this she will not become weak. ... she eats the foods I think she should eat because they are necessary for her health [father of four, living in a Hindu joint family]
>
> During pregnancy she should eat less, but it has to be good and healthy food; if she were to eat more food, she will have problems, and the child too, like the child growing in an unhealthy way [father of one, living in a Hindu joint family]

The last quote above shares a sentiment that was more commonly voiced among husbands – over a third (37.5 per cent) of the husbands indicated that during pregnancy, women ought to not consume too much food, as this could cause harm to the fetus, or cause the baby to grow too big, making birth treacherous. This would suggest that pregnant women's food consumption would be restricted in these households, with potential health consequences. Previous research in other parts of India has documented the concept of 'eating down,' of restricting food consumption during pregnancy.[48] Yet many men (50 per cent) thought that there should be no difference in the amount of food women consume during pregnancy compared to when non-pregnant. A significant minority (25 per cent) suggested that women should increase their food consumption during pregnancy as a way to avoid weakness and improve the health of mother and child. The diversity of opinions voiced by husbands underscores the importance of understanding domestic spaces, of how cultural food and health norms are digested in specific spatiotemporal contexts, shaping how maternal bodies are produced and managed.

Maternal bodies are not simply wrought in a hierarchical domestic space, but in negotiation and resistance, women create their own embodied experiences. In many nuclear households, it seems women have relative freedom to make their own dietary choices. Women are traditionally depicted as subservient to their husbands, as evident in meal seating and serving patterns and the quantity and quality of food consumed.[49] Yet despite some men indicating that women should eat after men have taken their fill, it was common for husbands and wives to eat together in this community. Many women modified their dietary habits according to their own ideas and past reproductive experiences.[50] Thus, the dynamics between husband and wife were not that of a simple hierarchy, but rather contingent on everyday practices within a range of family contexts and the idiosyncrasies of the individuals involved.

Health of pregnant women is also shaped by gender roles and responsibilities. Women participants defined themselves as 'housewives'. Part of these domestic responsibilities required heavy physical labour (elaborated upon below). The primary gender role that men articulated was as economic providers for their families. Most men equated economic provisioning with happiness, an association that cut across religious affiliation and family organization differences, as evident in these quotes:

> Men should earn the money [needed] to take care of his family. [In this way] he should give happiness to the family. [Muslim man, living in a nuclear family]
>
> Husbands should earn the money and take care of the family, and [so] should bring happiness to the family. [Muslim man, living in an extended family]
>
> Men should take care of their family, earning money for happiness and to maintain the house. [Hindu man, living in an extended family]

Yet earning money was a challenge for these men, as one Muslim man reflected that 'the husband should provide education to his children if possible, and he should earn the money, although nowadays it is very difficult to earn money'. Most were daily labourers, selling their bodies, their strength, for small earnings. On average, monthly household incomes were Rs2564 (US$ 56.98 in 2001) – hovering around the economic poverty line as defined by the Government of Delhi.[51] Recall that the men who were interviewed emphasized their roles as family providers. How then, is their identity affected when not able to meet the basic needs of their families? Almost half of the men (43 per cent) noted the economic difficulties of trying to provide healthy foods for their wives during pregnancy. While some would make every effort to provide these foods, as one father of three said, 'green vegetables, fruits, juice, milk, meat, eggs, and other healthy things – these foods give her energy that she needs in these days ... These are good for her health, they are very expensive but I have to buy them because they are necessary for her health.' But another man, a father of two children, explained that 'sometimes she eats these foods, green vegetables, milk, meat, fruits, but sometimes she can only take what is possible at home; because this food is very expensive, I only buy this food sometimes.' Because men's gendered identity is closely connected with economic provisioning, their concepts of gendered selfhood are potentially threatened. Such possible tensions are reflected in this Hindu man's statement: 'A man should earn money. If I have no money, I can't give, provide happiness, clothes and food. If I don't earn the money, no one will like me.'

How may these incapacities match idealized masculine roles affect health and well-being within the family? I was told by non-governmental organization workers and some local residents that alcohol consumption and gambling amongst the men of the community were problematic. On Sundays, the rest day (it was a six-day work week), I observed groups of men relaxing in the alleys, playing cards, smoking, and did occasionally run into an obviously intoxicated man. As my research at the time focused on pregnant women's health, I did not address men's health issues, although here I suggest that more work is need to situate men's health, to understand the ways men embody and cope with economic adversity in specific contexts, and the ramifications this has for their families. Spending even small amounts of money on alcohol or gambling may very well affect the quantity and quality of food and healthcare available to all family members, and consequently have negative repercussions for maternal health.

Living on the edge of the poverty line arguably did affect women's health. Inscribed on women's bodies were histories of stress. Height has been used as an indicator of quality of life, for growth is a response to environmental factors. When environmental insults, such as nutritional stress, are severe or repeated, growth slows or even ceases, and stunted height is the result.[52] Average height of women was $146 \pm .06$ cm – only 1 cm above the global cutoff for stunted height.[53] One of the health consequences of such small bodies is the increased risk of pregnancy complications. The average amount of weight gained during pregnancy was 7.07 kg; this is about half the recommended weight gain, especially when women's undernourishment prior to pregnancy is considered, in combination with the common practice of breastfeeding while pregnant among this group of women.[54]

Many women found that bearing responsibility for domestic duties was made more difficult during pregnancy, as their bodies changed, and especially if women faced bouts of nausea and vomiting. The physical discomfort of pregnancy was compounded when ill, yet having the responsibilities of running the household remained constant. Being ill made physical labour all the more arduous, and women spoke of the changes in their bodies as 'strange' (*ajeeb*), a heaviness, which could be debilitating making everyday tasks difficult to complete.[55] There was little to no relief from everyday duties, such as carrying heavy jugs of water. Women did not want to work so hard and were conscious of the risks that heavy work could entail, including miscarriage. However, they pointed out that there was no one else to do such work in the household. Only six men (17.5 per cent) indicated that housework is something that men should do as part of their family responsibilities and roles as husbands and fathers. For many women then, the dislocation of being in the city, separated from female kin who could provide assistance, shaped their sense of self and place.

Although maternal mortality was relatively low in this study population, many women voiced concerns over facing their own mortality with each delivery. Everyone knew someone who had suffered or died, even if she herself had not had an anxiety-ridden pregnancy or delivery. If the pain was especially intense, or if there were fears that something was going wrong, women's fears escalated.

Women's qualms about childbirth were especially compounded by the trepidation of potentially having to go to the public hospital – a place that reflected the effects of macro-level political-economic factors on healthscapes. Not only was the hospital an expensive venture, but many poor people's experiences of public hospital care were appalling. Stories of verbal and physical abuse at the hands of medical personnel were familiar. One woman explained 'I am scared about going to the hospital because I heard the nurses give beatings and child changing also happens.' In this scenario, the healthy child born to a poor woman is removed, and in its stead a wealthy woman's unhealthy baby substituted. Another version of this story was the substitution of a poor women's boy child with a wealthy woman's girl child. In such stories, the collective experience of poverty, disenfranchisement, and insecurity is demonstrated, indicating the nature of class relations, and the expectations of maltreatment poor women fear and expect to suffer.

These stories are exacerbated by the chronic underfunding of public hospitals, linked earlier to the rise of economic liberalization. People recounted stories about being turned away because of the lack of beds.[56] So, a perilous trip to the public hospital due to complications was exacerbated by the risk of it all being for naught. Furthermore, basic supplies such as blood required for operations, including caesarian sections, must be provided by relatives. However, this was not always utilized, but was also not returned to the family, leading to concerns over the collection and misuse of body parts and fluids.

Localizing Women's Biologies

To emplace maternal health, the spaces and the times which women inhabit must be deconstructed. These spaces include global, national and local political, economic, and social contexts embedded in a particular timeframe – in this case at the end of the first decade of economic liberalization and introduction of structural adjustment programmes. The associated political and economic changes were variably implemented, not only across India, but also within one urban centre. Government-controlled pricing of food was not necessarily beneficial to the poor, as seen in this community where prices in the local fair price shops were comparable to open market prices. Furthermore, the quality of food that was available to the poor, both in the fair price shops and in the produce stalls, was obviously inferior. This mirrored the substandard quality of health care offered in public hospitals.

The lower quality of care in the foodscapes and healthscapes available to those of lower status mediate health in a place-specific manner. Women's abilities to cope with the stresses associated with living in poverty are dependent on their immediate social locality. This includes the specific kinds of food and health resources locally available, as well as social support from kin and community. To emplace maternal health, domestic spaces – past and present – must be considered. Women's historical status within the family (e.g. as a girl, young daughter-in-law, and mother), whether she lived in a nuclear or extended family structure, and her relationship with her husband or in-laws, all shape local gendered subjectivities. These factors combine to produce a locally specific social context in which to emplace biology and health. In other words, understanding maternal health requires considering individual life histories of growth and development (e.g. how a particular girl was valued or neglected within a family), their body size and strength, as well as reproductive histories (e.g. birthing sons or daughters, histories of loss such as miscarriage or stillbirth).

To summarize, I hope to leave you considering the implications of global political-economic policies on nation-states, and how such policies have a major influence in shaping Government food and health policies and programmes. The residents of the squatter settlement faced specific local constraints in food and health care that shaped their 'local biologies,' their well-being, and particularly women's health and wellness. Women's sentiments that were shared here tell us how vulnerable this population is, for women do not have financial resources to provide themselves with adequate food and health care, and often do not have autonomy over their own bodies, leaving many of the women feeling angry, frustrated and vulnerable to the health hazards of living in poverty. Yet women simultaneously cope as best they can, and their specific position within the family is an important element in understanding an individual woman's resources of resiliency. Improving maternal health cannot displace women from their domestic spaces. Gender and age relations must be considered, and working with families as well as individuals is critical to improving maternal health.

Acknowledgements

I am grateful to Christopher Fletcher and Erika Dyck for the opportunity to participate in *Putting Region in its Place: An Interdisciplinary Conference on Health, Healing, and Place*, and for C. Fletcher's thoughtful comments that improved the presentation of ideas in this paper. There were many people who provided invaluable support and advice during my work in India, including Geraldine Moreno-Black, Sunil Khanna, Anita Weiss, Dr Sunil Mehra and the staff of MAMTA. A special thanks to my research assistants, Ravi Dahiya, Pinky Sharma, Veena Massey, and Umar Kumar, and most importantly those who gave their time to share their ideas and experiences. This research was funded by a National Science Foundation Dissertation Improvement Grant, a Sasakawa Foundation International Trade and Development Fellowship, two research grants from the Center for the Study of Women in Society, University of Oregon, and a scholarship from the Graduate School, University of Oregon.

2 PUTTING MEDICINE IN ITS PLACE: THE IMPORTANCE OF HISTORICAL GEOGRAPHY TO THE HISTORY OF HEALTH CARE

Jonathan Reinarz

Introduction

Reports on the economy, environment and identity often initiate debates concerning globalization, migration, devolution and displacement and usually the erosion of place in the modern world. In academia, with the decline of grand narratives, many scholars unanimously accept theoretical approaches that preach 'multiple sites of belonging'.[1] Identities are no longer rooted in single, stable locales and individuals once regarded as out of place are now more easily situated in a world of process and elasticity.[2] In historical studies, a preoccupation with place is associated with the rise of cultural history and a proliferation of micro-studies, most scholars engaging with their own unique places. Though always overtly and appropriately contextualized, these studies do not always speak to each other, even when situated within the same region. As a result, historians have been overwhelmed by detail and greater efforts are required by scholars to identify commonalities in studies of different places.

There is no better time for historians to engage with the work of geographers. Almost all historians study particular places, and place is the geographer's principle object of study.[3] The subject, however, is unfamiliar territory to many scholars, and remains a slippery subject, even to the specialist.[4] Most academics, for example, use the terms place and space interchangeably.[5] Often, place is simply regarded as a set of coordinates, or a point on a map. It is therefore crucial to commence this paper with a definition. In this case, I have borrowed one proffered by Tim Cresswell, who defines place as 'space with meaning'.[6] This definition is appropriate because it does not just emphasize location, but the relationship between place and people and the way individuals endow a space with meaning. As implied, place is socially constructed and its meanings change with time. It is the historian's task to chart historical variations accurately. It is the object of this chapter to trace a few of these changes in the history of medicine.

Scholars in science studies undertook what might be described as a geographical, or 'spatial', turn more than a decade ago.[7] It is an approach that more effectively highlights commonalities between individual projects, arguably with the potential to link subjects and studies, like isolines on maps, which connect areas that share similar flora or fauna.[8] The most important and innovative work has been elegantly summarized by David Livingstone in his treatise, *Putting Science in its Place*, from which this chapter borrows its title.[9] Livingstone reminds scholars that science is not 'placeless' and that scientific knowledge is inherently geographical. In particular, Livingstone demonstrates that place influences both the generation and consumption of knowledge.[10] The space and place of every inquiry, if not always evident, conditions the investigations carried out by researchers. It also offers a way for scholars to synthesize some of the findings of disparate and detailed micro-studies. In other words, by engaging with geographies of medicine, one might bring about some sort of 'global order out of local averages'.[11]

This chapter is an attempt to put medicine in its place by focusing on one particular nineteenth-century setting, the English manufacturing town of Birmingham. While location often explained epidemics in these years, place influenced numerous medical issues, including prevention and practice. In Birmingham, as elsewhere, it encouraged regional experiments in medical education. It also justified the appointment of local men to medical posts, due to the notion that they were better equipped to deal with manifestations of disease specific to the region. Though these ideas declined in importance with the rise of germ theory in the last years of the nineteenth century, the concept of place should remain an important consideration for historians of medicine. As others have reminded us, as placeless as science, or in this case medicine, appears to become, ideas are always clearly rooted in a particular time and place. Whether carried out in a laboratory or private practice, medicine bears traces of the parochial or contingent. Just as historians speak of Chinese, Islamic or Jeffersonian science, historians of medicine should be encouraged to discuss Paris, London and even midland medicine.[12] In an effort to do just this, the chapter concludes with a section that highlights three key aspects of place in the context of Birmingham medicine. Above all, these final examples underline medicine's geographical nature. Though tools and techniques in medicine inevitably change, the sites in which these are implemented determine the way in which these spatially-specific stories unfold.

Painting the Local Landscape

The regional distribution of disease was often emphasized in the publications of English practitioners. One example of this phenomenon is Edward Jenner's pamphlet on the cowpox, the second, less quoted, portion of his famous work's title specifying the disease's distribution in the 'Western Counties of England' and 'particularly Gloucestershire'.[13] Other diseases were linked to specific locales and given regionally appropriate names, such as Devonshire colic and Derbyshire neck,[14] domestic equivalents of Delhi belly or Malta fever. Contemporary guides often described the need for periods of 'seasoning' when travellers encountered new climates,[15] while individual epidemics demanded regionally appropriate rules, primarily because diseases were modified by location. Moreover, some therapies were tolerated less well depending on region. For example, in the eyes of John Harley Warner's southern doctors, Londoners tolerated bleeding less well than the robust inhabitants of the American south.[16] Finally, when sickness struck, the medical armamentarium with which practitioners confronted disease was always varied, comprising primarily local *materia medica*.

Over time, this system became known as the principle of specificity and justified the decision to study local disease manifestations. In some contexts, the principle was extended and used to support cases for regional medical education. Such was the case in the southern United States, but also in Birmingham in 1828. Medical instruction in the early nineteenth century, whether in England or America, was based on regional circumstances and the needs of local populations. Without a doubt, most inhabitants, whether in Birmingham, England, or Birmingham, Alabama would have concurred with the view that: 'Medicine, like disease, must spring from the very elements, soil, sunshine, moisture, etc., that produce disease'.[17]

While Warner alone developed these ideas extensively, other medical historians have placed region at the centre of their work. Historians Ian Inkster and Jack Morrell set an agenda in the early 1980s and charted the development of scientific culture in various metropolitan and provincial contexts, contrasting London with a range of provincial settings.[18] Their study encouraged multiple historical geographies of science, indicating that the reception of science in the English provinces could variously be enthusiastic or muted.[19] Aware that metropolitan events were often used to represent the state of medicine nationally, English medical historians also began to argue that generalization had run ahead of evidence, with ambitious regional studies, for example, exploring the development of healthcare in Yorkshire and Manchester.[20] Many other British studies have recently emerged, the histories of medicine in Scotland and Wales having noticeably flourished.[21] In the context of the English Midlands, perhaps no historian did more to bring out medicine's regional dimension than the eighteenth-century historian, Joan Lane.[22] Even her textbook, *A Social History of Medicine*, reveals a noticeable preoccupation with Warwickshire and the surrounding counties.[23]

The Place of Birmingham

This chapter shifts the focus of medical-historical inquiry to a particular place, and begins to chart a specific, local medical story, in Birmingham, England. Geographers remind us that places are founded through acts of exclusion.[24] From the eighteenth century, Birmingham contrasted with many English towns and cities – especially to old, established chartered towns, where guilds and similar institutions controlled the local economy – by carefully regulating the conditions of trade, the new manufacturing town was characterized by minimal regulation and exclusion, primarily because it lacked a town charter until 1838.[25] It therefore attracted migrants from a wide variety of religious backgrounds and a broad hinterland, eventually developing, without the usual commercial restrictions, into a town of 1,000 trades.[26]

In terms of healthcare, though a free market, Birmingham attracted fewer doctors than other manufacturing towns, and less than the smaller resorts and spa towns, such as Bath and Cheltenham, which possessed a greater proportion of middle-class inhabitants. In 1767, with a population approaching 40,000, it was nevertheless home to twenty surgeons, three university-trained physicians and an unspecified number of druggists, chemists and quacks.[27] It also supported a workhouse infirmary for sick paupers. By 1779, a group of enterprising individuals, led by one of these physicians, also established the town's General Hospital, a charity founded to treat the 'respectable' poor.[28]

Known as an industrial town, Birmingham also possessed a distinct landscape, as depicted in several landscapes produced during this period. Located on a hill, it offered its eighteenth-century inhabitants a good view of the surrounding countryside; this circumstance also ensured an efficient system of drainage and minimized outbreaks of waterborne diseases, especially in the first half of the nineteenth century. Though partially determined by geography, place, as geographers remind us, is also an event in the sense that places are always becoming, or changing, both figuratively and literally.[29] Described as the 'toy-shop of Europe', as well as London in miniature, the terms used to describe the town changed and determined the way in which the public understood both the place and the hazards it posed. Even the landscape was subject to change. In some cities and countries, transformations of the urban environment may be accelerated by natural disasters; however, in Birmingham the inhabitants themselves dramatically altered their natural environment. The exact way in which this influenced the health of the population will be discussed later in this section.

The importance of place to medical practice in eighteenth- and nineteenth-century Birmingham is revealed in numerous contemporary documents. One of the earliest works to situate Birmingham medicine in its local context was that of a relatively unknown local practitioner, Thomas Tomlinson. Besides being recognized as one of the most competent surgeons in the midlands in the late eighteenth century, Tomlinson delivered one of the first series of anatomy demonstrations in provincial England.[30] Together with numerous articles and book reviews, his anatomical lectures were published in a volume entitled *Medical Miscellany* (1769), a collection of writings originally intended as a quarterly, regional medical journal.[31] Like his contemporaries, Tomlinson was sensitive to the influence of environment on health. Evident from his writings, for example, is the fact that he kept a weather journal. Echoing ideas expounded by Sydenham, *Medical Miscellany* expressly states that the seeds of disease lay in the body, emerging with specific changes in environmental conditions. Though urban and industrial, Birmingham, according to Tomlinson, was ripe for economic growth, not epidemics, which were rare and even in decline.[32] As a result, the London-educated surgeon regarded manufacturing towns as healthy places. Interestingly, over the next century, few practitioners in the town challenged this view. Joseph Hodgson, another local surgeon, who attained a national reputation for his work on aneurism, expounded similar views in 1840.[33] Instead of epidemics and famine, the inhabitants of Birmingham appeared to face a new and equally formidable threat, namely that of luxury.[34]

Another relatively unknown practitioner who elaborated on the health of Birmingham was John Darwall (1796–1833). A local physician who studied in London and Edinburgh, Darwall was a promising young practitioner who died while in his thirties as the result of an infection contracted while performing an autopsy. Interestingly, coming from a non-medical family, Darwall was noticeably out of place throughout his short career as a practitioner in Birmingham. Following a local apprenticeship, Darwall walked wards and attended anatomical classes in London before completing his medical studies in Edinburgh. At a time when MD theses were remarkably generic and unoriginal, Darwall produced a particularly novel study on the 'Diseases of Artisans' (1821), comprising research undertaken while assisting his former master locally in private practice.[35] Returning to Birmingham to build his own medical practice following qualification, Darwall spent his spare hours engaged in medical journalism, one of his first articles being a medical topography of the town.[36] He also made a name for himself teaching botany to local medical students, regularly taking students herbarizing, or collecting local *materia medica*.[37] Recognized as one of the town's rising stars, he was appointed physician to the town's dispensary in 1831, and then consultant physician at the General Hospital shortly before his death. While treating hundreds of poor patients at both institutions each week, he continued to contemplate the link between illness and locality, as articulated in his thesis.

In Darwall's time, local concepts of disease were beginning to have less impact on regional medical practice. For example, despite Darwall's original work on industrial medicine, in 1840, seven years after Darwall's death, medical staff at the dispensary directly contradicted the correlations between industry and illness. In that year, the institution's annual report explicitly stated that it 'does not appear that any of the trades of the town are liable to excite particular disease ... nor is there any locality in the town which is especially productive of disease'.[38] For whatever reason, medical staff emphasized alternative causations. Much of this has been linked to the subsequent rise in germ theory in the late nineteenth century. It is also associated with a tendency among physicians to view the human being as an isolated physiological system, subject to physical and chemical laws which operated without apparent dependence upon environmental factors.[39] Interestingly, the dispensary physician who contradicted Darwall, Joseph Hodgson, eventually left Birmingham to commence practice in London, his less regionally specific approach to medicine having freed him from a career restricted to local practice. A generation later, greater numbers of practitioners would similarly abandon the region, literally and as an explanatory concept. Another consequence of these developments was that locally trained medical men were no longer the natural heirs to vacant medical posts and competed less successfully with better-qualified outsiders for coveted consultancies in their towns.[40] Conducted in laboratories, investigations into bodily systems would henceforth be described as 'placeless', allowing the results of researchers to be replicated by practitioners regardless ●cality. These new methods encouraged what historians have described as science's 'triumph over place'.[41] Alternatively, scientists and doctors were liberated from the influences of environment.[42] Working in laboratories where conditions could be regulated and recreated, practitioners sought to communicate their findings across the globe. Not coincidentally, hospital practitioners in these same years began to compare their statistics unproblematically, whether located in Birmingham or any other regional capital. More recently, historians appear to have similarly embraced these enlightened ideas. As a result, the context of place has often been obscured in histories of medicine, which often appear as placeless as the medical science they address.

Geographies of Medical Knowledge:
Three Birmingham Case Studies

The rise of the medical school in Birmingham offers an obvious example of this local medical tradition. Although a national curriculum was introduced at English medical schools from the second decade of the nineteenth century, regional elements continued to emerge throughout the century and provided schools with unique characteristics. This tendency encouraged, for example, the emergence of industrial medicine in Birmingham and Sheffield and tropical medicine in the port cities of Liverpool and London.[43] Medical schools were also defined by their geographical location. Birmingham, for example, was described by local practitioners as a safe place, while London, like other national capitals, was beginning to be regarded as 'a dangerous place', largely due to its size and the inability of medical instructors to police every aspect of students' lives.[44] Attempts to label places were also contested and often challenged if not occasionally discarded as conditions and circumstances changed. For example, less clear is when Birmingham ceased to be 'a safe place'. The remainder of this chapter will concentrate on three case studies of hospital medicine in Birmingham in order to emphasize three final ways in which place determined medical practice at the regional level.

The first of these examples deals with the General Hospital, Birmingham's largest voluntary hospital for nearly two centuries. More specifically, this example demonstrates the way in which place is both socially and literally constructed. As noted above, the meanings of a particular place regularly change, but occasionally the actual landscape changes, and not only over the *longue durée*. In the case of the General Hospital, Birmingham's changing physical environment in the eighteenth century determined the type of patients admitted to the town's first voluntary hospital. The second example will examine the realities of industrial medicine in the midlands by documenting cases treated at the Birmingham Skin Hospital, a specialist institution. While historians of industrialization and occupational health appreciate the dangers and benefits of industry, the relationship between work and illness in more general histories remains hypothetical, often influenced by the sensational accounts of accidents and injury recounted in newspapers and novels. For example, discussions of health and industrialization often conjure up images of male workers involved in spectacular accidents involving machinery. A glimpse at patient data from the skin hospital is intended to demonstrate the (not always predictable) influence of industry on labourers and will hopefully encourage scholars to rethink the nature of workplace hazards in industrial places. Finally, this section concludes with an examination of the patient records of the Children's Hospital, one of Birmingham's largest specialist hospitals. Among other things, this example has implications for the way in which historians of medical specialties frame their studies. In particular, it examines the potential for historians to compare patient data for medical institutions, such as children's hospitals, in different locations. In the case of Birmingham's Children's Hospital, patient records appear very closely to mirror local circumstances and developments. These variations need to be accounted for before any attempts at comparing institutions can be undertaken. Moreover, the reasons behind these differences can only be understood by engaging more closely with place.

An unusual feature of Birmingham's General Hospital is its relatively late appearance compared to other provincial institutions. Though a vibrant hive of industry, Birmingham was among the last major British towns to acquire a voluntary hospital in the eighteenth century. Commenced in 1765, the General Hospital did not admit patients until 1779, fourteen years after its foundation, or forty-two years after voluntary general hospitals appeared in other provincial centres, such as Bristol and Winchester.[45] As one might expect, unlike these institutions, the General Hospital in Birmingham was justified as an institution suited to an industrial town. More specifically, it was established for those without legal settlement in what was, until 1838, a large manufacturing town administered on the lines of a much smaller parish.

An investigation of the patients admitted to this institution is facilitated by the survival of nearly all of the hospital's records since 1779. Despite being inaugurated as an institution for individuals without settlement in the parish of Birmingham, or those residing there for less than a year,[46] the hospital always admitted primarily locals. In addition to patients' parishes of settlement, registers record each patient's name, age, disease and occupation. While historians are only beginning to undertake sustained work on the history of hospital patients, the potential research avenues, as should be obvious from the categories listed in ledgers, are numerous. Information available for the General Hospital, Birmingham, for example, would allow researchers to link occupation and illness regionally.

Birmingham was linked to a broad hinterland, the natural resources of which supported its industrialization in these years. With an underdeveloped road network, trade was augmented through the construction of a network of waterways. Nearly every history of Birmingham, not to mention contemporary sources, mentions the town's canals.[47] In terms of the development of healthcare in Birmingham, the canals had serious repercussions for local inhabitants in the late eighteenth and early nineteenth centuries. For example, their construction delayed the completion of the General Hospital. The undertaking diverted much financial support from the charity due to a perceived need to develop other aspects of the town's infrastructure, including roads, bridges and even leisure facilities, such as theatres.[48] Besides requiring considerable funds, resources and labour, the canals also literally changed the landscape of land-locked Birmingham in the last decades of the eighteenth century. Simultaneously, it changed the hospital's patient population. While historians have yet to uncover the physical toll resulting from the canals' construction,[49] it is evident that the existence of man-made waterways in subsequent decades resulted in numerous hospital admissions. Between 1803 and 1823, for example, hospital staff admitted 140 cases of drowning.[50] This alone should explain why the charity soon doubled as the regional branch of the London-based Humane Society.[51] Also included among the hospital's patients were a large number of canal-boat workers. In the decade from 1839 to 1848, staff treated 159 people engaged in this work, 104 for medical reasons, and 55 surgical cases.[52] Whilst consuming scarce funds, this branch of medical work provided hospital managers with a new charitable incentive. It was not long before the hospital began specifically to target the owners of the Canal Navigation Company during their annual fundraising campaigns.[53]

The relationship between industry and illness is clearly more complicated than identifying a locality's potential hazards and counting injuries. A healthy local economy is equally important in order to improve healthcare services, especially if one can identify industries whose workers utilize services disproportionately. Local industry is also often directly connected to innovations in medicine, many doctors having borrowed industrial technologies or adapted them for medical uses. Finally, one must not overlook the relationship between occupational health and illness, even if this potentially threatened to alienate those who funded medical services. Where records exist, the symbiotic relation between places and cases, not to mention the evolution of medical services, is often very easy to uncover.

The Birmingham Canal Navigation may have been the first company targeted by the General Hospital's collectors due to the numbers of their workers who benefited from hospital care, but they were not the last. In subsequent years, business subscribers regularly appeared on all hospital subscription lists. Business or corporate donors comprised only 5 per cent of subscribers in 1790–1820, but more than doubled in number by 1870 and accounted for 32 per cent in 1900.[54] Similar relationships existed between other industries and individual hospitals. As one of the largest manufacturing towns in England, Birmingham had a strong concentration of specialist institutions. Besides an orthopaedic hospital, it supported an Eye Hospital which was particularly well attended by miners and metalworkers and remained one of the most popular medical charities among all other trades, as its impressive late-Victorian premises alone should suggest.[55] The centrally located Queen's Hospital, the town's second general hospital, was equally popular with Birmingham's working community, due to its central location.[56] Its transition into the Accident Hospital in 1941, a century after its foundation, appeared appropriate to most locals given the needs of local industry.

The emergence of Hospital Saturday in the 1870s is another example of the strong links between industry and Birmingham's healthcare services. Established to allow the voluntary hospitals to meet the medical demands of mass society, Hospital Saturday involved local working people sacrificing one half-day's earnings, once a year, to medical charity.[57] Though seemingly insignificant when considered on an individual basis, the scheme demonstrated what locals later referred to as 'the power of the penny', following the placement of collection boxes in 1,200 workshops and 1,800 public houses.[58] By the third decade of the twentieth century, this charitable effort became the hospital contributory scheme, which noticeably changed the profile of hospital donors, who, not surprisingly, developed a sense of entitlement to care.[59] While this added to the demands placed on hospitals during the 1930s, the earnings multiplied and facilitated the regional integration of hospital services and arguably rationalized medical provision before the introduction of a National Health Service.

Though the dangers of industrialization are more familiar than such financial innovations, more research is required to reveal the complicated relationship between industry and illness at the local level. The hazards of industrialization, as identified by historians, are as often imagined as they are real. Much research has uncovered deaths of careless workers who were dragged into and devoured by machinery, whether described in the polemical diatribes of Marx and Engels or local newspapers.[60] The reality, at least as reported in the pages of Birmingham's hospital archives, is often very different, as the General Hospital's links to the Humane Society have already indicated. It bears reminding that the spectacular, if tragic, incidents involving workers ground into hamburger meat were less common than many other injuries, such as eye infections and eczema. The unrivalled popularity of the Eye Hospital among local workers, many of whom suffered from such routine ailments, has already been noted. Another specialist hospital that was generously supported by the town's workers was the Birmingham Skin Hospital, founded in 1881.

Although the institution's patient registers have disappeared, existing annual reports chart some of the hospital's work. Besides the usual information, reports present annual summaries of patients' occupations and diseases. They also challenge historians' general assumptions about healthcare in an industrial setting, for local housewives, at 26 per cent of patients, not industrial labourers, outnumbered all other patients suffering primarily from severe forms of dermatitis.[61] Among the next most common occupations were jewellers and brassworkers, whose percentages were nearly proportionate to their numbers within the local community.[62] Domestic servants, though underrepresented, remind us once again that more work in this area needs to be carried out in order to fully map the gendered history of industrial injury. The dozen or so cases of machinists appearing in the reports, though limited, equally demonstrate the real dangers faced by those working with heavy machinery, namely chronic dermatoses often resulting from contact with industrial lubricants.

Table 2.1: Occupations of patients at Birmingham Skin Hospital, 1885.

Occupation	Number of Patients
Housewives	296
Jewellers	38
Labourers	28
Brass-workers	20
Domestic Servants	20
French-polishers	18
Machinists	14
Total	1142

Source: BCLLS, Skin Hospital, Annual Report, 1885.

Over the next decade, the numbers of women treated at the hospital only increased, with charwomen gaining a place on this list. Workers engaged in heavy industry, on the other hand, were becoming less common, while those from the clerical sector were also beginning to appear among patients.

Table 2.2: Occupations of patients at Birmingham Skin Hospital, 1895.

Occupation	Number of Patients
Housewives	1183 (29 per cent)
Labourers	137 (3.3 per cent)
Servants	91 (2.2 per cent)
Charwomen	57
Shop assistants	57
Clerks	56
Brass-workers	53
Total	4120

Source: BCLLS, Skin Hospital, Annual Report, 1895.

The final case study in this section relates to the history of child health in the late Victorian period. Founded 1861, the Birmingham Children's Hospital was among the first dozen British children's hospitals. The hospital, like many specialist institutions, commenced on a small scale through the initiative of Thomas Heslop, who also founded the town's Skin Hospital. Originally opening its sixteen beds to children between the ages of two and fourteen,[63] the Children's Hospital grew gradually, moving into a disused lying-in hospital in 1870 and offering forty beds to Birmingham's youngest patients, sixty-two in 1900.[64] Modelled on London's Great Ormond Street Hospital, it was frequently compared to the pioneering children's institution.[65] Despite the efforts of early medical staff, it had one of the highest annual death rates of local hospitals, averaging 10 per cent during the second half of the nineteenth century.[66] Not surprisingly, it was this statistic that managers at most hospitals regularly compared in order to measure individual rates of success. Historians of paediatrics, like the medical officers of these institutions, have similarly adopted this approach, often comparing hospital statistics across regions.[67] Hospital historians, however, long ago identified the complex reasons behind variations in death rates, let alone other hospital statistics.[68]

Medical institutions, like Birmingham Children's Hospital, are not generic institutions comparable with institutions for like specialties across regions. This is, however, how they are often treated by historians. Their records clearly reflect local contexts and fluctuate in direct relation to changes in existing conditions. Only when the nature of these changes is examined in more detail, however, does this usually become apparent. At Birmingham Children's Hospital, this phenomenon is particularly noticeable in terms of fluctuations in the numbers of patients admitted with fever, as well as the incidence of orthopaedic and skin cases.

During the four last decades of the nineteenth century, scarlet fever was one of the few infectious diseases admitted into the Children's Hospital, which possessed a special fever ward, modelled on that existing at the children's hospital in Glasgow, not Great Ormond Street.[69] Cases of scarlet fever at the hospital averaged approximately 100 annually and declined only after Birmingham Council opened its own fever hospital in 1874.[70] A steady drop in cases at the hospital is noticeable from this date, declining more rapidly when the disease was made notifiable by the Registrar General. Though never disappearing entirely, the story of the disease's elimination from the hospital was a very local one, dependent as it was on the construction of a fever hospital locally. A similar decline is therefore not apparent in Edinburgh, for example, for at least another decade, much longer in other provincial centres.[71] Any comparison of cases at institutions must recognize this, though historians of children's hospitals have not always done so, whether comparing patients' illnesses, or hospital death rates.[72]

Table 2.3: Scarlet fever cases at Birmingham's Children's Hospital and Isolation Hospital, 1875–1900.

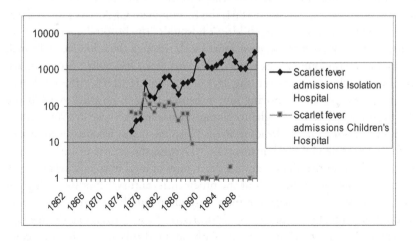

Source: BCLLS, Birmingham Children's Hospital, Annual Reports, 1875-1900[73]

Similar circumstances must be considered when explaining other developments at the institution. Among the most common of cases at all children's hospitals, comprising a third of admissions at GOS in the 1870s and 1880s,[74] orthopaedic cases in Birmingham were rarely prevalent throughout the late nineteenth century. This was due to the establishment of an orthopaedic hospital in the parish in 1817, making Birmingham one of the first towns in Europe, let alone England, to support such a charity. The existence of this institution consistently moderated the number of cases of club feet, spinal disease and other bone and joint diseases admitted to the Children's Hospital during its existence.

Table 2.4: Inpatients' diseases at Birmingham Children's Hospital, 1873 and 1883.

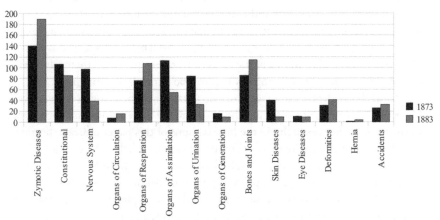

Source: Birmingham Central Library, Local Studies, Birmingham
Children's Hospital, Annual Reports, 1873 & 1883

A similar pattern is noticeable for skin cases. Forming a large portion of cases at most children's hospitals,[75] skin diseases at Birmingham Children's Hospital were common in the 1870s, but declined into insignificance by the 1880s. As one might expect, this decline was the result of another local charitable initiative. Home to one of the first orthopaedic hospitals in England, Birmingham also supported one of the earliest skin hospitals in provincial England. The fact that the charity was founded by Thomas Heslop, who established the Children's Hospital, only ensured that dermatological cases presented at the children's charity were efficiently directed to the town's dermatological institution from its foundation. While this practically ensured their disappearance from the children's charity in Birmingham, skin cases only increased at other children's institutions, including the Children's Hospital in Sheffield, where a specialist skin clinic was founded in these same years.[76] As should be apparent, given these very specific regional developments, comparisons between similar specialist hospitals, while often attempted, are almost meaningless should the specificities of place remain unexplored.

Conclusion

The history of medicine in Birmingham over the last two centuries underscores the importance of place in historical research. The Birmingham cases remind us that, as placeless as medical science appeared to become in the late nineteenth century, medical histories always contain a local dimension. In the case of Birmingham, the town was constructed through a process of naming, described by historians as an open community, resembling London in miniature, but generally more healthy. These meanings were also reconstructed, as occurred in the 1820s when John Darwall claimed that the industrial town was a potentially dangerous place, or even earlier, when a system of canals was first cut across the town, linking it to coalfields and markets, but also bringing new hazards to the local population. Local surgeons and physicians, including Tomlinson, were only some of the medical practitioners who concentrated on these specific aspects of place in their publications. In doing so, however, they provided themselves with considerable authority, claiming key medical positions in Birmingham.

While the work of geographers can help us take such local studies to new levels, historians engaging with place also need to employ more traditional approaches to the settings they research. As the final sections of this paper indicate, hospitals and their statistics may invite easy comparisons; nevertheless, by changing locations, the stories we research invariably change, often significantly. The reasons for these variations only become apparent upon more detailed investigations of local settings. Health and illness over time clearly reflect the regions being studied, as do studies of hospital development and medical treatment, among many other areas of current research. However, the relationships are not always obvious. Though these examples also serve to warn scholars of the perils of comparative research, hopefully they will not discourage such collective studies. They should merely emphasize the need to contextualize comparative studies more effectively.

In any case, historians of medicine must begin to engage with the work of geographers, who have considered the intricacies of place more thoroughly and critically than most scholars. Being informed by place, however, involves far more than simply writing about this town or that city. Neither does it end with locating particular places and their people in their respective cultures. It involves thinking about the implications of the idea of place for the town, city or region that is being researched. Only in this way can we avoid being inundated with yet more local stories. By engaging with the work of geographers, historians can finally begin to confront the plethora of micro-studies that are only set to increase and establish some 'order out of local averages'.[77] By considering what makes our particular places unique, we can also begin to compare them more effectively, whether working on hospitals, laboratories or asylums in Birmingham, or anywhere else.

Acknowledgements

I would like to thank Graham Mooney for his help with Table 2.3. and Rupert Millard for his help with Table 2.4.

3 FINDING PLACE IN *THE BIG-LITTLE WORLD OF DOC PRITHAM*: TELLING MEDICAL TALES ABOUT NORTHWOODS MAINE, 1920s–70s

Sasha Mullally

In *The Big-Little World of Doc Pritham*, readers are treated to a rousing tale of the life of an intrepid country doctor. Frederick John Pritham of Greenville Junction, Maine, is a practitioner firmly ensconced in the northwoods of his home state. The dust jacket tells how the doctor

> has traveled thousands of miles through the Maine wilderness on horseback and on foot; ridden cars, boats, planes, buggies, snowmobiles, lumber trucks, trains, and railroad handcars; gone on skates and snowshoes; jumped trains; swum rivers; waded through mud and snow and slush; skated over thin ice; plunged his car to the bottom of Moosehead [Lake] – all to provide medical service to an area of some five thousand square miles.[1]

It's small wonder that he pronounced 'getting there and back was the biggest obstacle to my medical practice'.[2]

This chapter explores the intersections of region and place in the medical life-writing by and about Dr Fred Pritham, who, by the late twentieth century, became very well-known in the rural and remote communities and towns of the Maine's northern counties. At the heart of his local celebrity is a biography, cited above, written by well-known Maine author Dorothy Clarke Wilson and published in 1971 when she was at the height of her career. Within the genre of physician auto/biography, 'country doctor tales' comprise a small but distinct body of literature.[3] And within this literature, physicians' travels dominate the texts. Because of their ubiquity as narrative devices, travel tales, in fact, become a defining characteristic of the rural medical life-writing genre.

Although the literature is still undeveloped, historians who utilize published life-writing have noted in general how healthcare providers on the 'periphery' often frame their work narratives as 'adventure tales';[4] the point where the adventure of rural and remote medicine is made most evident is in the travel: to see a patient, returning from delivering care, or out on rounds in the wilderness. This offers a point of contrast to historical work that has centred on unpublished life-writing, such as diaries. In such narratives, historians like Judith Leavitt have noted the physician's preoccupation with the domestic sphere, an orientation that defies traditional gender norms.[5] In published texts, travel tales speak to the masculine health and energy of these practitioners as men who can both swim rivers and jump trains in the course of attending to rural medical emergencies. At the same time, such stories emphasize professional dedication at a time and place when such physicians largely provided health services by going out into the homes of their rural patients. Although a detailed theoretical discussion of life-writing as a genre and historical source is not possible in the scope of a brief chapter, I will demonstrate how published narratives of country doctoring, replete with travel tales, provide an opportunity to explore and discuss the importance of 'place' and 'region' of early to mid-century rural medical practices. But, as their narrative divergence from Leavitt's diaries suggests, a careful analysis of such published texts is required for successfully unpacking the meanings of region and place in the history of medicine.

Historians, Region and Place

Historians of medicine have long recognized that considerable differences in the practice of health will often reveal themselves along regional lines. North American health history has benefited from longstanding and rich debates over the use of region as a category of analysis, which in turn has generated a valuable scholarly focus on region in the history of medicine.[6] Of particular note is a robust literature on southern health and healing in the American historiography, where southern medicine is a distinct medical practice, with distinct environmental concerns and a distinct professional evolution.[7] There is ample room, however, to expand scholarly attention to other regions of North America.

   In this chapter Pritham's work as a country doctor engages with a place-based vocabulary that references mountain and lake topography, cold weather and remote wilderness as key elements to master in making a success of rural practice during the interwar period. This may not have been the case in every rural area across America, but it was true for him. But place is equally important here in how it defined this physician's social environment and framed the cultural connections made in his early years in medicine. The Maine northwoods in the 1920s and 30s were defined by specific economies, namely lumber-based industries and wilderness tourism. Therefore, certain economic and industrial relations influenced the social and cultural contexts of northern Maine. Fred Pritham's combined private practice with company contracts.[8] For rural physicians such as he, both their authority at the bedside and the type and quality of assistance they provided related to the physical, social and cultural geographies of their rural region.

The Making of a Country Doctor

Frederick John Pritham was not originally from the northwoods, he was a transplanted from a farm in Freeport, Maine. Born in 1880, Pritham became interested in medicine because of a relationship struck up with a local physician, who treated him for a debilitating case of hayfever, a condition that compromised his future on the family farm. Dr Gray took him on as an assistant when Pritham was in high school, and working under the tutelage of this preceptor, he spent several years of his late teens following the Freeport doctor on his rounds. Although most of his jobs were menial, he learned to give ether and was introduced to the rhythms and practice of turn of the century medicine.[9] Upon his graduation from high school, he enrolled in the Medical School of Maine at Bowdoin College in nearby Brunswick, from which he graduated in 1906.[10] This was supplemented with a four-week post-graduate course in Obstetrics at the Harrison Avenue branch of the Boston Lying-In Hospital.[11] Concluding his medical education, he answered an ad for work as a medical assistant in Greenville, Maine. Conflict with the senior physician in town ended his assistantship earlier than planned, but the northwoods seemed to agree with Pritham. He decided to remain in the area and hang his own shingle in nearby Greenville Junction, located down the road on the railroad tracks. This decision coincided with his engagement and subsequent marriage to Sarah Ring. Together, they raised a family in Greenville Junction and would make their entire lives in the small community.[12]

Pritham's career spanned a marathon of over fifty years; the doctor treated patients right up to his death in 1972 at the age of ninety-two. *The Big-Little World of Doc Pritham*, published one year before the venerable doctor's death, is written as a life-and-times memoir. As such, it spans the doctor's career, but most of the action in the book revolves around incidents from the first two decades of practice. The bulk of text focuses on the inter-war years, when roads were poor and travelling difficult. Certainly, Pritham claimed an extremely large practice encompassing hundreds of square miles, including isolated lumber camps, which required much overnight travel. The doctor had only tenuous access to hospital services before the end of the Second World War, and the lack of year-round hard surface roads often meant the doctor got about his district by rail, by boat, by horseback or even on foot.

Travel as the basis for adventure narratives is foreshadowed on the very book jacket. The cover of *Big-Little World* is simple, featuring a black mortar and pestle on a green background, but the dust jacket bills the story contained within its bindings as a 'wonderful adventure story ... much more than a yarn about a country doctor.'[13] We read on the inside cover that this biography includes pictures of a 'wild, fresh and vivid life on an American frontier' where 'colorful characters of the region' veritably "swarm"' in the pages of the book.[14] And this colourful region is revealed through the exploits of a singular heroic individual: 'Doc Pritham'. The book is about a place and a time in Maine history, but '[r]ising out of the pages and the plot of these texts is the character of the doctor, [a] towering life figure.'[15] The physician, as hero at the centre of this epic, is likeable, endowed with a 'blunt, salty humour' but also a 'selfless dedication which make him not only a unique character but one beloved, almost worshiped, by hundreds of friends and patients'.[16]

Visual renderings emphasize the heroic scale of Pritham's work. The first printed page of Pritham's life story shows a map of his 'big' world, which encompasses most of the three counties of northern Maine: Piscataquis, Aroostook and sometimes northern Penobscot and Somerset counties. From this map, we understand that because country doctors alone bear the burden of care for communities who have few healthcare personnel upon which to rely, they go out and brave difficult terrain and weather to tend patients alone in far-flung practices. But his world is also 'little' in that the big world is thinly settled, and he tends a relatively small population up in the American borderlands. In selling Pritham's life story, publishers wrap the life of the country doctor in the vigourous self-sufficient language of pioneering. And thus, marketers for McGraw-Hill situate this Maine physician in a 'northwoods' American frontier.

Wilson Writes a Biography

Dorothy Clarke Wilson was intrigued by the northwoods, as were many 'flat-land' or 'southern' New Englanders of her day. Raised on Bible stories Wilson sought to transform human lives into parables for mass consumption. Wilson's books devote a lot of text to the details of her main characters' moral virtues, such as service, sacrifice, perseverance and courage in the face of life's challenges. The author enjoyed a wide readership, and she built her writing career by focusing on the lives of inspirational women.[17] Before her work on Pritham she had written about 'courageous Christians whose lives became legends', including America's first woman doctor Elizabeth Blackwell, social reformer Dorothea Dix, and 'American Indian princess' Susette LaFlesche, who herself became the first Native American woman physician.[18]

In many ways, writing the biography of Fred Pritham was a change of pace for the writer, who was looking for new subject material over 1968–9. In a memoir of her career, Wilson recalled friends had encouraged her to explore the life of an old doctor up in Greenville, Maine. Greenville was a community she and her husband Elvin had visited through his parish work and while on vacation, so she was familiar with Pritham's reputation. Encouraged by the 'tales of his exploits' offered by friends and intrigued by articles about the doctor in newspapers, she decided to explore his local celebrity in a biography.[19] Her husband advised against the project, arguing that the language of the lumbering country might prove 'too rough.' Nonetheless, Wilson decided she was capable of learning and representing 'the backwoods idioms of my native Maine' as well as the idiosyncrasies of a northwoods country doctor.[20] This is how Wilson came to write not only her first book about an inspirational man, but also her first book set in her home state. In an interview in the summer of 1999, Wilson explained to me that until that point, she had not fallen on an adequate subject that she thought would epitomize the spirit of Maine. In Fred Pritham, she found a life through which she thought she could tell that story.[21]

Wilson contacted Pritham and was surprised when he first refused her offer. He cited a failing memory of 'those days when I traveled' and did not wish to participate in any more retrospectives of his career.[22] Wilson persevered. Writing a second time, she suggested he consider the positive message his biography might send to new members of the medical profession: 'Surely ... his experience might inspire some adventurous young doctors to fill the dire need for medical service in our neglected rural communities.'[23] This new tack – playing to his sense of professional duty – worked. Pritham almost immediately replied in by telegram: 'I will cooperate.'[24]

Over time Pritham and Wilson developed a working relationship. Once a level of comfort had been established, Wilson wrote that Pritham quickly warmed to his subject, and 'As he rambled on coherently and in pithy detail about his early life I tried to scribble notes.' Eventually, the doctor pulled out a looseleaf scrapbook, whose 175 pages contained 'a most wonderful array of incidents covering perhaps the first half of his life'. The scrap book was complete with photos and newspaper clippings he had collected and that friends had sent him. It also contained travel notes Pritham had kept over the years. The material in the scrapbook was a jumbled assortment of memories, 'as rough as uncut diamonds,' but Wilson began her work by building the doctor's life story from this source.[25] She later recalled, 'If it weren't for that scrapbook, I couldn't have written any book at all.'[26]

This emphasizes the ways in which Wilson framed the context of her work. The story of the doctor would be, in many ways, her version of the history of northern Maine. She familiarized herself with the town, visiting the old YMCA whose top floor had served as a makeshift hospital prior to the First World War. She spent time in the town and took pictures of the Pritham residence. Upon exploring her research files, one finds that Wilson immersed herself in secondary source research about the economic history of the county, especially the lumbering industry, which had driven almost all local commerce for the first decades of the twentieth century. Determined to master the vocabulary of the northwoods, her notes are full of references to lumber songs, glossaries of lumbermen's terms for tools of their trade, aspects of their work and the wilderness where they lived. 'I assembled an album of thirteen geological maps,' she wrote, 'which were to prove invaluable in tracing Doc's incredible travels.' She took a ski lift to the top of Squaw Mountain, hired one of the town's pilots to fly her in a small plane out over the 5000 square miles of lake and mountain wilderness where outpost lumbercamps and the towns in service to this industry had been a part of Pritham's patient load.[27] Deeply impressed by the geographic scope of Pritham's work, the writer in Wilson began to play with the idea of this physically small man[28] situated within a geographically immense area.

At this juncture, the writer attempted to round out the anecdotes mined from the doctor's personal archives. She interviewed close friends and relatives to supply character development for the physician. By the end of her time in Greenville, there were enough anecdotes to fill far more than the length of a 300-page biography. Wilson wrote, 'It seemed as if everyone I met knew Doc and had some tale to share.'[29] At first it seems as though Wilson was encouraged by this flood of stories about the doctor, but the tales shared so freely actually contained little information about Pritham as a person. Interviewing the doctor's family yielded nothing further. Fred Pritham's wife Sadie was diffident about their personal lives, perhaps because of unsavoury interactions with journalists over the course of their later years.[30] The doctor's son Howard Pritham, who was at the time working as a physician in Panama, simply described his father as a perennial 'sober-sides' who seemed 'pretty straight-laced in comparison with the more rough and ready denizens of Greenville.' The son offered little more beyond this insight.[31] Perhaps it was family solidarity or simply a particular Pritham taciturnity that stymied the writer. Perhaps Wilson had overestimated her ability to get beneath the surface of the Pritham household and Greenville's small town amiability, or perhaps she simply did not care to press the matter. Travel anecdotes were invariably the responses offered to her questions. Greenville residents, as well as the doctor and his family, could effectively avoid personal confrontations by defaulting to a limitless supply of travel narratives about the doctor's active life.

In the end, the anecdotal string of travel manifests itself clearly in this biography and Wilson makes extensive use of Pritham's peripatetic exploits. Pursuing the travel tale as an organizational device required her to change publishers, as her first choice desired a greater character analysis than was present in the final version.[32] Of all her books, this is the only one that was billed 'an adventure story.' The spirit of Maine did not turn out to be a physician burdened with the duty of his calling, but a matter-of-fact adventure-embracing medical man on snowshoes. Retrospectively, Wilson acknowledged that the formula was quite evocative of Pritham. She suspected that he had probably wanted the book written this way all along.[33]

Framing State o'Maine Medicine

Big-Little World captures several dramatic moments in the physician's life. Pritham's version of events was invariably less dramatic, and less romantic and heroic, than the version that went to print in newspapers and magazines or the versions told in the oral history collected by Wilson. The physician was a 'stickler for details' and insisted on correcting all travel and medical details for accuracy.[34] Wilson maintains that when presented with content conflict, she deferred to the doctor's version. She remembers, for example, 'If I was asked once, I was asked ten times, "Have you heard the story about the time Doc's snowmobile went in the lake?"' Over the course of her time in Greenville, she collected at least ten versions of this travel tale. The most extravagant version had Pritham swim for miles in icy winter water with his black bag hung around his neck to get to a patient needing an emergency operation. In the end, she opted for the version created at the time of the incident, a version where he simply extracted himself from the ice and walked most of the way: 'Doc's [account], chronicled in his notebook, was the simplest, and I used it.'[35]

Although the physician dictated and limited the information available to Wilson, ultimately she wrote the book and she used a great deal of imagination in adding colourful details in order to heighten drama and keep the reader engaged. When she sent a first draft to the Pritham family, soliciting their comments, she remarked, 'You will find that many of the incidents have been dramatized – in other words some conversation has been introduced, words put in people's mouths which they may not have actually uttered, thoughts and emotions which may be slightly imaginative'. She asked them to state if any of these 'went contrary to fact', but added 'it is these elements, I am sure, which have made my biographies as popular as they have been.'[36]

Of particular note is the description of one of Pritham's most difficult cases, a kitchen table appendectomy performed in 1928 in a remote cabin northern cabin near the community of Rockwood. As biographer and artful narrative dramatist, Wilson details the difficulties travelling in the spring. Moosehead Lake was full of treacherous ice, and the muddy roads were impassable. Pritham, we learn, undertakes a laborious journey by railroad, although not by train. Instead, he pumps his way along the track using a 'jigger', or handcar apparatus. For the final several miles, he continued on foot. In *The Big-Little World*, Pritham arrives in time to take out the appendix of a ten-year-old boy, the son of woodsman Harry Johnson. The book describes a room full of fearful locals who crowd in to watch the operation; the boy's father meekly agrees to the surgery while looking at Pritham 'with eyes like a trusting dog's'. The emergency appendectomy occupies their attention so much that no one moves when Pritham orders more wood to be put on the fire after it dies down and the room cools to dangerous levels. 'Superstitious about something,' Pritham observes. These characters are no help to the doctor, but luckily, one competent volunteer assists Pritham. A local entrepreneur steps in on request to administer anesthesia. But, throughout, the doctor is in control. His orders are 'crisp,' his preparations provide 'as meticulous [care] as in the hospital'. His attention remains on the surgery at hand. Pritham's actions become 'lightening swift' when, because of the cold, the boy stops breathing, and he administers cardio-pulmonary resuscitation. Ultimately, thanks to the physician's quick decision-making and skill, we read how the kitchen-table surgery is a success, and the boy makes a full recovery.[37]

In this vignette of kitchen-table surgery, Wilson depicts the people of northern Maine as simple woodsmen, described as 'superstitious' onlookers frozen in awe of the doctor's skills. The physician, by contrast, is the only character with agency. The flat depiction of local people as little more than parts of the scenery was a regional packaging that the publishers hoped would have mass appeal. McGraw-Hill wanted to sell these stories nationally and sent promotional trailers for the book across the United States. The singular heroism of Pritham that is emphasized in this story of the backwoods appendectomy is not only reiterated throughout the book, but also foregrounded in promotional materials. One advance notice for the biography used such cases as evidence that 'they don't make men like Big-Little Doc Pritham anymore' and his life of 'tough compassion' in a 'fast-vanishing northern frontier of past-century America' would inspire young people to take up the challenge of rural medicine.[38]

Perhaps Wilson's narrative framework could be read as inspirational for some young readers, but eyewitness accounts, including one from the doctor, tell a somewhat different tale. The first record of the event saw printed pages in the *Portland Daily Herald* and *Sunday Telegram* in 1928, the year the surgery took place.[39] Local journalist Alfred Elden wrote a human-interest portrait of Pritham as 'Maine's Most Remarkable Country Doctor' and this story became part of the tribute piece. Interviewing a fire warden who was present, we learn that a man described as a hunting guide escorted the doctor to the home. Pritham did not actually have to travel through the northern wilderness by foot alone once the rail track ended; he had someone familiar with the terrain show him the way. This hunting guide dropped the ether. During the procedure, the wood fire in the cabin began to die down. Although the camp guide (not the doctor) called on one of the bystanders to put fuel on the fire, the people in the room were indeed 'scared to death' and did not move to assist. However, they were not immobilized because of the tension of the proceedings as much as the flammability of ether. The local fire warden was of course present as one of the onlookers. The fear of a larger conflagration is why Pritham had to complete the appendectomy in a cold room. 'In the city I suppose that would have killed the patient', the fire warden mused, but in this instance, 'the boy came through all right'.[40] State newspapers delighted in highlighting the ingenuity of the Maine physician, but also in the physical toughness of his backwoods-bred young patient. These versions make much more of the role played by the guide, who acted as Pritham's surgical assistant. And, the people in the cabin deferred to the fire warden over the physician (and his guide-attendant) by refusing to stoke the fire when asked. Overall, a different picture of rural medicine emerges from the framing of these contemporaneous, journalist accounts.

In a speech given to the Maine Medical Association to mark his fiftieth year in practice, Pritham largely concurs with these earlier versions. In his own retrospective account, Pritham indeed recalls how he felt he should accommodate the onlookers by allowing an audience to stay for the operation. He complained, however, that this did interfer with his sterile field in ways he regretted, but could not avoid.[41] He also impressed upon his medical colleagues how skilled the hunting guide was in dropping ether. Surgery was common in Pritham's practice, and he explained that the guide, his longtime friend Walter Maynard, had, over the years, assisted the physician on a fairly regular basis. He had been present to administer anaesthesia at several demanding and serious abdominal operations when Pritham had been on surgical calls in the north.[42] Moreover, the doctor fully recounts the resuscitative efforts, crediting Maynard as an active participant in saving the boy's life. In Pritham's own account, therefore, the activities of the physician as well as the role of community and family onlookers are cast in a different light than that put forth in the published biography.[43]

The first-person accounts of Pritham's 1928 appendectomy are more useful historically, especially since they are in agreement with each other on the place of the physician and the role of bystanders. But Wilson's biography provides a long view of the physician's life and work that provides context not available in other narrative accounts, whether retrospective or journalistic portrayals. The Johnson appendectomy is significant because it represents an expansion of Pritham's scope of practice into major surgery, including abdominal, for which he did not receive training or accreditation. In 1913, when the first real hospital with an operating theatre opened in Greenville proper, local physicians gained access to facilities where they might perform major surgeries. Previous to this, they had more often sent such cases down to Bangor. For this reason, Pritham had never undertaken a major surgery himself. But we learn in *Big-Little World* that he learned to perform an appendectomy after observing his colleagues, Maynard and Hiram Hunt complete such a case shortly after the new facility opened. The following week, he was performing them himself. Because of the scarcity of physicians in the area, made worse when Hiram Hunt entered semi-retirement, Pritham adopted a wide scope of practice as a matter of course. According to Wilson's biographical treatment, he 'developed a skill equal to almost any emergency', including a ruptured appendix.[44] Before a year had passed, he had also learned, without any specialized radiology training, how to operate the small portable X-ray equipment donated to the hospital and apparently became adept at interpreting the slides. The remote location of Greenville provided justification: '[w]ith the nearest radiology department in Bangor, seventy-five miles away, the need was exigent.'[45] A maverick adaptor of medical technology, his move into abdominal surgery seemed to excite neither comment nor censure from local doctors. Neither did his haphazard application of operating room antisepsis. Although Wilson quotes nurses who were impressed by Pritham's attention to what, in his medical school days, went by the name of 'sanitation', they also remembered his more idiosyncratic practices.[46] Pritham refused to scrub in with rubber gloves, preferring instead to coat his hands with 'a hand lotion somewhat resembling shellac'. This was a compound he took with him 'for emergency situations in the wilds' and was a fixture in his practice, and so was likely deployed on the occasion of the Johnson appendectomy a decade later. Standing on a stool so he could reach the patient on the operating table, he adopted surgical garb and cap, but did not wear a mask.[47] Wilson's biographical narrative is an important piece of life-writing, even for all of its dramatizations and regional stereotyping, as it shows how the remoteness of Greenville created space for physicians to experiment, adapt or resist standardized practices in the early decades of the twentieth century. These details about his larger surgical career would be lost to posterity without the biographical treatment. And without them, we lose insight into how place, in this case the remoteness of the northwoods, encouraged the physician to develop the skills and the capacity to perform the Johnson appendectomy in the first place.

The biography remains the most complete rendering of Pritham's life and work, and proved to be a great success locally. The physician had enjoyed many community tributes in his later years, and he seemed to enjoy the launch of *Big-Little World*. The elderly doctor accompanied Wilson to book signings, such as one in the summer of 1971 at the Shaw Public Library in Greenville. Wilson remembered that, although she had been to many launches over the years, she had never experienced such a success: 'Of course, it was Doc's party, not mine. People came, hundreds of them – friends, patients, people Doc had delivered, treated, operated on, advised, scolded, traveled over lakes and mountains, mud and snow and rain and ice to save.'[48] Wilson and Pritham signed books for hours. The book sold well at community celebrations even after Pritham's death. Otherwise, Wilson writes, 'The book did not set the world afire.'[49] None-theless, Wilson was pleased to point out that while her Boston publisher had little faith in the long-term appeal of Pritham's life, the book went through three printings because of sales in her home state of Maine.[50]

Region, Place and Representation

The research methods employed by Wilson, and the evolving relationship with Pritham, inform the narrative process in such a way that led her to render people and place in stereotypical ways. From her research notes and memoir, it seems clear that Wilson changed certain details not only to heighten drama, but also because, failing to extract the kinds of personal details she felt were necessary to craft her original idea for a book about Pritham, she came to rely on sources of information from outside the local community.[51] Examining the iterations of this tale in the print archive used by the writer, we see how in 1929 when the story about the Johnson appendectomy was released to Associated Press, the narrative shifted to emphasize the doctor's professional isolation in a backwards region. Along with accompanying pictures of Pritham jauntily dressed and pos-ing in a flannel shirt, woollen knickers and moccasins, accompanied by photos of snow-laden Maine cabins where the doctor is often 'forced' to perform opera-tions, the appendectomy story is recast as one of Pritham's countless 'adventures and narrow escapes.'[52]

The depictions were not ultimately flattering for the physician, for they end up casting him as an anachronistic figure. Yet the juxtaposition of the small town of Greenville acting as a gateway to the wild wooded areas reached through the inland sea of Moosehead Lake impressed Wilson. Pritham becomes part of a geo-graphical biography, so embedded in place that he is as static as the mountains of the Moosehead region. The replacement of the lumber camps with mechanized forestry industry, the emergence of a burgeoning tourist trade in the post-war years, the building of roads and the construction of a hospital in Greenville were built into the narrative as signs of progress bringing the isolated town into the fold of the twentieth century. Pritham remains an idiosyncratic practitioner as he changes to accommodate these advances; as the promotional materials said, he is the kind of doctor 'they don't make anymore'.

We can see how Pritham's practice, his work and relation to both the environ-ment and local community, is subjected to a kind of tailoring that also emphasizes the physician's role as singularly heroic, as well as historically static. This kind of heroism that Wilson crafted drew currency from the New England heritage industry.[53] Pritham is situated on a 'frontier' where the physician's rugged deter-mination epitomizes Yankee grit, the kind necessary for community-building in wilderness conditions. Regional tourism in the United States saw a shift by the last two decades of the nineteenth century toward nostalgic depictions of rural New England life. Old New England is a place where application of ingenuity, self sufficiency, and an honouring of family and community connection provide a foundation for small-town prosperity.[54] And by the twentieth century, Joseph Conforti argues that northern New England, including rural Maine, becomes a region most strongly associated with these values.[55] In *Big-Little World*, Wilson attempts to make Pritham the embodiment of the self-sufficient 'Old New England,' and all but reduces others in the narrative to 'scenery'. Northwoods people are recast as passive benefactees of the doctor's care and skill, but in framing this kind of depiction – one that disagrees with the physician's own accounts – Wilson overlooks the community connection that made Pritham himself reciprocally dependent on the people of northwoods Maine. It also overlooks how the place itself shaped him.

Historians spend much time and energy unpacking 'local colour' when it comes packaged as regional stereotype. Rural historians, such as Ruth Sandwell, have long emphasized that rural lives and communities often reveal themselves to be surprisingly complex, despite common twentieth-century depictions that suggest lives of rural people are somehow more rooted in past folksways, and somehow 'simpler'. Careful scholarly attention is required to help problematize 'that curious intellectual sleight of hand that has allowed "modern" to stand in contrast to "rural".'[56] The social and cultural geographies uncovered about Pritham's work, such as the Johnson appendectomy in 1928, reveal many hidden complexities. A combined understanding of geography and weather as well as inventive use of transportation technologies underpinned Pritham's successful prosecution of a northwoods medical practice. The willingness to expand the scope of practice and learn new techniques while 'in harness' were key characteristics of this event, and common throughout his life's work, pointing to a dynamism within rural medicine that remained an inter-war legacy bestowed by the traditions of home-based practice. Scientific technologies and techniques, such as anesthesia, asepsis and major invasive surgeries, were integrated into Pritham's practice in ways that would certainly run counter to the precepts of standardized, scientific medicine of his day. As social historians of technology have noted, the agency of rural consumers in determining the uses of new twentieth-century transportation and communications technologies was very strong during the inter-war period.[57] This study suggests the same may be true for technology in medicine between the wars. The complexities of rural practice meant physicians like Pritham did not rely on their authority to secure any necessity to cope. A deep reading of his travel tales reveals how the doctor cultivated relationships with the people who provided key services and resources, like handcar transit on railway lines, or training a hunting guide to drop ether. He adopted practices of creatively utilizing and moulding his practice to make use of new facilities, technologies and incorporate whatever forms local assistance took. These activities required knowledge of local culture; they required that he compromise and become part of an interconnected web.

Place is a part of rural medical practice. Pritham's own travel tales do not flaunt his singularly heroic contributions; they are testaments to successful country doctor strategies, which utilized the physical, social and cultural geographies of place to serve the needs of his practice. Pritham's narrative about his practices, the narratives generated by eyewitnesses and participants, and the narrative that went to press, all demonstrate the influence of place. It is important to note that Pritham was among the last medical generation to practise before widespread adoption of health insurance schemes. Scholars investigating later decades of the twentieth century may well come to different conclusions about the power of place in the lives and practices of general physicians like Pritham. The centralization of general medicine, and the decline of peripatetic models of care, may also mediate the importance of place or change the terms of place for later generations of practitioners. But in this study of inter-war Maine medicine, region and place continue to be defined by navigating both the big and little worlds of a country doctor.

Acknowledgements

I gratefully acknowledge the support of Associated Medical Services (Hannah Foundation), Toronto, who funded the doctoral work upon which this research is based. Members of an interdisciplinary writing group at the University of Alberta, Lianne McTavish, Anne Whitelaw and Julie Rak, provided important insights and comments on an earlier draft. Finally, I am grateful for the editorial work and guidance of Erika Dyck, and the suggestions of an anonymous peer reviewer, which helped to focus the content and arguments made in this article.

4 PUTTING HYPERACTIVITY IN ITS PLACE: COLD WAR POLITICS, THE BRAIN RACE AND THE ORIGINS OF HYPERACTIVITY IN THE UNITED STATES, 1957–68

Matthew Smith

when the bears
        hurled a spaceball
                into heaven
                        from left field
        us got real scared
us expanded our spaceball program
us expanded our vocabulary too
us expanded everything
        'till us then got the man in the moon
hah!
        us beat them bears
yep!
        us showed them bears
                a giant leapfrog for all mankind[1]

Introduction

In the late 1950s, the first American children were diagnosed with hyperactivity. They would not be the last. By 2006, the National Institute of Mental Health conservatively estimated that two million American children were afflicted with hyperactivity or Attention-Deficit/Hyperactivity Disorder (ADHD), a disorder characterized by hyperactive, inattentive, impulsive, defiant and aggressive behaviour. During the last five decades, these children have represented a major portion of the patients seen by American paediatricians, child psychiatrists and general practitioners, have been the subject of thousands of medical articles, textbooks and self-help manuals and have contributed significantly to the profits of pharmaceutical companies such as Novartis through sales of hyperactivity drugs such as Ritalin. Hyperactivity has also become a cultural phenomenon, identified with cartoon characters such as Dennis the Menace, Calvin (from the *Calvin and Hobbes* comic strip) and Bart Simpson, and a topic featured in television shows ranging from *The Simpsons* to *The Sopranos*.[2]

The presiding opinion of most paediatricians, psychiatrists and other physicians that hyperactivity is merely a neurological condition fails to shed light on why educators, politicians and physicians during the late 1950s increasingly believed that hyperactive and distractible behaviour was pathological and warranted medical attention. It also overlooks why hyperactivity became problematic in the United States long before other countries. While thousands of papers in American medical and education journals had been written about hyperactivity during the 1960s, the disorder did not become widespread in the United Kingdom until the 1990s. The first mention of hyperactive behaviour in the *Lancet*, for example, did not occur until 1970, and was a letter to the editor written by American psychiatrists. The only response to the letter was also by an American psychiatrist.[3] Hinting that American preoccupation with hyperactivity was rooted in something other than neurology, a 1973 editorial in the *Lancet* asked: 'Are the Americans ahead of the British, or behind them, or do their children's brains dysfunction in such an ostentatiously exotic transatlantic fashion that they require drug therapy?'[4]

Although hyperactivity is now regularly diagnosed in the United Kingdom, and many other developed countries, it emerged first in a particular place, namely the United States during the 1950s. Just as David Livingstone has argued that science has not developed in 'placeless places', sites 'where the influence of locality is eliminated,' medical knowledge, and medical concerns, have also been shaped by regional circumstances.[5] These regional circumstances are often political. With regards to psychiatry, ideas about mental illness may not be typically rooted in physical geography – although anyone affected by seasonal affective disorder would beg to differ – but they have often been enmeshed in the political, cultural and ideological features that are also essential to defining and understanding a geographical space. In some cases, the social climate can encourage a liberal approach to the development of medical knowledge. As Erika Dyck has argued, the activism, optimism and stability of the Cooperative Commonwealth Federation government in Saskatchewan during the 1950s and 60s created a political climate in which it was possible for scientists to launch a bold programme of therapeutic LSD experimentation.[6]

In other circumstances, however, notions about mental health have been commandeered by broader political pressures, particularly during times of conflict. Military, economic and ideological threats to the integrity of nations have often played a role in expanding the number of behaviours that have been thought to be pathological and in need of psychiatric treatment. Mark Jackson has demonstrated, for example, that, during the first decades of the twentieth century, notions about and responses to feeblemindedness were fuelled in part by fears emanating out of the Boer War that young British men were unfit, physically, mentally and intellectually, to defend the British empire.[7] Similar concerns emerged in the United States after World War 2 when it became known that two million individuals were rejected for service by the military for neuropsychiatric reasons.[8]

The pressures and demands of the Cold War also had a significant impact on how Americans perceived mental health and, in particular, the mental health of schoolchildren. While numerous changes to the structure and function of American families, schools, workplaces and medical care undoubtedly and substantially contributed to the emergence of hyperactivity as a major medical problem, the roots of the disorder are found in the politics of the Cold War. Put another way, the origins of hyperactivity are rooted not in human genetics, but in a specific, political place, namely, the United States during the middle years of the Cold War. As the Soviet Union developed hydrogen bombs and launched the first satellites and humans into space, many influential Americans became convinced that the United States was losing the 'brain race' and, unless the scholastic performance of all American children improved markedly, they would lose the Cold War altogether.

This persistent perception contributed to the growth of hyperactivity diagnoses by: 1) demonizing behaviours seen to interfere with high educational achievement, such as hyperactivity; 2) demanding that all children, especially those who underachieved academically, stay in school as long as possible where behaviour such as hyperactivity was liable to be problematic; and 3) urging that school counsellors be hired to identify hyperactive children, label their deficiencies and refer them to physicians for treatment. As such, the hyperactive child became symbolic of perceived American intellectual inferiority and the target of politicians, physicians and educators who saw improvement in academic achievement as essential to national security.

Putting the History of Hyperactivity in its Place

While some historians and physicians suggest that hyperactivity dates back to the nineteenth century, often citing the observations of physicians such as German Heinrich Hoffman and Englishmen Thomas Clouston and Sir George Still,[9] prior to the late 1950s research into the disorder was sporadic and typically limited to children confined to mental institutions, rather than schoolchildren.[10] Moreover, when the research of these physicians, such as Still's 1902 articles in the *Lancet*, is examined, it is evident that hyperactivity was only one of a great number of behaviours that were cited, and that other, more disturbing behaviours, such as extreme violence, self-harm and criminality, were more central to the researchers' concerns.[11] In other words, during the first part of the twentieth century, hyper-activity was not perceived as being pathological in and of itself. Finally, the labels used to describe behaviour similar to hyperactivity, terms such as post-encepha-litic disorder and minimal brain damage, indicated that earlier researchers were usually concerned with children suffering from the residual effects of fever, infec-tion or head injury.[12] As such, the depictions and causes of so-called hyperactive behaviour found in the medical literature of the early twentieth century bear little resemblance to what is recognized as hyperactivity today.[13]

In 1957, however, a pair of articles on 'hyperkinetic impulse disorder' by psychiatrists Maurice Laufer and Eric Denhoff, along with Gerald Solomons in one instance, described behaviour virtually identical with what is currently associated with hyperactivity.[14] Laufer *et al.*'s depiction of 'hyperactivity; short attention span and poor powers of concentration; irritability; impulsiveness; variability [of behaviour and school performance]; and poor school work' was only marginally different to modern conceptions, descriptions and understand-ing of hyperactivity today, according to paediatrician Howard Fischer, in a 2007 edition of the *Journal of Pediatrics*.[15] Soon after the 1957 publications of Laufer *et al.*, dozens and then hundreds of researchers began studying hyperactivity, and by 1968, when the disorder was included in the second edition of the *Diagnostic and Statistical Manual of Mental Disorders*, it was recognized as a disorder of epidemic proportions in the United States.

Laufer *et al.*'s depictions of hyperactive behaviour facilitated this explosion of interest in three key ways that distinguished their conception of the disor-der from that of earlier researchers. First, and most importantly, Laufer *et al.* restricted their attention to a narrower range of behaviours than their predeces-sors, and chose the term 'hyperkinetic impulse disorder' to reflect the primary features of this condition.[16] In so doing, Laufer *et al.* drew special attention to hyperactivity as a core cause of behavioural and scholastic difficulty. The label enabled subsequent researchers to focus on a more specific, yet easily recogniz-able, constellation of behaviours that they could then identify, diagnose and treat. Second, unlike previous researchers, Laufer *et al.* stressed the ubiquity of hyperactivity among the general school-age population.[17] Finally, Laufer *et al.* concentrated on children who presented no evidence of brain damage, chil-dren for whom there was no apparent cause for their hyperactivity, and left the question of the aetiology of hyperactivity largely unanswered.[18] Described in such a way, hyperactivity was not restricted to severely disturbed, brain-injured children, but could be applied to a significant percentage of the school-aged population in the United States.

The 1957 papers of Laufer *et al.* provided a point of departure for modern conceptions of hyperactivity by depicting the disorder as one that could be applied to millions of children. This notwithstanding, sweeping categories and novel labels do not attract patients as moths to a flame. As historian Joan Jacobs

Brumberg has demonstrated with anorexia nervosa, and anthropologist Allan Young has shown with post-traumatic stress disorder (PTSD), popular psychiatric disorders tend to reflect contemporary politics, concerns and circumstances.[19] So what were the circumstances that catapulted hyperactivity into medical and cultural prominence? What led hyperactivity from being not mentioned in Leo Kanner's seminal textbook, *Child Psychiatry* (1957) to becoming so prevalent by the mid-1960s that 'mere mention of the term "hyperkinetic syndrome" [was] guaranteed to stir up vigorous discussion in medical, psychological, social work, and educational circles.'[20] And why did the disorder first emerge in the United States? Although many of the profound changes to American society during the 1950s and 60s played a role in the origins of hyperactivity, the prime catalyst had much to do with the Cold War and the launch of *Sputnik* in 1957.

Cold War Kids

The United States during the 1950s, as depicted in television programmes such as *Leave it to Beaver* and *Father Knows Best*, was a place characterized by confidence, calm and contentment, a nation buoyed by the thriving economy, a relative thaw in the Cold War (following the end of the Korean War and Stalin's death in 1953) and the rise of the suburban nuclear family. Historian Irving Bernstein has cautioned against this idea, however, proposing that only the four middle years of the decade (1953–6) can accurately be described as indicative of such a self-satisfied atmosphere.[21] The political picture of the early 1950s, for example, were characterized by McCarthyism, the Korean War and the Soviet Union's emergence as a nuclear power. By the late 1950s, Khrushchev had won supreme power in the Kremlin and determined that the Soviet Union would outstrip the Americans militarily and technologically. During that pivotal period he received his wish, as the Soviets put two *Sputnik* satellites into orbit and tested a powerful hydrogen bomb.

The notion that the United States was failing to keep up with Soviet scientific and technological advances and, thus, was losing the intellectual battle of the Cold War, encouraged many politicians and educators to look to the schools for both explanations and solutions. As authors Barbara Ehrenreich and Deirdre English put it, 'Sputnik hit like a spitball in the eyes of American child-raising experts, educators and Cold War propagandists ... Communist children were co-operative and good-tempered to a degree that was almost eerie compared to the Dennis-the-Menace personality deemed acceptable in American kids.'[22] Contemporary educators echoed such observations, complaining that 'American public education was the object of vigorous and widespread criticism and attack without parallel in our history',[23] that 'our schools have been, and are, under terrific fire'[24] and that 'the Soviet firing of Sputnik into space seemed to unloose a veritable Pandora's box of criticisms of us'.[25]

Fear that 'the Soviets have gone far ahead of us in the production of trained minds in science and technology',[26] precipitated scathing critiques of American education, including Arthur Bestor Jr's *Educational Wastelands* (1953), Admiral Hyman Rickover's *Education and Freedom* (1959), Max Rafferty's *Suffer, Little Children* (1962) and James Conant's *The American High School Today* (1959).[27] Admiral Rickover, well known as the 'Father of the Nuclear Navy', stressed that 'the schools are letting us down at a time when the nation is in great peril. To be undereducated in this trigger-happy world is to invite catastrophe'. Educator Asa S. Knowles echoed these sentiments, warning that 'this sphere [Sputnik] tells not of the desirability but of the URGENT NECESSITY of the highest quality and expanded dimensions of the educational effort ... the future of the twentieth century lies in the hands of those who have placed education and its Siamese twin, research, in the position of first priority'.[28] Others, such as physicist Lloyd Berkner, were equally convinced that 'brainpower [was] the resource upon which our nation must depend for its future economic and social health'.[29] In other words, the United States could 'no longer ignore the early school dropout on the excuse that we need a large labour force of uneducated muscle men'.[30]

The message in such publications was clear: education was to be the battleground on which the Cold War would be won or lost and, as of 1957, the dominant view was that the Soviets were winning.[31] For most critics the solution to this perceived catastrophe was to reject the 'fun and games' approach of child-centred progressive education, which had dominated pedagogic philosophy since the 1930s, and to institute a more rigorous, academic and standardized system in which firm, federally established objectives would be set out for students to achieve. [32] Crucially, dropping out of school to find unskilled work, a choice made then and now by many hyperactive students, was no longer considered an option. [33] Instead, substantial efforts would be made to identify struggling students' barriers, address them through various remedial measures and encourage them to stay in school and reach their academic potential.[34] Such recommendations, largely, though not universally, endorsed by educational administrators and supported by federal legislation such as the National Defense Education Act (1958) and the Elementary and Secondary Education Act (1965), established a framework in which hyperactive, inattentive and impulsive schoolchildren were increasingly identified as disordered and referred by school counsellors to paediatricians and psychiatrists for diagnosis and treatment.

Future Scientists and Underachievers

It might be argued that the relationship between the Cold War and the rise of hyperactivity is one of correlation, rather than causality. However, educational publications of the 1950s and 60s reveal that hyperactive, impulsive and inattentive behaviour was increasingly associated with academic underachievement and, by extension, the intellectual shortcomings of the United States. An example of this is illustrated in a study published in the periodical *Exceptional Children* intended to address the 'great concern about the use of talent in our society' and the 'wastage in the [educational] system'.[35] The authors compared impulsivity rates in 'underachievers' and 'future scientists' (students who had been accepted into a summer space camp) and discovered that the 'future scientists' were not only much less impulsive than their underachieving classmates, but also more able to control their motor activity or, in other words, less hyperactive.[36] The study's conclusion was that the impulsive, hyperactive behaviour displayed by the underachieving students was the key distinction between them and the 'future scientists' desired by critics such as Conant and Rickover. Other researchers also argued that impulse control was essential to 'our survival as a nation', and insisted that 'the ultimate and highest goal in so-called control comes not from the teacher or group domination, but with the establishment of self-control within the individual'.[37]

Concern about impulsivity and hyperactivity echoed a shift with respect to which behavioural characteristics were deemed to be most pernicious by American educators, physicians and politicians. Whereas shy, withdrawn and neurotic children who tended to be inactive were of greatest concern prior to the late 1950s,[38] the increased premium on intellectual achievement following the launch of *Sputnik* meant that the most acute apprehension swung to excessively active children. As child psychiatrist Gregory Rochlin noted, commenting on the previous trend, 'motor activity in the young child, even if excessive, is more favourably regarded than its opposite. Although the child who is hyperactive may be as emotionally disturbed as the shy inhibited child, the latter is apt to receive more attention than the former'.[39] Another indication of this shift in perception is evident in Katherine Reeves's 'The Children we Teach' series in the education periodical *Grade Teacher*, which changed its focus on shy, withdrawn children to concentrate on children like 'Charles' who 'slips from one interest to another, intense in his preoccupation of the moment, absorbing the essence of each, but moving insatiably from one activity to the next'.[40]

The increased concern about hyperactivity was also reflected in subtler ways. A series of Kellogg's breakfast cereal advertisements in *Grade Teacher*, for instance, featured a trio of troublesome children, all of whom displayed different symptoms of hyperactivity. While 'Window-Watchin' Wendy, who 'skips class right in her seat' represented the inattentive child, hyperactive children were characterized by the 'restless and irritable' 'Lemon-Drop Kid' and the 'Clockwork Kid', who was liable to be the 'mainspring of a classroom rebellion', embodied the impulsive, defiant child.[41] According to Kellogg's, however, these children did not need a revamped educational system; all they required was a better breakfast, ideally one found in a Kellogg's Corn Flakes box. That a company such as Kellogg's had picked up on the concern about inattentive, hyperactive and impulsive schoolchildren indicates how problematic such behaviours were thought to be by the late 1950s.[42]

Changes in child development theory during the 1960s also contributed to the notion that the behaviours of the Kellogg's trio needed to be identified and corrected. Specifically, paediatricians and child psychiatrists were beginning to question developmental theorists such as Eric Erikson who believed that many of the pathologies of childhood and adolescence were transitional in nature. Instead, many psychiatrists began to fear that disorders such as hyperactivity would persist into adulthood and hinder the individual's employability and work performance, perhaps becoming as debilitating as chronic depression and schizophrenia. [43] According to James F. Masterson, Erikson's 'dangerous [ideas] prevented a thera-peutic intervention', an intervention that could be 'a crucial encounter for the adolescent'.[44] Educators also recognized that the 'cost of prevention is far less than the cost of breakdown and its treatment' and that they, too, were involved in identifying problems such as hyperactivity and impulsivity.[45] Hyperactivity in schoolchildren, therefore, became seen as a precursor of not only academic underachievement, but also subsequent mental health problems.

No Place in Society for the Dropout

One circumstance educators intended to prevent through such 'therapeutic intervention' as identifying hyperactive children was the phenomenon of the school dropout. There was 'no place in society for the dropout' according to many education critics who were also adamant that a sizeable improvement in high-school completion rates was a necessary condition of a competitive, tech-nologically-sophisticated workforce.[46] As President Lyndon Johnson stressed in 1965, 'jobs filled by high school graduates rose by 40 per cent in the last ten years. Jobs for those with less schooling decreased by nearly ten per cent'.[47] Although the proportional rates of early school leavers were actually falling, the percep-tion was that school dropouts was not only a national problem, but a matter of 'national security'.[48] Palmer Hoyt, publisher of the *Denver Post*, in seeking a 'reevaluation of the whole education program', warned that 'the Russian corps of skilled technological brains now totals 2,700,000' and that the United States was not keeping pace.[49]

In order to train more scientists, engineers and technicians, critics such as Rickover not only demanded more high-school graduates, but also wanted higher standards for high-school graduation, including more hours of classes, more homework and the attainment of higher levels of education in a shorter amount of time.[50] The former Harvard President and Ambassador to West Germany, James Conant, also believed that not only should more American youth complete high school, they should also attain higher standards, especially in core subjects such as English, mathematics, foreign languages and science.[51] That such recommendations became a reality is demonstrated in a letter to the editor of *Science* in which the author complains that

> after Sputnik, the educators suddenly became infected with the idea that the day of reasonable [homework] assignments was over; from then on, students had to complete at least 100 problems per assignment in addition to increased reading assignments. Each instructor seemed to take the attitude that his assignments should occupy all of a student's waking hours.[52]

New York Times education columnist Dorothy Barclay concurred:

> The school picture ... in 1958, reflected almost entirely a tightening-up. But in some classrooms or communities, unfortunately, it was more like a cracking down. Concern about college admissions and general anxiety about America's technical ability, as highlighted by the space race, combined to produce demands for higher standards of achievement in the upper elementary grades and in high schools. The switch has given new incentive to some youngsters, but, where misapplied, its sudden severity has put a strain on others who have been unable, thorough lack of adequate preparation, to meet the new demands. ... Even more significant to the average family, however, is the amount of attention being given to smoking out and stimulating the efforts of the under-achievers. These youngsters of varying abilities who are not working up to their potential.[53]

Writing in 1959, two years prior to when Ritalin was first marketed to children, however, Barclay was not likely aware of the irony inherent in her phrase 'smoking out and stimulating the efforts of the underachievers'; indeed the behaviours most often associated with underachieving youngsters during the post-*Sputnik* period were those which would increasingly be treated with stimulant drugs. Nevertheless, Barclay did recognize that higher educational standards highlighted the academic difficulties of those students who, in previous decades, would have left school for employment in their early to mid-teens. Such students, whose penchant for being active and energetic was viewed as positive in many labour-intensive careers, were now expected to stay still in their seats and attend to lectures. Indeed, researchers recognized that hyperactive, inattentive children showed 'extremely poor advancement' with respect to the 'increasing emphasis placed on abstract concepts' that emerged in the latter years of schooling.[54] The situation was exacerbated by the fact that 'multiple [academic] failures ... undermine individual children's ambition and causes a profound sense of failure and lack of motivation – facts hardly conducive to learning'.[55]

Conant's particular concern about the dropout rates in slum-area schools, 'where as many as half of the children drop out of school in grades 9, 10, and 11', while reflecting admirable aims, also thrust a spotlight on the behavioural problems deemed to contribute to such rates.[56] By the late 1960s, many educators were concerned about how many children from poor neighbourhoods were being labelled as hyperactive, and that little effort was being taken to invest in 'the total environment of our children from inadequate homes and backgrounds'.[57] Some, such as psychologist Howard Adelman, went as far as accusing schools of labelling failing students as disordered in order to salvage the school's reputation, arguing 'whenever a youngster's learning problems can be attributed to deficits in the instructional process, that child should not be categorized as learning disabled'.[58] Nevertheless, schools were dealing with many more students who, in previous decades, would have abandoned academic pursuits for occupations where hyperactive, energetic behaviour would be viewed as positive. Unfortunately for such students, these behaviours were not conducive to learning in the classroom.

The Counsellor, the Physician and the Hyperactive Child

Despite Adelman's concerns, schoolchildren during the 1960s were ever more diagnosed with hyperactivity. One important cog in the diagnostic machine was represented by a relatively new profession in American education, the school counsellor. Counsellors played the role of mediator between the educational sphere, where hyperactive behaviour was increasingly recognized, and the medical sphere, where such behaviour was diagnosed as a disorder and treated. Moreover, education critics of the late 1950s were adamant that counsellors had an essential role in improving American education. Conant, for example, stressed the establishment of a comprehensive counselling infrastructure (at a student to counsellor ratio of 250:1) and believed counselling to be an essential part of any 'satisfactory' elementary or secondary school.[59] He especially called on school counsellors to 'be on the lookout for the bright boy or girl whose high ability has been demonstrated by the results of aptitude tests ... but whose achievement, as measured by grades in courses, has been low'.[60] This description of the underachieving student of average or above-average intelligence would become the stereotype of the hyperactive child.[61]

Historian Alexander Rippa has confirmed that many schools did follow Conant's recommendation, hiring large numbers of counsellors who specialized in identifying the problem.[62] His view is reflected in education periodicals where it is also apparent that these counsellors were instrumental in identifying hyperactive, inattentive and impulsive children and viewing them as a discrete category of problem children, separate from the 'mentally retarded' and '"pure" emotionally disturbed'.[63] Teachers were also an important part of identifying such behaviours, for example, by learning 'the difference between serious symptoms in child behaviour and simply annoying behaviour', but were expected to cede responsibility for rehabilitating hyperactive, inattentive children to counselling staff.[64] While some teachers resented this intrusion into their domain, it was also believed that others sought 'diagnostic solace as a means of rationalizing her own programming inadequacies'. In other words, teachers unable to control the behaviour of hyperactive, impulsive children in their classroom were now able to rely on counsellors to determine 'some medical or psychological malady' and absolve themselves of blame for the student's difficulties.[65]

Whatever the teachers' motivations, the emergence of the counsellor as an additional resource in American schools undoubtedly facilitated the process by which problem students were labelled as hyperactive and referred for treatment. Although counsellors often recommended educational interventions, the low success rates of such measures compelled them to refer hyperactive students to physicians for medical treatment.[66] Indeed, counsellor John Peterson admitted that his colleagues sought 'a panacea for our non-performing students, a magic that will stir the laggard and salve the distressed.'[67] For many hyperactive children the panacea provided by physicians was stimulant medications, such as Ritalin. In an era where scientific advancement was thought to take priority over everything, it was somehow appropriate that the solution for the problem of the hyperactive child, the symbol of American academic underachievement, was to be found in the highly scientific, highly technical setting of a pharmaceutical laboratory.

Conclusion

Although the United States essentially ended the space race in 1969 by placing men on the moon, this triumph of American education ironically paralleled a tightening of federal education expenditure, as monies were instead allocated to fight the Vietnam War. Although the National Defense Education Act had won its primary objective of surpassing Soviet technological prowess, returns were diminishing for many American students, especially those struggling to cope with raised expectations for academic and behavioural performance. As John Gardner, Secretary of Health, Education, and Welfare put it, a 'crunch between expectations and resources' was occurring, especially with regards to 'early childhood education, work with handicapped children, [and] special education for the disadvantaged'.[68] Despite this 'crunch', concern about hyperactivity remained and even increased during the 1970s, as pharmaceutical companies, physicians and parent advocacy groups took the lead in condemning such behaviour and marketing pharmaceutical solutions.[69] Echoing the political, ideological and cultural place from which it emerged, the disorder has remained a controversial, contested and confusing entity for parents, teachers, physicians and children.

Much has changed in the United States since the late 1950s, but many of the concerns that spurred interest in hyperactivity have re-emerged in the last decade. The United States is once again involved in an intractable, divisive and ideological conflict, not with global communism, but with the equally problematic concept of 'terror'. Concurrently, American economic supremacy is under threat from China, India, Brazil and the European Union. As it was the case at the height of the Cold War, to define the United States as a place in 2010 is to evoke the political situation it finds itself in and the numerous social, cultural and political ramifications that have resulted. For example, when the National Defense Education Act reached its fiftieth anniversary in 2008, fears that the United States' position in the world was slipping spurred calls for a new such Act. The Association of American Universities warned that 'as the scientific and technological advantage that the US has held over other nations is slipping away ... [to] rapidly developing economies, particularly in Asia' a new Act is required 'to enhance the pipeline of US students trained in fields vital to our national and economic security'.[70] The fields mentioned mimicked those identified in 1958, namely, 'science, mathematics, engineering and languages'. As during the Cold War, the geopolitical situation facing the United States threatens to dictate education and, perhaps, mental health policy.

The philosophy of the American Association of Universities, along with their Cold War predecessors, explicitly indicates their belief that childhood is nothing more than a period of investment that is returned in the form of American national and economic security. Similar thinking in the context of New Labour Britain has led historian of childhood, Harry Hendrick, to observe that in such circumstances, 'children ... are too valuable in terms of human capital to be given any say in shaping their own lives. Rather, they are to be possessed in order to maximize their potential as investments in *our* future'.[71] Although thinking of children as human capital might be excused as being sensibly utilitarian, this rationale, as Hendrick implies, obscures the fact that it is those in power, and not the disadvantaged members of the whole, who benefit from such accruement.

In the case of hyperactivity this has also been the case, as the perceived needs of the state have subsumed those of the child in the process of identifying certain behaviours as being pathological, and then attempting to medicate them out of existence. This does not mean, however, that the United States has always or will always benefit from the suppression of behaviours associated with hyperactivity. The overenthusiastic diagnosis and treatment of hyperactivity, when perceived differently, ceases to be a matter of simply inhibiting behaviours perceived as detrimental to learning, and instead becomes the constraint of potentially positive behaviours, behaviours which could be of benefit to both children and the state:

hyperactivity becomes dynamism and energy; distractibility becomes creativity and inventiveness; impulsivity is seen as taking initiative; and, possibly most importantly, defiance becomes courage and the willingness to question. The task for educators, politicians and physicians, therefore, becomes not to limit the range of childhood behaviour to guarantee academic success and national security, but to channel such behaviours in positive ways that benefit both the child and society.

5 WHY CANADA HAS A UNIVERSAL MEDICAL INSURANCE PROGRAMME AND THE UNITED STATES DOES NOT: ACCOUNTING FOR HISTORICAL DIFFERENCES IN AMERICAN AND CANADIAN SOCIAL POLICIES

Alvin Finkel

Why does Canada have universal medical insurance while the United States has a mixture of private and public programmes that leaves 70 million Americans without insurance for at least part of the year?[1] More generally, why is Canada's welfare state more advanced than its American counterpart? According to Seymour Martin Lipset, Americans are heirs to a revolution that embodied individualist values. Canadians, heirs to the North Americans who stayed within the British fold, developed a more 'toryish' or organic approach to society, an approach that eventually allowed socialism to emerge as an important, if minority, ideology. While socialism became a 'foreign' ideology to Americans, it gained respectability in Canada. 'Red Tories' became the backbone of a social consensus in Canada decidedly left of its American counterpart.[2]

The historical record contradicts Lipset's theory. As late as 1960, the American welfare state trumped its Canadian counterpart. Progressive social interventionism in Canada is a recent phenomenon for which events in the 1770s provide little explanation. This chapter argues that Lipset confuses cause and effect regarding social policy variances between the two countries. He provides little evidence that Canadians favoured social intervention more than Americans in the period *before* their major social programmes were implemented. He merely establishes that today's Canadians support their country's social programmes while Americans seem happy enough with the limited social welfare state that characterizes their country. As we shall see, in the period when Canada was implementing social programmes, American public opinion also favoured such programmes. So, if Americans historically were willing to embrace collectivism, why did their governments produce a tepid welfare state relative to most countries? Why did they fail to create universal medicare?

Historian Penny Bryden, focusing on Canada, and political scientist Antonia Maioni, comparing the two countries, both suggest what Maioni calls 'the dynamic impact of parties and institutions'[3] as an alternative explanation to the political cultural thesis of Lipset. Bryden focuses on struggles within the Liberal Party to explain the development of universal medicare.[4] She largely ignores the influence of the social-democratic New Democratic Party. By contrast, Maioni argues, 'the presence of a party of the Left profoundly shaped the health insurance debate by focusing on the role of government in health care financing, and by influencing the federal and provincial governments to fulfill this role'.[5] This observation begs the question why, if 'political culture' is unimportant, Canada produced an influential Left party while the United States did not. This chapter emphasizes that place influences the development of political ideas about healthcare rights and equality. A comparison of rights movements in Canada and the United States shows how people who start with many common premises can nonetheless diverge dramatically in the political practices they choose and eventually end up with fewer common premises than they started with. For example, the two trade union movements considered here start with the premise that universal social programmes are worthwhile. Both support Cold War ideology. But the Americans, because they stand on American ground, see their Cold War allegiances as trumping almost everything; so they unionize political support to Cold War party, which ends up disappointing workers in the area of medical care and social insurance more generally. Then the American union movement starts to reassess its original support for universal medical care altogether, abandoning social welfare commitments to workers in favour of commitment to an idealized Cold War version of the place called America. The Canadians, standing on Canadian ground, do not see themselves as operating in territory that has to lead in the Cold War. They stick to their social welfare principles as their top priority, somewhat following their government in a passive and inconsistent support of 'free world' policies, which they gradually start to view as imperialism since, in Canada at this time, the debate between whether the US is defending democracy or international plunder is not as taboo a subject as it is in the United States.

In turn, for the women's movement, which in both countries, gradually becomes anti-imperialist, the sense of place plays a decisive role in determining whether they can work with a government that purports to speak for all who live there. In both countries the women's movement starts with the premise that there should be greater equality of women and men, and that indeed all citizens deserve greater equality of both opportunity and condition. In Canada, the government is constructed by the women's movement as pliable; it appears credible that it can be converted from a patriarchal tool to an instrument that can, at least in part, benefit women by providing them with social programmes that work towards women's liberation. In the United States, by contrast, the women's movement is aware of their government as not only a tool of patriarchy at home but of unspeakable exploitation abroad. So, while they begin, like the women's movement in Canada in believing in greater equality for all citizens, both formal and economic, they believe that much of this has to be achieved from the ground up because it is inconceivable that the government of the place where they live can be turned into a positive force. At best, they can try to campaign for it not to allow formal discrimination against women.

This paper argues that social agency, rather than values, explains why Canadians more successfully triumphed over elite resistance to social programmes after World War 2 than Americans. Specifically, Canadian trade unionists and feminists, the organized representatives of class and gender, developed better strategies for turning public support into legislated programmes than their American counterparts. They steered public discourse about social policy and influenced the political system to deliver at least some of their demands. While public opinion measured by surveys is important, it cannot alone predict the development of social policy. Absent overwhelming social pressures for reforms that benefit the less advantaged, there is tremendous bias built into state structures in both countries to maintain elite privileges. There is no single explanation for why mass movements in the two countries, which had similar collectivist social values, chose divergent strategies. But the far greater global power of the American state has caused social movements in the US either to identify closely with that power, thereby weakening their ability to act as effective opposition movements, or to be so repulsed by their government as to seek to effect change mainly via non-electoral means. In Canada, by contrast, social movements generally regard government institutions benignly and seek changes within the parliamentary framework.

Some argue that the United States is a laggard in social policy because its state institutions are biased in favour of inaction. Impediments to change include the president's veto, Congress's ability to ignore the president's initiatives, and the House and Senate powers to tie each other's hands. Meanwhile, the states and the federal government can checkmate one another in many areas of jurisdiction.[6] But the Canadian political system is equally marked by fragmentation of power. Observes constitutional scholar Alan Cairns:

> The combined Canadian state at both levels is characterized by a centrifugal scattering of public authority. This fragmentation manifests itself in federalism, in the more than 260 cabinet ministers and their departments of its eleven senior governments, and in a proliferation of government agencies and corporations only loosely connected to the traditional responsible government focus of executive authority. Countless programs, mostly old, occasionally new, and frequently contradictory, are applied by thousands of separate bureaucratic units of the eleven governments. The result is a fragmented state with a frightening impact on society.[7]

Yet, for all the fragmentation of authority in the two countries, each has had a period of rapid advances in social policy led by the federal government. In the

United States, the New Deal period of the 1930s witnessed the greatest social advances while in Canada the crucial period was that of Liberal government from 1963 to 1968.

Social Policies in Canada and the USA

By World War 2 the US had legislated unemployment insurance, employment-related old-age pensions, and Aid to Dependent Children. Canada's only federal social programme was a means-tested, modest old-age pension cost-shared between federal and provincial governments. Both countries had workmen's compensation and mothers' allowances programmes at the state/provincial level,[8] but in both areas the Americans had led the way. Yet, by the early 70s, Canada left the United States in the dust in social provision. Universal family allowances were introduced in 1944, federal sharing of social assistance costs with provinces culminated in the Canada Assistance Plan (CAP) of 1966, requiring the federal government to pay half of all social assistance costs, and every province established a publicly-funded hospitalization insurance and medical insurance programme after the federal government provided generous funding for the former in 1957 and the latter in 1968. The poorer the province, the larger the health insurance grant.[9] Unemployment Insurance (UI), introduced in 1940, was under federal control and in 1971 became nearly universal, with maternity benefits added to the mix.[10] American UI was controlled by the states and restrictive.[11] American medicare for the aged and medicaid for the destitute introduced in 1965 left most Americans to find medical insurance in the private market; federal government direct aid for the destitute, apart from medicaid, was restricted to food stamps and the Aid to Families with Dependent Children programme. During the 1980s and early 90s, the Canadian 'safety net' proved considerably more effective in stemming the rise of poverty than its American equivalent, though both countries had weak welfare states relative to other industrialized nations. Canadian family allowances and CAP disappeared in the early 90s, while the modest guarantees of federal social assistance for the poor in the United States were minimized even further. Canadian medicare, introduced in 1968, was never broadened to cover pharmaceutical or dental costs as did many European public healthcare programmes.[12] Nonetheless, levels of income equality in Canada were closer to European norms than American.[13]

A Divergence in Class Politics

The mainstream of the Canadian trade union movement in the 1940s consisted of affiliates of American-based unions that belonged either to the American Federation of Labor or the Congress of Industrial Organizations. The AFL forced Canada's Trades and Labour Congress to purge CIO unions in 1939.[14] In the late 40s, it forced the TLC to abandon support for the independent, Communist-led Canadian Seamen's Union.[15]

The CIO unions joined the small All-Canadian Congress of Labour to form the Canadian Congress of Labour. CCL affiliates generally operated autonomously from American headquarters.[16] Politically, the CIO and CCL took divergent paths during the war with important consequences for political developments in each country. Both union centrals were responding to what they perceived as available political opportunities. The CIO leaders retained their dependence on the Democrats, hoping that their influence within the party would produce social democratic reforms. The CIO regarded an alliance with the Rooseveltian wing of the Democratic Party as essential to countering 'the new power of big business and the aggressive anti-union politics of the congressional and entrepreneurial right wing'.[17] Mike Davis, however, suggests that the trade union leadership's smothering of efforts from below to create independent labour policies reinforced other leadership initiatives that entrenched centralized bureaucratic control, defeating rank-and-file attempts to produce democratic local unionism. He denounces the 'barren marriage of American Labor and the Democratic Party'.[18]

By contrast, the CCL rejected Canada's bourgeois parties. In June, 1943, it announced its support for the socialist Co-operative Commonwealth Federation (CCF). Core CCL activists were usually either CCFers or Communists and while the latter fought to keep the union movement non-partisan, the CCFers were better organized and enjoyed greater working-class support. Indeed, the CCL decision to endorse the CCF coincided with rising CCF support. The party, formed as a coalition of socialist, labour, and progressive farmer parties in 1932, had won only a handful of seats in the federal elections of 1935 and 1940. It formed the official opposition however in British Columbia and Manitoba, where it had solid working-class support, and Saskatchewan, where its roots were in the farmers' movement.[19]

The CCL's willingness to support the CCF might be seen as simply following rank-and-file opinion which, during the war, was increasingly pro-socialist, while the CIO leadership's coolness to the idea of an independent labour party could be explained in terms of the hostility of American workers to socialism. But a wartime Roper survey of American public opinion suggested that a quarter of the population was favourable to socialism. Another 35 per cent indicated an open mind regarding socialism while 40 per cent said they opposed it.[20] Canadian surveys indicated somewhat greater support for socialism – somewhere between 35 and 40 per cent of the population – when this is defined as public ownership and operation of the major corporations.[21] This is unsurprising in light of Canada's having a socialist party with representatives in Parliament and a federal government that, while anti-socialist, had found it expedient, in wartime, to establish twenty-eight Crown corporations that did everything from building war-time housing and bombers, mining uranium, and refining fuel.[22] That 25 per cent of Americans supported socialism and many more were open-minded on the issue despite having no mass-based non-Communist socialist party in their midst nor a government practising quasi-socialism in the name of the war effort suggests significant potential for a Labour party.

Why then was the CCL more open to labourite politics? The most plausible explanation is that the CCL was not tempted by a Franklin Roosevelt to stifle plans for independent labour politics. The CIO had made its initial appearance in peacetime, encouraged by the Roosevelt administration's relatively pro-labour stance.[23] Its Canadian equivalents, by contrast, faced hostile federal and provincial governments before the war, Conservative and Liberal. Socialists within the CCL therefore had little cause to mimic the American CIO leadership's strategy of working closely with the left wing of the Democratic Party to form a progressive political bloc made up of a plurality of social classes.

The strategy of accommodation to the Democratic Party led the American CIO in 1945 to embrace a programme designed to create a progressive capitalism in which the trade union movement joined private companies and the state to create economic stability. While the CIO supported a range of welfare state measures, it believed the capitalist system was capable of reform.[24] The same year the CCL adopted a manifesto that came to opposite conclusions and embraced public ownership and vast social spending.[25]

Despite its minority status, the CCF had a decided impact on political developments in Canada. The party came a close second in the Ontario provincial election of 1943 and formed a government in Saskatchewan in 1944 that lasted twenty years. The Saskatchewan CCF government became Canada's first to recognize the right of public service workers to join independent unions with the right to strike.[26] The federal Liberals, in response to rising CCF support, introduced family allowances in 1944 and promised health insurance, universal old-age pensions, and federal support for all unemployed persons. Even the Conservatives promised Canadians extensive social benefits in the 1945 federal election. The apparent conversion of the bourgeois parties to left-wing perspectives along with a well-financed anti-socialist campaign weakened the CCF's electoral advance in 1945.[27] The CCF won only 15.6 per cent of the vote and carried just 28 of 245 federal seats.[28]

Still, the CCL maintained its link with the CCF, and while both organizations drifted rightwards during the Cold War, gradually dropping their emphasis on public entrepreneurship, they remained within the orbit of post-war social democracy on the European model with its emphasis on social policy. When the CCL and the TLC merged in 1956 following the parallel merger of the CIO and AFL, the new labour federation, the Canadian Labour Congress (CLC), adopted

CCL political strategies. With support for the CCF declining under the twin pressures of the Cold War and post-war prosperity, the CLC supported the creation of a new social democratic party with formal labour support. The result was the New Democratic Party in 1961 with its large bloc of labour delegates ensuring a significant role for trade unionists in the making of party policy and the choosing of leaders. Though the NDP largely elected middle-class professionals as party representatives, it maintained an organic link with the trade unions.[29]

Meanwhile, in the US, the post-war labour movement remained embedded within the frayed New Deal coalition whose ability to deliver social programmes declined. Though Harry Truman supported national medical insurance, the combination of southern Democrats and northern Republicans in Congress stymied his plans.[30] The labour movement accepted the congressional defeats and focused on collective bargaining efforts to win employer-paid comprehensive medical coverage for union members. The resultant plans were rife with high deductibles and co-insurance payments that caused many nominal subscribers to avoid seeking medical care. Only 60 per cent of Americans had coverage in 1959. But labour leaders largely abandoned calls for a universal programme.[31]

Within Canada, the Liberals also initially failed to implement their post-war social promises, using an alleged lack of provincial cooperation as an excuse to mask the conservative wing of the party's lack of enthusiasm for major social spending programmes.[32] The labour movement, because it was clearly an opposition movement in the political arena, was not constrained in its efforts to press for social legislation.

While the leadership of the Canadian labour movement proved only slightly more resistant than its American counterpart to purge Communists, it faced less pressure to reject all socialist ideas as 'un-Canadian'. By contrast, the American union movement operated within an environment in which right-wingers happily branded their liberal and left-wing opponents as 'un-American'. The United States's leading position within the Cold War alliance placed pressures on all elites, including trade union movements, to participate in subversion abroad to deflect the growth of Communist and anti-American nationalist movements.[33] There was little such pressure on Canada's trade union leadership, since Canada played a rather junior role in waging the Cold War.[34] While the impact of the Cold War on Canadian thought and behaviour should not be minimized, the bipolar world model of the post-war period had less impact on the lives of most Canadians than on Americans. Canada's minor position in world affairs made it impossible for the equivalents of Senator McCarthy or Congressman Nixon to emerge as serious figures in Canadian political life and CCL leaders defended the rights of Canadians and potential immigrants to espouse unpopular views.[35] So, labour's opposite strategies in Canada and the United States led to two opposed discourses on social issues. While American labour de-emphasized social class

and trumpeted a liberal agenda within the framework of an enlightened capitalism fighting tyrannical Communism, Canadian labour called for a measure of
economic democracy to accompany political democracy.

Perhaps because labour in Canada followed a class-based strategy, Canadians
are far more likely than Americans to identify themselves as working class.[36] Such
class consciousness, in turn, acts as a restraint against Canadian politicians following the example of many American states and introducing 'open shop' and
'sunset' laws that destroy unions. Certainly, some strikingly anti-labour legislation
has been passed in Canada, but Canadian labour has not had to face an all-out
assault by the state on its right to exist. Indeed, the Parti Québécois regime in
Quebec in the late seventies introduced the continent's first anti-scab legislation.
While union densities in Canada and the United States were similar in the early
1970s, by 1994 the rate of unionization of the labour force stood at 14 per cent
in the US while in Canada it was 36 per cent; the rate dropped to 32.3 per cent in
Canada in 2003 while the US rate rose marginally to 14.3 per cent.[37]

Labour and CCF/NDP pressures contributed significantly to Liberal government decisions to implement the spate of progressive reforms introduced
during the Pearson years from 1963 to 1968, viz. the Canada Pension Plan,
national health insurance, and the Canada Assistance Plan. When the Liberals
formed the government in 1963, they had committed themselves to introducing
these programmes. But, as in 1945, the conservative wing of the government
urged a go-slow policy. The liberals within the government triumphed by
emphasizing that theirs was a minority government dependent upon NDP votes
to survive Conservative votes of no-confidence. The road to an eventual parliamentary majority, they argued, lay in establishing the Liberals as a social-minded
party that could attract votes away from swing voters for the NDP.[38]

Confident that social insurance programmes would be introduced eventually, Canadian labour maintained constant pressure on the Liberals and
Conservatives to implement their promises to Canadian workers and farmers.
It deserves credit, in particular, for its long fight for national medical insurance.
Federal governments in the 50s were cool to the idea, though a consensus among
the federal and provincial governments was reached in favour of hospital insurance in 1957.[39] The Canadian Medical Association did not object strongly to
hospital insurance but lobbied hard against schemes that would make doctors
employees of the state. Saskatchewan's CCF government fed their worst fears
when it introduced a provincial medicare scheme in 1962 that covered all visits to physicians. By then, the Conservative government of John Diefenbaker,
responding to continuing pressures for a national medicare scheme, had established a Royal Commission to investigate the need for such a programme.

Though stacked with Tories, the Commission, reporting in 1964 to the new
Liberal government, proposed a universal, prepaid medical insurance scheme.

The report repeated the labour movement's arguments against market-led medical provision. This was unsurprising because labour led the fight for medicare before the Commission with richly-documented briefs and rebuttals of the claims of medicare opponents. In particular, labour cast doubt on the physician/medical insurance industry claim that growing enrolments in private insurance plans obviated the need for a state plan. The CLC dissected many of these private plans and found them wanting. It rebutted the propaganda of both the Canadian Medical Association and the Canadian Chamber of Commerce in favour of voluntary private insurance. Social workers' elaborate briefs demonstrating the substandard medical care received by the poor and uninsured added to labour's indictment of the treatment received by the insured led the Commission to conclude that only a national, public medical insurance scheme would guarantee access to quality health care for all Canadians. The many briefs of these two well-organized groups were vital because ordinary Canadians, while telling pollsters they wanted socialized medicine, were unwilling to appear before the Commission and explain why.[40] While the Canadian government implemented a programme that ignored some of the Commission's objectives – doctors' visits and laboratory tests were covered but visits to dentists and the costs of prescription medicines were not – in 1968 Canadians enjoyed as a matter of right a degree of medical coverage that Americans to this day do not. The labour movement and its New Democratic Party ally deserve much of the credit.[41]

In the United States, the labour movement must take some of the blame for the nation's failure to legislate national health insurance. Polls during World War 2 suggested that almost three Americans in five wanted 'a tax-supported federal health care system'.[42] While this was modest support relative to Canada and Great Britain,[43] it demonstrated that a majority of Americans embraced state medicine. A poll in 1945 indicated that a slight majority of Americans were prepared to have Social Security cover doctors' visits and hospital care even if it meant higher social security taxes.[44] The Wagner-Murray-Dingell bill introduced in 1946 attempted to implement the wishes of the majority, proposing a national contributory medicare scheme without user fees. While both the AFL and the CIO supported the bill, John L. Lewis, president of the United Mineworkers and a maverick on many issues, was opposed, arguing that his members had won a better medical plan through collective bargaining than the legislators were offering.[45] Harkening back to the AFL's line on all social insurance programmes before 1932, he claimed that the proposed bill would make it less attractive for workers to unionize and win benefits from their employers through their own struggles. This was a minority voice in the labour movement which worked with the Democrats to try to produce a congressional majority for national medical insurance.

Liberal Democrats, with the southern flank of their party totally opposed to social insurance programmes, could not mount the voting bloc necessary to pass

Wagner-Murray-Dingell, and by the 1950s had largely ceased to press the medical insurance issue except with respect to the elderly. Big business, the American Medical Association, and the Republicans happily linked proposals for state medicine to communism and Soviet tyranny.[46] Such a discourse was muted in Canada,[47] where the trade union movement defended socialism while attacking communism. The American movement, by contrast, was on the defensive, and by the late 1950s had abandoned its demand for a universal medical insurance programme, calling only for public medical coverage of the elderly.[48] As Jacob Hacker puts it, 'Unions turned to private health insurance as an alternative to national health insurance.'[49]

Medicaid and medicare in the mid-60s, providing free medical care to the destitute and the aged respectively, were, arguably, steps in the right direction, though it was left to the states to determine eligibility for medicaid.[50] Once these programmes were legislated, some elements of the labour movement supported a campaign for a universal national medical insurance plan. The United Autoworkers, among other unions, was instrumental in getting the Democrats to include support for a national plan in their 1976 platform. The UAW viewed the private insurance system as too expensive and looked to a public system to contain costs for their members.[51] But Democratic Party platforms were notoriously unsatisfactory guides to what a Democratic administration might do, and Jimmy Carter's government largely ignored the medical insurance issue. While the UAW continued to press the issue, the larger labour movement demonstrated only minimal interest. Indeed, the unions proved willing during collective bargaining in the 1970s and 1980s to weaken their members' medical benefits in return for job security.[52]

The prospect of universal medical insurance was revived in a special Senate race in Pennsylvania in 1991. Democratic candidate Harris Wofford used the issue to turn an initial 40 per cent lead by his Republican opponent into a 10 per cent Democratic victory.[53] The next year, Bill Clinton, running for president, suggested that he would implement a universal health plan. In 1993 President Clinton proposed a complicated medical insurance bill that would provide private insurance for most work-force family members. It emphasized managed competition with large insurance purchasing alliances to be created to negotiate with corporate insurers for the best plan for their members. As Milton Fisk observes, managed competition

> calls for coinsurance (the insured pays part of the premium) and co-payments (the insured pays part of the cost of each service until a certain sum of those out of pocket payments have been reached). It also calls for deductibles (the insurance begins to pay only after the insured has paid a given amount) as a disincentive to free choice of physicians.[54]

If passed, the Clinton proposal would have given the United States the most mean-spirited national medical insurance programme of the developed countries. Still, it was too interventionist for the health insurance industry and it was defeated by Congress.

Labour had become too weak and unprincipled to mount an attack from the Left. Colin Gordon summarizes the dilemma of American labour:

> The inattention and insincerity of the Democrats underscores a pervasive organizational skew in American politics. Quite simply, those who need health care reform are woefully disorganized and those who oppose it have the resources and the political power to deflect real reform. Organized labour has found it hard enough to battle concessions, let alone press more comprehensive political goals. The AFL's support of the 'play or pay' plan reflects both the weakness of organized labour in a capital-intensive political system and the peculiar conservatism of the AFL. Some progressive unionists have rallied union locals and pressed State-level reform, but with little hope of translating popular support for national health insurance into political action.[55]

In short, American labour leaders' decision from the 1930s onward to tie working-class politics to the fortunes of the Democratic Party, in contrast with Canadian labour's decision to support an oppositional social-democratic politics, has created the kind of labour political impotence that insures minimal progress in the struggle for social insurance. Of course, the gains that Canadian labour has made by backing the NDP can be exaggerated. While Canada's three New Democratic Party governments of the 1970s implemented significant extensions to social programmes during periods of relative prosperity, their equivalents of the 1990s and 2000s have accepted neo-liberal discourse and its fetish with balanced budgets and 'free' markets untrammelled by state intervention.[56] Labour has proven, especially in Ontario and Saskatchewan, to have limited control over the directions that NDP governments would take. A similar case can be made for Quebec, where the labour movement supports the Parti Québécois, a party whose main aim is to achieve sovereignty for Quebec but which also claims to be social democratic in its social policy orientations.[57]

Nonetheless, the decision by Canadian labour to create a labour political vehicle has served Canadian working people far better than American labour's path of supporting a bourgeois party with a liberal wing. The latter made this decision partly because they felt that individualist values within their society limited the likely success of a democratic socialist party. But their rejection of independent labour politics has simply strengthened the anti-statist, individualist beliefs among Americans over time.

Two Contrasting Women's Movements

Like the trade union movement, the Canadian women's movement appears superficially a carbon copy of its American counterpart. The American women's suffrage movement preceded the Canadian; the General Federation of Women's Clubs formed in 1890, three years before the National Council of Women of Canada (NCWC); Canadian women pressed for a Royal Commission on the Status of Women only after President Kennedy's Commission on the Status of Women had reported; and the women's liberation movement in Canada took its inspiration from the American movement.

Beneath the surface however lie two very different feminist histories with important implications for the impact of the women's movements on the history of the welfare state. Once again, if one looked only at the period before World War 2, the American movement appears more successful than the Canadian. Mothers' pensions and minimum wages for women were introduced by many American states before Canadian provinces gradually followed suit, and there was no Canadian equivalent to the Children's Bureau, which American feminist pressures brought into being in 1921. Though the bureau was disbanded in 1927, many states established equivalent organizations. It is misleading, though, to assert, as does Theda Skocpol, that, in contradistinction to European paternalist welfare states, the United States 'came close to forging a maternalist welfare state'.[58] Women in several countries, particularly France and Australia, received far better benefits in recognition of their maternal role than American women.[59] There is less exaggeration in Kathryn Kish Sklar's claim that middle-class women's activism 'served as a surrogate for working-class social activism' in the US.[60] With the early male-dominated trade union movement hostile to social programmes, organized women's political interventions influenced the passage of the modest reforms of benefit to women and children before the New Deal period. These were no match for the public funding for childcare, universal medical care and maternity insurance that paternalist France funded by 1920. As Linda Gordon has suggested, the priorities of American feminists before World War II partly explain the American social welfare landscape. 'Female welfare activists', she writes, 'designed programs that would benefit women directly when male wage-earners failed them', but did not promote economic independence as such.[61]

Successes of the Progressive period and the early 1920s gave way to a period of anti-feminist and anti-statist reaction in the late 20s. The women's movement began a long process of splintering[62] from which it has never really recovered. Largely ineffectual from the 30s to the early 60s, the women's movement largely accepted the hegemonic Cold War ideology of the post-war period,[63] and was wary of the state. While one wing of the movement continued to support protective legislation that recognized women's gendered disabilities in the labour force because of the social role assigned to motherhood, an 'equal rights' wing opposed protective legislation and fought to remove all gender bias from state and private employer policies. The individualist bias of the latter group reflected the long-established anti-statism of American discourse, a position that the Cold War would only enhance. The women's liberation movement that had roots in the New Left in the late 60s embraced the New Left's antipathy to statism. The American state, after all, was slaughtering millions in Indochina. Both the New Left and the women's liberation movement were ultimately pessimistic about the possibilities of reshaping an imperialist, racist, patriarchal state to serve the needs of the people; they called for new people's institutions from the bottom up, unlike the old Left's emphasis on seizing state power.[64]

Hence the major campaign of the American women's movement of the 70s and 80s was for an Equal Rights Amendment rather than for social programmes.[65] In 1986, a section of the women's movement, including the leadership of the National Organization of Women, fought California legislation requiring employers to grant pregnant women four months' pregnancy leave.[66] NOW insisted such legislation was discriminatory unless it affected all employees with disabilities that prevented them from working rather than simply pregnant women. It was unconcerned that such legislation had no impact on women's employment opportunities in other countries. Its gut reaction was the traditional 'equal rights' individualist reaction. Other feminist organizations supported the California legislation but this split in the American women's movement caused 'amazement' among Canadian feminists for whom 'the different economic and social context ... has fostered an entirely different feminist climate'.[67]

American feminists in the New Left tradition continue to question whether the welfare state has done more than create dependency of women upon a patriarchal state acting as a stand-in for fathers and husbands. While the US government merrily trashed the small gains that poor and disproportionately non-white women had won over many years, Wendy Brown could ask in *Feminist Studies*:

> Does the late twentieth-century configuration of the welfare state help to emancipate women from compulsory motherhood or help to administer it? ... Do female staff and clients of state bureaucracies ... transform the masculinism of bureaucracy or do they become servants of it, disciplined and produced by it? Considering these questions in a more ecumenical register, in what ways might women's deepening involvement with the state entail exchanging dependence upon individual men for regulation by contemporary institutionalized processes of male domination and how might the abstractness, the ostensible neutrality, and the lack of a body and face in the latter, help to disguise these processes, inhibiting or diluting women's consciousness of their situation qua women, thereby circumscribing projects of substantive feminist political change?[68]

Unsurprisingly, most scholars of the interactions of the welfare state and women reject such a rigid and functionalist view of state provision of social services. But it is the widespread acceptance of such a perspective[69] that causes Linda Gordon and Frances Fox Piven to emphasize the need to view the state as an entity shaped by social interactions rather than an immutable abstraction whose elimination would create Nirvana.[70] There is little parallel for their work along these lines in Canadian scholarship because no one supposes that the Wendy Browns compose a significant ideological cohort within Canadian feminism.

Within the mainstream movements of American feminist activists during the 1970s and 80s the need to balance the views of social interventionists and libertarians dampened efforts to introduce social policies more favourable to women. Historian Sonya Michel notes: 'Out of a principled aversion to "mainstream" and "establishment" politics, feminists tended to eschew conventional politicking in favour of local action and grassroots, community-controlled (and community-funded) provisions. They were, as a result, no match for the highly mobilized and politically sophisticated lobbying machinery of their conservative opponents.'[71] In the case of daycare:

> Although the women's movement challenged the prevailing prescription for motherhood, it failed to mobilize a viable campaign for public child care. The rights-based orientation of the most visible branch of second-wave feminism – liberal organizations such as the National Organization for Women and the Women's Political Caucus – focused on formal aspects of gender equity such as access to education and employment but generally ignored the implication of women's lack of social citizenship epitomized by the absence of public child care.[72]

The Canadian women's movement before World War 2 followed a similar trajectory to the American. The dominant organization was the NCWC whose leaders employed a maternalist discourse and led campaigns for mothers' pensions and protective legislation, as well as temperance.[73] In Canada, unlike the US, equal rights feminists continued to work closely with feminists emphasizing gender differences. If there was acrimony within the women's movement, it was mainly on a class, ethnic and regional basis. Quebec Catholic francophone women formed their own organizations while farm and labour women's groups felt estranged from the NCWC because its bourgeois leadership appeared uninterested in promoting the interests of workers and farmers.[74] On the whole, though, the women's movement in Canada did not divide into hostile camps.

While the Cold War affected the women's movement in Canada, feminists, like unionists, looked to the state for solutions to inequalities. Political scientist Jill Vickers suggests that Canadian feminists did not buy into the American anti-statist message. Canada's New Left was weaker than its Old Left, both social democratic and communist, and younger activists participated within electoral political parties. They were not as marginalized as the youthful activists in the United States. Women activists who reacted against the patriarchal character of Canadian politics, including the politics of the Left, also maintained the idea that political change meant, in good part, putting pressure on the state to implement progressive legislation and participating in electoral contests to put feminist politicians in office.[75]

Canadian women's campaigns in the 1950s, led by the NCWC, and later supported by the trade unions, had caused the federal government to end most discrimination against women in the granting of unemployment insurance by 1971. Paid maternity leave for women would be funded by UI after 1971. Women's movement campaigns for childcare yielded some provincial successes from the 1970s, and during the 1984 federal election, when the three major national political leaders discussed women's issues in a televised debate hosted by the National Action Committee on the Status of Women, all three promised a national daycare programme. The election winner, Conservative leader Brian Mulroney, had lied. But his decision to make such a promise demonstrated the success that the women's movement had had in framing public discourse around the daycare issue. Their victories on the daycare front relative to the American women's movement have caused Sonya Michel to note: 'a Canadian-style coalition of feminists, labor, and child care professionals, never materialized in the United States'.[76] The women's movement also won significant concessions with regards to the Canada Pension Plan.[77]

As noted earlier, organizations of social workers and national welfare organizations played a significant role in persuading the Royal Commission on Health Care to propose a national medicare scheme. These organizations, largely dominated by women, reflected the views of Canadian feminists of the time in favour of free healthcare for women and children.[78]

Apart from successes on the welfare front, the Canadian women's movement won the prize that eluded the American movement: the equivalent of an Equal Rights Amendment. The Canadian Constitution was 'patriated' by the Liberal government of Pierre-Elliott Trudeau from Britain in 1982 after a deal with the provinces minus Quebec. A Charter of Rights and Freedoms was included in the new constitution, somewhat equivalent to the American Bill of Rights. Lobbying by the women's movement produced two sections that guaranteed women equal rights. Section 28 reads simply: 'notwithstanding anything in this Charter, the rights and freedoms referred to in it are guaranteed equally to male and female persons'. The women's movement was powerful enough to force the premiers to agree to exempt this provision of the Charter from another provision that allows provinces to exempt some laws from the rights provisions of the Constitution.[79]

If Canadian feminists have been more inclined to fight battles with the state rather than focus on the creation of grassroots, non-state structures, it is first of all because the post-war political climate in Canada, with its socialist third-party movement and relatively progressive trade union movement, encouraged such a strategy. In turn, the effectiveness of the women's movement in winning legislative victories for women, including poor and nonwhite women, has reinforced this strategy. Notes political scientist Jill Vickers: 'Generally then, most Canadian feminists perceive the state more as a provider of services, including the services of regulation, than as a reinforcer of patriarchal norms, and most seem to believe that services, whether child care or medicare, will help'.[80] They are 'committed to the welfare state that Canadian women helped to create'.[81]

Neo-liberalism since the 80s has eroded some earlier gains made by the women's movement. But the reaction of the Canadian women's movement has been to fight back rather than to retreat into privatism and voluntarism. The women's movement has taken the position that government social service cutbacks not only mainly throw women out of their jobs but that they make women in the home unpaid care providers substituting for the women who have lost their jobs.[82]

Perhaps the greatest advantage of the women's movement in Canada over the American movement is simply that it has historically been more united. While roadmaps are required to chart the formation, splits and break-ups that have characterized women's organization in the US, Canadian women's organizational history can be encompassed within the story of three umbrella groups, the National Council of Women of Canada (formed in 1893), the Fédération des Femmes du Québec (1966), and the National Action Committee on the Status of Women (1972). The NCWC has mostly represented the volunteer sector, while the latter two groups reflect the politics of modern feminism. NAC, formed to pressure governments to implement the recommendations of the Report of the Royal Commission on the Status of Women (1970), has demonstrated a political sophistication capable of placating the different perspectives of almost 600 organizations ranging from the women's sections of parties as diverse as the Conservative Party and the Communist Party, as well as women's labour groups and organizations of Native women and women of colour. In the 1970s, its presidents included both Laura Sabia, a free-enterprise feminist with a long association with the Conservative Party, and labour leader Grace Hartmann, a left-wing New Democrat.[83] The NCWC played a key role in the battle, ultimately unsuccessful, to prevent the free trade agreement between Canada and the United States, an agreement which threatened and continues to threaten the viability of Canadian social programmes.[84] Shortly afterwards, Judy Rebick, a Marxist feminist who might have been dismissed as a fringe figure in the United States, became president of NAC and insured that women's issues, including social programmes, were central in constitutional discussions of the early 90s. Her successor, Sunera Thobani, made issues affecting poor women and women of colour the central focus of NAC's work.[85]

The FFQ, a member of NAC until 1981, left the Canadian umbrella organization when NAC, having won an equal rights provision in the constitution, supported the formula for patriation agreed upon by Prime Minister Trudeau and nine premiers. Relatively good relations were later re-established between the FFQ and NAC though the former, reflecting the growing sovereigntist thrust of Quebec, has been unwilling to rejoin the Canadian umbrella organization. Within Quebec, the FFQ plays much the same role as NAC and its provincial affiliates play elsewhere in the country, pressing upon legislators women's demands, and organizing demonstrations and public meetings around feminist issues.[86]

Of course, most feminist activists in the US are liberals or socialists and the Canadian women's movement is certainly not without divisions. American feminists have had victories, and Canadian feminists were unable to prevent federal governments from scrapping family allowances and ending earmarking of social assistance in federal payments to the provinces. Still, the Canadian movement has been more united and less reticent about making the traditional political arena, rather than identity politics, its focus.

Conclusion

In some countries, there is a well-developed sense of entitlement to social programmes that is unmatched in other countries. Notions of entitlement are weakest in the United States.[87] But it is easy to exaggerate Americans' rejection of universal social programmes. Surveys suggest that most Americans, when provided with a relatively accurate description of the Canadian medical system, would like their country to copy it. 10 per cent of Americans described themselves as socialists in the last days of the Cold War even though there is no credible mass socialist party in their country.[88]

Choices made by the labour and women's movements as well as an all-pervasive racism have contributed a great deal to American 'exceptionalism' with regards to the development of the welfare state. Canadian unionists and feminists have made different choices despite the powerful impact of American institutions and American thought in Canadian life. Their choices have played a large role in creating a somewhat more egalitarian bent in Canadian public policy than the US. Of course, even Canada's progress in this regard pales against most continental European countries. The choices made by Canadian and American social movements, however, while hardly predestined, were conditioned by several key factors. Both the Cold War and racism defined limits to American reform in the post-war period far more than Canadian reform. But it seems one-sided to suggest that prevailing ideologies determined the discourse and possible successes of social activists. The comparison between Canada and the United States demonstrates that the discourse and successes of the activists play an important role in shaping the dominant ideology. In Canada, where trade unions and the women's movement have won a variety of universal social programmes, popular opinion holds that the federal government should insure that individuals receive a basic set of services regardless of income. In the United States, where trade unions have fallen victim to the neo-liberal climate whose creation they did too little to combat and the women's movement lacks cohesion, popular opinion is less accommodating to the poor. Still, in both countries, there is a sufficient support for social justice upon which movements for social change can build. Human agency, rather than iron laws of the limits of North American socialism and liberalism, will determine the extent of reform in both countries.

6 ALBERTA ADVANTAGE: A CANADIAN PROVING GROUND FOR AMERICAN MEDICAL RESEARCH ON MUSTARD GAS AND POLIO IN THE 1940s AND 50s

Susan L. Smith and Stephen Mawdsley

In the mid-twentieth century, Americans turned to Canada as a proving ground to help save the lives of North American soldiers and children. To American medical researchers and government officials, the province of Alberta in western Canada provided ideal conditions for scientific experimentation in military and civilian field trials with human subjects. During the 1940s, American military personnel worked closely with their Canadian counterparts to learn from mustard gas open-air field trials and gas chamber tests conducted on more than 2,000 soldiers at the Suffield Experimental Station in Alberta. These human experiments were part of Allied preparation for potential chemical warfare during World War 2. A decade later, American scientists and leaders of the National Foundation for Infantile Paralysis invited Canadians to enrol children in a massive clinical trial in the US of the Salk poliomyelitis vaccine. The testing of over 1 million children, including approximately 50,000 in Alberta, Manitoba and Nova Scotia, was part of the battle against polio in the 1950s. How did Canada contribute to American medical research through testing in Alberta? Why was data generated in this Canadian province of interest to American researchers?

These two very different historical case studies demonstrate an American interest in the 'Alberta Advantage' promoted to medical researchers.[1] They reveal some of the key themes in the history of US–Canada health relations, an emerging area of scholarship.[2] These case studies show that in times of crisis, Canadian officials were eager to collaborate with Americans in order to save lives, offering Alberta as an ideal location for research. They also show that Canadian officials knowingly exposed individual soldiers and children in Alberta to added health risks in anticipation of political gains and public health benefits, key issues in military and medical history.[3]

US–Canada health relations occurred within the context of a cooperative, yet asymmetric, relationship between the two nations. The longstanding imbalance of power has led some historians to identify these nations as 'ambivalent allies', especially after 1960.[4] Canadian military and health officials were eager to work with the US because they saw such international activity as in the interests of Canadians. Despite unequal power relations, Canada's participation was promoted and defined by Canadian, as well as American, officials. As these case studies show, Alberta's involvement in international efforts to save lives enhanced, as well as alleviated, risks to human health in the province. They illustrate the tensions between the needs of society in times of crisis and the necessity of safeguarding human health. By joining with Americans and sharing the short-term health risks, Canadian officials anticipated long-term benefits to the province and the nation.

Soldiers and Mustard Gas in Alberta

The experiments in Alberta with mustard gas, a vesicant or blistering agent, were not isolated events but part of a transnational programme of biomedical research in chemical weapons, led by American and British officials.[5] The history of the Canadian experiments reveals the intersections and interconnections across several national research programmes. The British conducted mustard gas experiments on their own soldiers at Porton Down in England and in Canada, Australia, India and New Guinea. Americans, in turn, ran experiments in the US and in Canada, Australia, and on San Jose Island off Panama. These projects were not just parallel developments, but closely coordinated wartime efforts taking place in several nations at the same time. This science in the service of alliance warfare included efforts to upgrade older military technologies and investigate the casualty-causing properties of chemical weapons.[6] In light of the terrifying and deadly poison gas, including mustard gas, used on the battlefields of World War I, Allied governments during World War 2 resumed their interest in the toxicology of mustard gas to find out even more about its effects.[7] Several nations, including Canada, had signed a 1925 international agreement to limit gas warfare, but it only banned first use of the weapons, not retaliatory use.[8] Although Allied nations ultimately did not use mustard gas in combat during World War 2, they were prepared to.[9] Thus, they conducted experiments for both defensive and offensive purposes: to learn how to best protect Allied soldiers from potential gas attack and how to create casualties to disable the enemy.[10]

In 1940, the United States, Canada and Britain created an advisory committee to share chemical warfare information. In the United States, scientists conducted mustard gas testing under the direction of the Office of Scientific Research and Development. Much of the US mustard gas research was run through the

US Army's Chemical Warfare Service and the Naval Research Laboratory. The US Chemical Warfare Service developed close connections with the Canadian Army's Directorate of Chemical Warfare and Smoke. The Americans sent materials, including mustard gas, and an American representative to Suffield in Alberta.[11]

Canadian officials at both the provincial and national level were eager to collaborate with the United States in chemical weapons research because such wartime activities provided enhanced status for a nation eager to assert its sovereignty and autonomy within the British empire.[12] Canada readily shared its resources, including scientific expertise and military technology, with Americans, as well as the British. Suffield's researchers met with scientists at several American universities, including the University of Chicago. Canadians also coordinated efforts with the chemical weapons researchers at the US Army's Dugway Proving Ground, located in Utah, creating a close relationship between Suffield and Dugway that continues to this day.[13]

Experiments with mustard gas in Alberta reveal how government funding in wartime reoriented medical research to meet military priorities. The militarization of medicine and the medicalization of defence research resulted in the imposition of short-term health risks that turned into long-term health problems for some of the soldiers.[14] World War 2 marked a time when government-funded research expanded human experimentation dramatically, especially in the United States, but also in Canada. In the US, medical scientists turned to a range of so-called 'volunteers', including soldiers, conscientious objectors, orphans, the mentally ill and prisoners.[15] As historian David Rothman notes, World War 2 was 'the transforming event in the conduct of human experimentation'.[16]

Scientists in the US and Canada conducted three types of experiments to evaluate the human body's response to mustard gas exposure and to develop protective clothing, ointments and respirators or gas masks. The first type was the drop test and patch test in which scientists applied a small amount of mustard agent to bare skin or to skin partially covered with an ointment to examine its protective properties. The second type was the field test in which aeroplanes sprayed soldiers with mustard gas while they were in open fields wearing various levels of protective clothing. Finally, in the third type of test, known as the 'man-break test', scientists placed men in gas chambers and released mustard gas in order to determine what types of injuries developed and how long it took before the men were incapacitated.

Important studies by journalists, politicians and film makers, including Karen Freeman in the US, John Bryden in Canada, Bridget Goodwin in Australia, and Rob Evans in Britain, have documented the alarming history of mustard gas experiments in their respective nations.[17] They have dramatized the harm experienced by soldiers and brought the experiments to the attention of the public. Meanwhile, scholars like Donald Avery in Canada and Jonathan Moreno in the US have analysed the significance of science to the conduct of war and issues of state secrecy and ethics. Finally, in 1993, a committee of the National Academy of Sciences in the United States published a landmark study called *Veterans at Risk* that identified the short- and long-term health consequences of the experiments.[18] These various studies show that Allied medical scientists conducted experiments with mustard gas on thousands of soldiers. Although the exact figures are extremely difficult to determine, current estimates suggest that the testing programme involved more than 2,000 Canadian soldiers, 3,000 Australian soldiers, 7,000 British soldiers and 60,000 American soldiers.[19]

American mustard gas tests on human subjects began in 1943 and included at least 4000 soldiers in gas chamber and field tests, while the rest of the 60,000 American soldiers faced patch tests and drop tests. The corresponding figures for Canada, Australia, and Britain would also be higher if all mustard gas exposures were included. Indeed, these figures reflect incomplete data because many of the government records about the experiments remain classified or, as in the case of the US, have been reclassified in recent years. The numbers also do not include civilians and military personnel who encountered mustard gas during production, transport and training exercises, not only during World War 2, but also in the following decades. In gas training exercises the military taught soldiers and sailors how to recognize mustard gas, and other types of chemical agents, in order to respond quickly to protect themselves. Thus, if such activities are included, more than 150,000 American servicemen and civilians were exposed to mustard gas and other chemical weapons during World War 2. [20]

Allied military and scientific interests, coupled with a hierarchical system in which soldiers were encouraged or ordered to 'volunteer', made these appalling experiments possible. Veterans report that they participated in the experiments for a wide range of reasons, including out of patriotism, intimidation, unbearable boredom, the promise of extra pay and special leave privileges, and sometimes when they learned that their military unit was to be shipped out to the front.[21]

Despite government claims at the time that soldiers faced no serious harm, there is plenty of evidence to the contrary, including in government reports of the Canadian mustard gas experiments at the Suffield Experimental Station in Alberta. The station, which opened in 1941, specialized in chemical weapons research. Although the superintendent was British scientist E. L. Davies, most of the staff were Canadians. The Canadian and British governments jointly financed the station until 1946 and the Alberta government leased the 2,600 square kilometres of land for one dollar per year for ninety-nine years.[22] The military organized Suffield into two camps: Camp A held the experimental laboratories and Camp B was the quarters for the military personnel who 'volunteered' to serve as human subjects. There was also a hospital where a few nurses treated the most severely injured test subjects.[23]

Although some soldiers experienced only minimal mustard gas exposure, especially those in drop tests on the forearm, others faced high dosages. The reports on experiments conducted during the 1940s at Suffield document the immediate health consequences of soldiers' participation in field trials, whose purpose, after all, was to create casualties among the test subjects. For example, in 1942 the Canadian military conducted six trials, each with sixty soldiers, in which aircraft sprayed men with mustard gas. The men were next forced to march for two miles, returned to the station by truck, and then required to sit in their contaminated clothing for four hours to see how much damage would be caused to their skin, despite wearing battle dress and respirators during the spraying. In this study, a few men were so severely burned that they were considered casualties and hospitalized.[24]

Americans were interested in the results of the mustard gas experiments on Canadian soldiers at Suffield for two key reasons: research opportunities provided by Alberta's geography and weather, and the Canadian military's willingness to conduct full-body exposures, especially in the open-air field tests. The province's sparsely inhabited, dry prairie land provided an ideal location to reproduce combat conditions in various types of weather in a very large test site. Like other western Canadian provinces eager for a share of the economic benefits of war, Alberta promoted the Suffield area as big, isolated and cheap.[25] Furthermore, in 1942 Suffield officials created new rules to expand experiments beyond mere arm tests to exposure of the entire body, likely at the request of the British military.[26] In 1944, Canadian officials even offered to send some Canadian soldiers to the US to participate in American mustard gas field trials because of the Canadian military's more permissive rules regarding exposures to soldiers.[27] Clearly, Canadian officials were willing to go to great lengths, putting the lives of their own men at risk, to ensure that Canada remained a key player in the war effort.

Suffield researchers often conducted trials at the request of the American military, providing human subjects as needed. In January 1943, just as some Americans were urging greater access to human subjects, an official with the US Chemical Warfare Service commented on the benefits of the Canadian approach. In identifying the value of a field trial at Suffield on 'The Casualty Producing Power of Mustard Spray', the American official noted: 'The results indicated the advantages of using human rather than animal subjects, particularly because, aside from the physiological differences, an animal tied to a stake is unlikely to behave in the same way as a soldier in the field, and this is a determining factor in the effectiveness of spray'.[28] He argued that the use of soldiers in laboratory and field tests more closely approximated human behaviour in conditions of warfare than animal proxies. Later that year, three officers from the US Chemical Warfare Service observed a five-day field trial of impregnated clothing, which meant it had been chemically treated to protect against gas. An aircraft sprayed sixty-eight men from 1,300 feet to determine the necessity of two layers of clothing, including impregnated underwear, for fighting in tropical climates. The test showed that two layers provided greater protection against mustard gas exposure, a finding no doubt not welcomed by soldiers fighting in hot weather.[29]

Many Allied soldiers later insisted that they had been given no warning of the level of the pain and suffering that they would face from such experiments or the fact that there would be little immediate care and no follow-up care. Evidence from a range of sources, including government reports of the experiments and testimony from veterans, shows that some men had experienced immediate and severe eye injuries and damage to lungs. Most frequently, men had burns and blistering on the skin, especially on the face, hands, underarms, buttocks and genitals.[30] The Canadian defence reports provide horrific textual and photographic evidence of men who not only developed blisters on their arms and back, but also had to be hospitalized with 'kissing blisters' on their buttocks, intense genital swelling and lesions on the scrotum and penis. Others faced systemic poisoning. For example, in October 1943, several of the thirty-five men who took part in a Suffield field trial, entitled 'Vapour Danger from Gross Mustard Contamination', became very sick and were hospitalized with a high fever, nausea and vomiting.[31] Many of the men who took part in mustard gas experiments were in agony for days, weeks and even months from the blisters and oozing sores on their bodies. There were also psychological consequences from the intense fear these young men experienced, especially when they begged to be let out of the gas chambers but were refused. Finally, there were long-term health consequences, such as post traumatic stress disorder, cancer, asthma, emphysema and eye problems, including blindness, as well as concerns about sexual function, reproduction and health problems in offspring.[32]

For decades, veterans of the mustard gas experiments said very little about their experiences in the experiments. The men had been sworn to secrecy by the military and threatened with jail for treason if they talked about them. Later, some veterans had confided to their physicians in hopes of getting help for ongoing health concerns, but were told that they were wrong about the cause because mustard gas was only used during World War 1. Thus, many men suffered the health consequences of the experiments in silence, not even telling their wives, or only doing so decades later.

Since the 1980s, veterans from the United States, Canada, Australia and Britain have spoken publicly about the effects of wartime experiments with mustard gas. One Canadian soldier remembered a bluish rain dropping on him and other men as part of field tests. 'They didn't tell us what it was or to put on respirators. They said they were just testing our uniforms', Norman Amundson recalled. As a result of the test, his lungs and lower body were burned by the gas. John Dickson, a nineteen-year-old Canadian soldier sent to Suffield, was one of six men put into a windowless bunkhouse or chamber that was then filled with mustard gas. The chamber at Suffield was a wooden hut about 11 cubic metres in size. Dickson explained that within one hour two of the men were unconscious. The researchers finally took all of the men out once everyone had lost consciousness. Dickson recalled that they placed him in the Suffield hospital where he saw about seventy other burned soldiers, many of whom had taken part in open-air field trials.[33]

The Canadian defence reports, although generally sterile accounts of the experiments, couched in neutral, scientific language, provide glimpses of the price that some men paid as human subjects. For instance, in 1944 the US Chemical Warfare Service requested Suffield researchers to conduct low altitude spraying of men with mustard gas. Four of the twenty Canadian men who took part in the test were badly hurt and required hospitalization for at least three weeks. One man became seriously ill. He had erythema or reddening of the skin from his neck down to his waist and his shoulders showed intense vesication or blistering. He developed a fever of 102 degree Fahrenheit, his scrotum became inflamed and swollen, and his penis was covered with small blisters. According to the report, 'On the 4th day after the spray this man was very distressed ... [and] complained of incessant pain and irritation'.[34] Although no doubt a gross understatement of the man's agony and emotional reaction, the inclusion of his complaint in this government report represents a reminder that these experiments were harming human beings.

For some men, severe injuries from mustard gas exposure contributed to a sense of personal humiliation and violation. Veterans remembered that it was especially embarrassing to have their burns treated by young female nurses. Enormous, grotesque blisters developed, especially in the armpits and on the genitals, areas where sweating was greatest. The wife of one soldier who had worked as a nurse at Suffield hospital recalled her husband's suffering and that the healing took a very long time because 'as soon as one blister broke and ran, underneath was another blister'. Dickson, who ended up blind in one eye, looks back on his experience with deep regret: 'We got into this mess ... because we did everything they said. We thought we were fighting for the country, but it was a useless scam. I don't know how human beings could do that and take a new bunch of men every two months and put them through that type of torture'.[35]

Some of these World War 2 veterans were politicized by their government's response to the health problems they faced. They grew frustrated when officials repeatedly denied that such experiments had taken place and refused to provide special healthcare and pensions. Like government treatment of other veteran groups in the twentieth century, Allied governments later refused to acknowledge the veterans' specific wartime contributions and provide appropriate assistance.[36] Although individual veterans had little political clout, collectively they waged political battles with their governments, which began to respond, if slowly. For example, in 1997 in response to Access to Information requests, the Canadian government declassified some of the records pertaining to the mustard gas experiments. Yet, compensation was still not generally forthcoming so in 2003 some veterans filed a class-action lawsuit against the Canadian government for physical and mental suffering caused by exposure to compounds in chemical and biological warfare experiments, including at Suffield. In 2004, only days before Canadian military ombudsman Andre Morin was to release a critical report on the experiments, the Canadian government offered a $50 million compensation package, providing a one-time payment of roughly $24,000 per veteran, in recognition of their service in the experiments. The veterans can also apply for a disability pension through Veterans Affairs Canada, although they are not guaranteed one.[37] In the early 1990s, the US Department of Veterans Affairs announced that it would make it easier for veterans to make claims for compensation and identified specific illnesses it would cover. Yet only in 2005 did the department begin to contact World War 2 veterans to inform those who had been exposed to chemical warfare agents in experiments that they were eligible for special benefits, and even then they were only eligible if they had experienced full-body exposures.[38]

Although Allied government experimentation did not result in the same level of injury and death as that produced by German and Japanese medical scientists during World War 2,[39] it did use and abuse individual soldiers' bodies in pursuit of medical knowledge for military benefits. Officials and scientists viewed the participation of soldiers as necessary to the war effort and sometimes treated the men much like animal subjects. Indeed, as one American veteran testified in his claim for healthcare compensation, 'I was placed in a gas chamber with several sheep. I was dressed in protective clothing and wore a gas mask. Mustard gas was vented in to the chamber and the sheep quickly keeled over'.[40] Likewise, in 1944 researchers at Suffield placed two caged rabbits in a gas chamber along with six Canadian soldiers. The rabbits died seventy-two hours after the exposure.[41] Such actions drove home the point to the men that they were expendable and merely another type of animal subject for research.[42]

Chemical warfare research has left a bitter legacy for many veterans, including those who served at Suffield. They later questioned the philosophy of wartime medical researchers for whom the ends justified the means. For instance, according to the chief of Canada's Chemical Warfare Laboratories at the time, wartime conditions justified risking the health of a few soldiers to save the lives of the many.[43] This view reveals how wartime necessity shaped medical research in disturbing ways. As veterans and journalists have pointed out, causing harm to human health was not merely an unintended consequence of the mustard gas experiments, but the very point of the research programme.[44]

After the war, American scientists insisted that medicine had derived benefits from its partnership with the military, including in Canada.[45] For example, doctors used nitrogen mustard derivatives in chemotherapy in the war on cancer.[46] Cornelius P. Rhoads, the head of the Medical Division of the US Chemical Warfare Service during the war, was also a major figure in cancer control research.[47] According to the authors of the official history of the US Chemical Warfare Service [CWS] during World War 2:

> While it is true that positive and immediate militarily useful results from chemical warfare medical research were relatively meagre in view of the great effort made, under the threat of gas warfare the CWS had no choice but to explore every toxic agent suspected of being of interest to the enemy and every known or conjectured aspect of gas casualty aid and treatment. To this end the full resources of medical science in this nation and in the British Commonwealth were made freely available, enabling the Chemical Warfare Service to command a degree of assistance never achieved before.[48]

According to the authors, even though the immediate military benefits of the experiments were few because the Allies did not engage in chemical warfare, the work was still justified because of the long-term rewards in basic scientific data and in progress in clinical medicine.

A dilemma remains in Canada, and elsewhere, regarding what to do about research on chemical and biological weapons. In 1988, as Joe Clark, then Secretary of State for External Affairs, observed in a letter to an Edmonton peace activist: 'One of the questions for Canada is the degree to which we prepare to defend ourselves against weapons we are trying to eliminate'. In Clark's view, 'The security of our citizens demands that we make some preparation'.[49] Hence, Canada has remained committed to working with the United States, and other nations, to conduct defensive research on chemical and biological weapons to protect military and first responder personnel. The website of Defence Research and Development Canada-Suffield indicates that the military is currently developing a new type of exposure chamber for 'research and validation studies involving protection of military and first responder personnel against highly toxic substances'.[50]

Furthermore, in response to the so-called War on Terror, the US has once more turned to Canada to assist with medical defence research. In 2004, the Bush Administration created 'Project Bioshield' and one of the numerous biodefence research ventures is the research network 'CounterACT: Countermeasures Against Chemical Threats.' CounterACT is funded by the National Institutes of Health (NIH) to produce 'new and improved medical countermeasures designed to prevent, diagnose, and treat conditions' caused by chemical weapons, such as mustard gas.[51] For example, in 2006, the NIH awarded a $1.7 million grant to PharmAthene, a private, biotechnology company in Maryland engaged in developing biodefense products. Its goal is the commercialization of drugs to prevent and treat military personnel and civilians from the effects of chemical warfare. The Suffield defence laboratories in Alberta are a major site for the company's research.[52]

Thus, Canada's mustard gas experiments in Alberta during World War 2 were not only tied to American medical defence research in the past, but are also linked to events today. The history of Allied mustard gas experiments shows us that the search for 'miracle weapons' has left a terrible health legacy, even when they were not used in combat.[53] What will the search for today's miracle biodefence drugs bring?

Children and Polio in Alberta

In the 1950s, children in Alberta joined a field trial sponsored by American researchers with the National Foundation for Infantile Paralysis (NFIP). Earlier in 1938, President Franklin D. Roosevelt and his law partner Basil O'Connor had formed the NFIP to fund medical treatment, education programmes, and research in the battle against poliomyelitis (polio).[54] Polio was a particularly feared viral disease, since it primarily affected children and could result in permanent paralysis or death. By 1953, Foundation patronage of medical science led to a significant breakthrough when Dr Jonas Salk and his associate Dr Julius Youngner developed a prototype polio vaccine.[55] To prove the efficacy of the new vaccine, the Foundation in 1954 sponsored one of the largest vaccine field trials in American history involving 1.8 million children, most of whom were in grades 1, 2 and 3.[56] While locations outside of the United States were not initially considered, NFIP officials eventually extended an offer for Canadian participation to Dr Robert Defries of Toronto's Connaught Laboratories in recognition of his assistance with development of the vaccine.[57] Defries relayed this offer to the Deputy Minister of the Dominion Department of Health and Welfare, Dr G. D. W. Cameron, who in turn notified each province.[58] Due to provincial jurisdiction over health issues, provinces had the authority to accept or decline participation.[59]

On 19 May 1954, Alberta Health Minister Dr W. W. Cross announced Alberta's inclusion in the study, making it the first province in Canada to officially accept the American offer and the only Canadian locality to have province-wide involvement.[60] The resulting international collaboration between Alberta and the Foundation proved to be a timely alliance. Alberta's participation served as an assertion of its authority over health and one that met the interests of its bureaucrats, citizens and politicians. Foundation officials welcomed Alberta as a proving ground because the NFIP had encountered unforeseen domestic complications and a need for more data. In spite of ethical dilemmas and safety issues, Foundation officials pushed ahead with the trial in Alberta through the tacit approval of the Canadian government and the trust of its citizens.

The Salk polio vaccine field trial proved to be a massive undertaking requiring Alberta health authorities to distribute parental request forms, ship the delicate vaccine, administer injections, keep accurate records and coordinate efforts with the Vaccine Evaluation Center in Ann Arbor, Michigan. Alberta public health officials considered the field trial a rare opportunity to gain international recognition and justify their prior expenditures in laboratories and staff.[61] Alberta's Deputy Minister of Health Dr A. Sommerville assigned the task of managing the study to Dr E. S. Orford Smith.[62] As the Director of the Poliomyelitis Survey, Dr Smith sought to demonstrate Alberta's scientific competency to Foundation officials and allay their concerns. As he explained to NFIP medical consultant Dr Thomas Dublin:

> I telephoned Dr C. R. Amies, the Virologist at the [Alberta] Provincial Laboratory of Public Health here, as soon as I had finished speaking with you, and he was very interested in your suggestion that the [Salk] vaccine trial should be made the opportunity for an immunological survey.[63]

According to Dr Smith, not only could provincial authorities conduct a vaccine trial under pressing time constraints, but they were willing to organize a further 'immunological survey' of blood samples on behalf of the Vaccine Evaluation Center. By promoting Alberta's scientific capabilities, Dr Smith situated the province as a foreign partner for an advanced American biomedical study.

Due to the power imbalance between the US and Canada, the field trial forced Alberta health officials to weigh the tradeoffs of foreign involvement against autonomy. Initially, provincial authorities upheld protectionist sentiments. This stance became evident on 25 May 1954, when Dr Dublin offered to send an American medical consultant to Alberta in order assist with organizing the study.[64] Dr Smith's reply to the NFIP confidently explained that sending a consultant 'would not be necessary' and that 'everything so far [was] running smoothly'.[65] Dr Dublin, evidently surprised with the response, informed his associate, Dr Harold Press that:

> Apparently, the Alberta authorities have changed their minds about consultation with us. It had been my understanding that they were very desirous of having you come up to Alberta. I had asked Dr Smith to request such a consultation by telegram but we have heard no further word from him.[66]

Alberta health officials perhaps chose to reject external support, because they felt sufficiently qualified to manage the trial on their own and wanted to retain their independence from the large American Foundation.[67] Yet health officials' protectionist attitudes shifted once they realized the magnitude, complexity and cost of the study. On 17 June 1954, Dr Robert F. Korns, a senior official at the Vaccine Evaluation Center, arrived in Edmonton to check on local developments and to speak with officials.[68] According to Dr Smith, Dr Korns's arrival was both desirous and timely, as he cleared up misconceptions concerning the vaccine registration schedules, as well as explained 'certain peculiarities in the situation of Alberta compared with that of placebo control areas in the United States'.[69] The importance of avoiding errors and generating accurate data for an international study apparently trumped Alberta officials' desire for operational independence.

Alberta citizens were likewise eager to participate in a test that promised to end the spectre of polio. In 1953 alone, the Royal Alexandra Hospital (RAH) in Edmonton treated hundreds of polio paralysis cases, including 107 in respirators.[70] As physician Dr Russell Taylor explained, the 'impact on the community was enormous'. He recounted that: 'one day in late November 1953 there was a total of fifty-five [polio] patients in the [RAH] Isolation Hospital, thirty-three of them on respirators attended by eighty-five nurses, and eight doctors!'[71] Due to the emotional, physical and financial toll brought about by epidemics, Albertans followed the development of the Salk vaccine closely and were enthusiastic to play a role in its evaluation. Even small rural newspapers, such as the *Drumheller Mail*, discussed the 'announcement of a new vaccine' and details of the pending inoculation schedule.[72] Parental support for the vaccine was so strong that it exceeded the expectations of provincial public health officials. As the *Edmonton Journal* reported:

> More grade two and three children have been authorized by their parents to take part in the polio vaccine test programme in Edmonton than there is vaccine to treat them, Dr G. M. Little, medical health officer, said Monday ... The extra 515 children cannot be included in the program, Dr Little said. 'We offer our regrets to these parents'.[73]

The momentum generated from years of public fear and powerlessness in response to polio led to grassroots endorsement of the vaccine trial.

Alberta politicians also backed the experiment, not only in reaction to public opinion, but also to uphold their commitment to the fight against polio and to improve their reputation among voters.[74] Earlier, in 1938, the governing Social Credit Party implemented the Polio Sufferers Act, which paid the majority of expenses associated with the treatment of polio cases.[75] Alberta was the only Canadian province to institutionalize government-funded polio treatment and after-care, resulting in major recurring costs and considerable criticism from opposition parties.[76] By 1954, the province budgeted a hefty $900,000 for the provincial management of polio cases alone.[77] Therefore, participation in the field trial not only complemented existing government policy, it promised an expedient financial solution as escalating costs could be brought under control if the vaccine proved effective. The popularity of the party was also at stake. Elected officials needed to show that they were receptive to new scientific solutions given the fear generated by polio epidemics. The party was already suffering politically through 1954 and provincial elections were only one year off. The failure to authorize the trial of a polio vaccine, when offered to the province for free, could prove disastrous at the polls. Governmental acceptance of the study, therefore, emerged out of pragmatism and political necessity.[78] By endorsing a progressive public health campaign, politicians hoped to enhance their status among the electorate.

Any fears surrounding the experiment were largely placated by Canadian officials in Ottawa, who implicitly vouched for the safety of the vaccine and negotiated for its timely shipment into the province. However, Albertans did not know that in the process of importing the vaccine, the Canadian Federal Food and Drug Directorate's conventional pharmaceutical regulatory role had been bypassed.[79] NFIP consultant Dr Foard McGinnes expressed appreciation for this absence of bureaucratic red tape when he acknowledged to Dr Cameron that: 'your notification of Dr C. A. Morrell, Director of Food and Drug Divisions, of your cooperation with us should be helpful in expediting shipment of materials into Canada'.[80] The vaccine was shipped into Alberta without any safety assurances or claims about its efficacy.[81] This purposeful oversight by Canadian regulators upheld trust in American practices, but ignored the significance of two largely unresolved vaccine concerns at the time: the quality control of US manufacture and the overall safety of the killed virus vaccine concept.[82]

Although evidence does not indicate which official in Ottawa sought to expedite the trial, what is clear is that the Dominion Minster of Health, Paul Martin Sr, was excited about the potential of the vaccine and confident in its safety.[83] His son's earlier bout with polio in 1946 added to his zeal to rid Canada of the affliction. Even though Dr Cameron advised against proceeding too quickly, it appears that political expediency and encouragement from Martin forced the circumvention of Canada's normal pharmaceutical evaluation processes.[84]

Canadian officials derived confidence in the trial vaccine from both Dr Defries of Connaught Laboratories and the verbal assurances of NFIP officials. In fact, Dr Cameron wrote to the Foundation's Dr McGinnis, stating that,

> with regard to the shipment of vaccine, I hope what you say [is true] about the care with which the material is being tested for safety and that Dr [William] Workman of the Biologics Control Divisions of the Public Health Service is collaborating with you.[85]

Although Dr Cameron was in no position to provide informed consent on behalf of Albertans without first instituting a method for vaccine safety testing, his actions were influenced by pressure to act during a time of crisis. Consequently, in bypassing normal testing procedures and assuming that the vaccine was safe, the Dominion Department of Public Health and Welfare implicitly legitimated an unregulated experimental substance for use in Alberta children.

The social and political climate of the United States by the spring of 1954 also made the inclusion of Alberta in the trial especially desirous. One of the primary motivating factors was ascribed to vaccine manufacturing delays and its effect on the inoculation schedule.[86] Since many of the American pharmaceutical manufacturers were initially unable to consistently inactivate the polio virus to produce vaccine, a temporary halt to production was called by Dr Workman at US Biologics Control.[87] While production difficulties were being resolved, precious time was being lost. The observed seasonal nature of polio, with rising incidence as temperatures climbed through the summer months, necessitated that southern states begin their inoculations earlier than northern states. Unless injections began on time, it would be difficult for statisticians at the Vaccine Evaluation Center to determine if the vaccine had any protective qualities. Consequently, by the time manufactures resolved the production issues, many of the southern test areas had to be dropped.[88] Alberta, as a northern region, proved appealing for Foundation officials to compensate for the loss of some of the original sites.

The role of the American media also shaped NFIP considerations. On 4 April 1954, popular radio personality Walter Winchell devoted part of his Sunday evening broadcast to an alarming account of possible dangers with the proposed Salk vaccine field trial in the United States.[89] After Winchell's broadcast, many frightened American parents contacted their local health officials, demanding that their children be removed from the field trial. Members of the Medical Society in Michigan, for example, asserted that they would not allow their children to participate until the NFIP provided 'further assurance' as to the safety of the vaccine.[90] Due to overwhelming public pressure, some northern districts withdrew from the trial, resulting in the loss of approximately 150,000 subjects (or 10 per cent of the planned test group).[91] The withdrawal of participants motivated NFIP officials to enroll new test sites as a method to maintain the statistical merit of the study.

Foundation officials were further attracted to Alberta due to its population's recurring polio epidemics. As polio typically had a low incidence, the inclusion of high incidence populations for study was desirable for statistical reasons.[92] The years 1952 and 1953 were among the worst polio epidemics in Alberta, exceeding the per capita incidence of many US locations.[93] In 1952, Alberta experienced 774 cases of polio with 81 deaths out of a total provincial population of 1 million.[94] By 1953, there were 1,458 polio cases and a recorded 111 deaths. Dublin alerted senior Foundation officials to Alberta's exceptional status, stating in part that 'Alberta had a province-wide outbreak of poliomyelitis [in 1953] accounting for the largest number of cases ever recorded in the province ... The severity of poliomyelitis was also noteworthy in that deaths from this cause exceeded those reported as due to tuberculosis'.[95] As a region with a high incidence of polio, Alberta was a valuable addition to the vaccine field trial.

The data produced through the participation of Alberta was also important to the merit of the final vaccine report. Approximately 59 per cent of the participating health districts (all located in the United States) followed observed control inoculations, which Basil O'Connor authorized in the early planning stages of the trial. Under this system, second-grade students were vaccinated and the first- and third- grade students were observed. No placebo was given and no randomization of the subjects was involved. Since it was clear who was getting the authentic vaccine, there was no complicated record keeping, which was both convenient and popular with the public.[96] Unfortunately, observed controls were considered by leading statisticians and the head of the Vaccine Evaluation Center, Dr Thomas Francis, as unacceptable for a proper assessment of the vaccine.[97] Realizing this lack of scientific rigour, Dr Francis attempted to salvage the field trial by instituting a double-blind placebo control group for the remaining 41 per cent of health districts, including Alberta.[98] In contrast to the observed control group, the placebo group drew participants randomly from all three grades, providing either vaccine or placebo through coded doses so that neither the child nor the vaccinator knew whether the real vaccine was being given. Only through tracking and later decoding the dose number at the Vaccine Evaluation Center would the true dose content be determined.[99] Dr Francis ultimately sought 'to use as much of this new [placebo vaccine] lot 513 in Canada as is possible'.[100] Considering the research and expenses involved, the nature of the data gathered in Alberta became important to evaluating vaccine efficacy.

Despite the benefits of expanding into Alberta, NFIP officials risked their carefully cultivated image as a medical philanthropy for Americans. They were offering expensive vaccine and materials to members of a foreign population who had never sent a single penny to its cause, while at the same time turning down the inclusion of some US communities.[101] However, NFIP officials remained confident in the advantages of including Alberta, since its public health authorities had prior experience with large-scale pharmaceutical and vaccine field trials. In fact, Alberta officials conducted field trials as early as the 1920s, including a major study of diphtheria anti-toxin in 1927.[102] In addition, provincial authorities cooperated with earlier NFIP polio preventative studies, including the 1952 gamma globulin (GG) trials on children.[103]

Given that conducting a complex vaccine field trial on short notice could be challenging for any health region, the NFIP was encouraged by Alberta's public health administrative structure and excellent laboratory facilities. Between 1950 and 1951, the Alberta Government created additional health districts that provided greater delegation of public health programmes to local authorities.[104] The existence of these districts enabled the Alberta Department of Health to quickly organize and administer the trial. Dr Dublin expressed further assurances, noting that Alberta maintained 'a laboratory with a well-qualified virologist' and facilities to exceed blood testing requirements.[105] In fact, Alberta's provincial virologist, Dr C. R. Amies, was personally known to Dr Francis, who sent him a letter during the field trial, explaining that he 'was pleasantly surprised to know that [Dr Amies was] in Edmonton.'[106]

On 12 April 1955, Dr Francis finished tabulating the field trial results and announced to the world that the Salk vaccine was 'safe, effective, and potent'.[107] Despite the optimistic finale, the history of the polio field trial in Alberta raises troubling questions about medical ethics. The safety of the vaccine, although monitored through triplicate testing, was never guaranteed by the Foundation.[108] Aware of this tenuous situation, NFIP officials created participation forms that utilized carefully crafted language, preferring that words such as *experiment* be replaced with *study* and requiring parents to *request* rather than *consent* to their children's involvement.[109] According to Foundation lawyers, such wording was important from a legal perspective in crafting the volunteer form as a kind of waiver.[110] Since most parents held only a superficial understanding of the trial, its objectives, or its risks, such forms did not provide a satisfactory level of information to make a truly enlightened decision.[111] In fact, a later incident in the US showed that there were legitimate reasons for concern, since a year after the trial an improperly produced Salk vaccine resulted in 164 cases of paralysis and ten deaths.[112] Evidence also suggests that the polio trial in Alberta may have resulted in long-term health risks to participants. In June 1959, Dr Bernice Eddy at the US Biologics Control discovered that the Salk polio vaccine contained a previously undetected simian virus (SV-40), which proved to be carcinogenic.[113] Alberta children, who were injected with the experimental vaccine, may have been exposed to a biological agent, which could increase their risk of cancer.

The Alberta government and the National Foundation for Infantile Paralysis cooperated on the Salk field trial because it fulfilled their respective financial, political and research objectives. Alberta health officials eagerly sought to test the vaccine on children in the province because they considered the trial to be an opportunity to evaluate a vaccine, increase their prestige and justify prior expenditures. Alberta parents were willing to sign the field trial request forms, as they were desperate for a way to protect their children against polio. They assumed that the Foundation, as well as their federal and provincial governments, had taken all precautions necessary to mitigate the risks. Alberta politicians remained supportive of the field trial as part of a continuing health policy commitment, a potential means to control treatment expenses, and a chance to boost their image among voters. The Foundation was pleased to include Alberta, as it had suitable research facilities, a population inundated with polio, and a willingness to follow the placebo control method. This international alliance realized the desires of each party, while furthering the collection of data for medical science.

Concerns about informed consent and the health consequences of pediatric field trials persist to this day. In fact, according to an article in the *Boston Globe* in 2006, there are 'relaxed rules ... surrounding the booming industry of experimentation on children'.[114] As a result, children in the United States and Canada could face serious heath risks by participating in pharmaceutical trials. The *New York Times* recently reported that pediatric trials for a new antibiotic should be stopped because Food and Drug Administration officials found it to be deadly in certain circumstances. The FDA's Dr Johann-Liang cautioned parents that 'the long-term consequences ... are unknown for the developing [immune] system'.[115] Testing pharmaceuticals for pediatric use remains fraught with ethical concerns due to unknown health consequences.

Alberta remains an active site for biomedical studies on civilians. In July 2005, the biotechnology company Altachem received approval to conduct a Phase 1 clinical trial on a dozen Edmonton volunteers of a compound to treat a pre-cancerous skin condition. Altachem president Dr David Cox explained that Alberta was an excellent test site for the new topical treatment, since as one of 'sunniest provinces in Canada', its residents may already face elevated risks to skin cancer.[116] Pharmaceutical companies have also allied themselves with post-secondary institutions and public health authorities to streamline the implementation of biomedical studies in the province. In June 2007, the University of Alberta, in collaboration with Capital Health, launched a new Phase 1 clinical trial facility housed at the Northern Alberta Clinical Trials and Research Centre. Deemed to be the 'most advanced facility of its kind' in western Canada, the new Phase 1 Unit will administer research studies for multinational corporations and local biotechnology firms. Although the risks associated with first-stage trials are carried by Albertans, promoters of the plan uphold the potential for economic benefits and international esteem. Capital Health President and CEO Sheila Weatherill believes that the Phase 1 Unit will 'leverage [the] health system as an economic driver for Edmonton' and broaden the local economy beyond the oil and gas sector. With similar gusto, Mayor Stephen Mandel contends that the facility is 'a natural fit' and will 'solidify Edmonton's position as the Western Canadian hub for biotechnology'.[117] Alberta politicians and public health officials continue to seek international scientific collaboration and offer up their population as test subjects in the hope of future recognition and investment.

Conclusions: Place Matters in Medical Research

The Alberta case studies of the mustard gas experiments in the 1940s and polio vaccine trial in the 1950s reveal why place matters in medical research. They show how Canadians promoted the 'Alberta Advantage' to further US–Canada health relations. In times of crisis, Canadian officials have joined with Americans to identify solutions to shared health concerns. Alberta, in particular, has contributed to developments in American civilian and military medical research. These field trials in western Canada were part of the history of 'big science, ' which is often associated with the wartime Manhattan Project to build the atomic bomb and Cold War scientific research programmes involving government funding of large research teams rather than work by isolated researchers.[118] The trials illustrate some of Canada's contributions to the history of American medical science.

As these historical case studies demonstrate, US–Canada health relations provided benefits to both nations. Canadian officials readily embraced opportunities for collaboration with American medical researchers because they viewed Canada as a junior partner not a pawn, an assessment supported by the historical record. Both testing programmes entailed large financial investments and through collaboration with the US, Canadian officials gained access to valuable additional resources. They also managed to retain control over most of the arrangements with the Americans. Therefore, Canadian officials were willing to accept some health risks for soldiers and children in Alberta, as local officials did elsewhere in North America, in order to save lives, alleviate public fears, and achieve political goals, such as winning a war or fighting an epidemic.

However, it was the research subjects who would pay the price if there were short-term or long-term health problems. In Canada, lax safety regulations and disregard for existing rules meant inadequate protection for Canadians. Although the polio vaccine proved to be successful for most children, there are still unanswered questions about how the research was conducted. As for the mustard gas experiments, there were dire consequences for a significant number of soldiers. Thus, transnational medical research necessitates public scrutiny and public debate in all participating countries to ensure that nations develop and enforce government regulations for transparency, accountability, and the safety of all people.

Acknowledgements

Financial support was provided by a standard research grant from the Social Sciences and Humanities Research Council of Canada and a research grant from the Institute for United States Policy Studies, University of Alberta.

7 PLACING ILLNESS IN ITS CULTURAL TERRITORY IN VERACRUZ, NICARAGUA

Hugo De Burgos

Introduction

It is now widely accepted in medical anthropology and in the social sciences in general, that illness is an embodied cultural experience.[1] Thus, rather than being an objective entity hovering over our human consciousness, illness is a cultural category. Feminist scholars, sociologists, medical anthropologists and many other social scientists have powerfully illustrated how the influence of moral values and subjective meanings is regularly imposed on information that is often presented simply as biological facts.[2] Furthermore, Good argues that *disease*, the presumably objective description of illness, belongs to the culture of biomedicine, and that 'culture is not only a means of representing disease, but is essential to its very constitution as a human reality'.[3] Illness belongs to the cultural territory where it is experienced and confronted by suffering bodies and treated by healers. Like any other cultural category, illness is culturally contingent; and therefore it is also a polysemic experience. Hence, due to its cultural contingency, depending on age, ethnicity, education, religion, social position, geographical origin, gender and place, people perceive, experience and configure illness in a multiplicity of fashions.

In this paper I examine the culturally contingent nature of illness in the context of place among the people of Veracruz del Zapotal, or Veracruceños, from the department of Rivas, in southwest Nicaragua. Veracruceños are a Spanish-speaking Indigenous community claiming to be descendents of the Nahua people who settled in the Isthmus of Rivas around AD 500, and came to be known as the Nicarao.[4] The Nicarao also inhabited the islands of Ometepe and Zapatera.[5] Their largest city was also their capital, called Quauhcapolca, situated near the city of Rivas and around nine kilometres northwest of Veracruz. A cacique or chief ruled in every city or chiefdom with the advice of the Monéxico, or the council of elders.[6] As an ancient institution, the Monéxico has historic value and practical importance for Veracruceños today. Currently numbering approximately 3,800, they inhabit the Veracruz del Zapotal valley and the mountain region between the rivers *Camarón, Guachipilín* and *Rio Grande* in the department of Rivas, in southwest Nicaragua. Locally, Veracruceños are governed by the *monéxico,* comprised of approximately 25 people.[7]

My analysis of 'placing illness in cultural territory in Veracruz, Nicaragua' builds on previous studies about the culturally contingent nature of people's perceptions and experiences of illness.[8] My contribution, however, is to examine the particular ways in which illness is articulated in the context of a cultural territory in Veracruz that is simultaneously both a conceptual system and a physical space. Theoretically, I draw upon Lakoff's definition of a conceptual system as the inherently metaphorical nature of human thought, particularly in how abstract concepts such as time, events, place and causation among others, are understood in terms of, or in relation to, concrete physical and interpersonal experiences.[9]

My approach to physical space, on the other hand, borrows from Gordillo's argument of place as 'produced in tensions with other geographies', and the ways in which 'these tensions are made tangible through the spatialization'.[10] Whereas Gordillo focuses on the spatiality of memory, I examine the spatiality of medical configurations – illness, etiological theories, treatments and healing, as embodied cultural experiences. Placing illness in cultural territory in Veracruz translates into how subjective meanings of illness/healing are grounded on both the land as physical space and on culture, as a subjective territory. The concept of cultural territory as local subjective meanings in Veracruz is marked by a sense of unity with the natural world, by a symbiotic relationship between culture and physical space, and by their interdependency in the production and understanding of medical experiences. I take the term *medicine,* and hence its derivative medical, to refer to a system of 'beliefs and practices that are consciously directed at promoting health and alleviating illness and disease'; and healing as the polysemic and therapeutic means through which we consciously or unconsciously free ourselves and others from naturally or socially caused suffering.[11]

I have chosen the metaphor 'territory' for three reasons: Firstly because Veracruceños use the same metaphor; secondly because of the 'boundedness' with which they perceive their cultural space; and thirdly because the embodied experience of illness grows out of perception, movement and physical experience of their landscape as cultural space.[12] Lived history, ancestors, notions of political struggles, sense of group identity, benevolent and harmful spirits, and the very sustention of life constitute the ideational spatiality embedded in the physicality of their land. As will become clear, the Veracruceño territory is simultaneously inhabited by both human and 'other-than-human' beings.[13] It is within the physical and subjective territory that people, spirits and place become meaningful landmarks of a historically produced medical topology in Veracruz.

Land as History and Identity

In March of 2002, during one of our many conversions, *Culturally Conservative Leader* (hence forth CCL), Esban Gonzáles stated the following:[14]

> Our Indigenous identity is inscribed in our genealogy; we are Nahua descendants by blood, which intimately tie us to our history, and land; and by our unique Indigenous institutions and customs, our monéxico, festivities, medicine, and many other aspects of our culture.[15]

Veracruceños understand their ethnic identity in essentialist terms. They believe it is indelibly written in their biology, and grounded on both the land as physical space and on culture, as a subjective territory. 'Indigenous identity' in Veracruz is understood as a primordial condition, one into which one is born.[16] As all 'imagined communities', Veracruceños instrumentally manipulate their culture to maintain a sense of group history and identity.[17] Sahlins argues that culture may set conditions to the historical process, 'but it is dissolved and reformulated in material practice, so that history becomes the realization, in the form of society, of the actual resources people put into play'.[18] Nowadays most Veracruceños tie notions of group history to their land 'as produced in tensions with' the mestizo geography, and define their Indigenous identity in opposition to the mestizo one.[19] Although the term *mestizo* originally designated the offspring of a Spaniard and a Native American, it is now generally applied to people who speak Spanish and observe cultural norms of Hispanic origin.[20] In Nicaragua ethnic identities are not defined only on the basis of physical characteristics or genealogy. Field argues how discursive narratives of mestizaje in Nicaragua can be holistically seen as encompassing:

> ... a process of biological miscegenation; as a process of nation building which requires that mestizos, as individuals and as collectivities, undergo 'de-indianization' in order to accommodate national identity in ways that Indians [*sic*] cannot; and a process that necessarily creates a panoply of divergent identity positions.[21]

Being a mestizo has become both an ascribed and an achieved status.[22] As noted by Field, Indigenous and mestizo identities in Nicaragua are fluid and overlap in a manner that shapes the historical emergence of different kinds of mestizos and different kinds of Indigenous people.[23] As a mestizo myself, I sometimes have trouble relating to my multiple identities, which include a partial Indigenous one, precisely because the boundaries dividing these social categories can get dynamically blurry and even ineffable at times.

Unlike most Indigenous communities in southwest of Nicaragua, Veracruceños hold legal title to their land. In 1847, twenty-six years after Nicaragua became independent from Spain, the land Veracruceños had traditionally occupied was confiscated using the legislative decrees of 5 March and 22 April

1830. These decrees stipulated that crown and ecclesiastic properties had to be proscribed and auctioned to private owners.[24] According to Veracruceños' oral tradition, under the protection of these rulings public notary José Ruíz fraudulently claimed ownership of their land. He was given legal title to the Veracruceño territory by the government sub-commissioner in Rivas, J. Martiniano. Thirteen years later, 3 July 1860, and after a long process of struggle and negotiation, Veracruceños legally purchased back their land. In December 2001, CCL Arturón Morales told me that for many years Veracruceño men and women, including youths, children and the elderly, donated many hours of their labour to purchase the land. Most males worked in agricultural fields and in indigo processing plants at hacienda El Camarón [The Shrimp], while the majority of females laboured in the kitchen and other domestic jobs of the same hacienda. Others went to the pacific coast to gather snails and sold them to be used as dyes for fabric in Rivas. The payments were arranged as 20 *pesos duros* (or *fuertes,* both terms were used interchangeably) in the summer, and 20 in the winter, making a total of 40 annually. It took the community around ten years to pay a total of 400 *pesos sencillos* or 320 *pesos Duros.*[25] Pedro Mata, Pedro Ponce, and Atanacio Pérez, representing Veracruz, signed the document that entitled Veracruceños as the 'rightful' owners of their territory.[26] Public notary Teodoro Granados did the legal paper work in the city of Rivas. On 9 August 1888 the community finally registered its property in el Libro de Registro de la Propiedad del departamento de Rivas (the Rivas's Department of Land Registry). It was then when their territory became a bounded space. The land title stipulated the actual limits of their territory, introducing a new spatial concept to the community.

Due to a presidential decree, twelve years after Veracruceños registered their land title it lost its legality. In 1910, the Liberal Party president Zelaya had abolished the 'Indians' of Nicaragua. He imposed Spanish as the official language and accepted as 'Occidental', all who dressed in European fashion. As noted by Hoyt, during this time 'many Indigenous people abandoned their dress and customs in order to participate in the economic life of the country'.[27] Throughout the Zelaya years, many Indigenous communities in Rivas underwent difficult times and unstable social situations. In the midst of all this, some communities regrettably became legally and *de facto* extinct. The Indigenous community of San Jorge, located at approximately nine kilometers northwest of Veracruz is an example of the vanishing community in the region.[28] Between 1914 and 1919, however, a new Liberal government in Nicaragua implemented a series of decrees known as *Las Leyes de Comunidades Indígenas* (Laws of Indigenous Communities). According to these laws, all municipalities in Nicaragua were required to recognize and respect Indigenous communities within their territorial jurisdiction, but only if these Indigenous communities were legally recognized by the government. Seeking protection under these new laws, Veracruceños registered their community. Theoretically, these new laws were to bring Veracruceños government support and the opportunity to reinstate their legal Indigenous status. Through a presidential decree on 4 June 1915, the community of Veracruz was officially recognized as a legitimate (ostensibly) autonomous, and a legally constituted Indigenous community. This 'legalization' took place during time of the liberal administration of Carlos José Solórzano. He reformed the 1906 and 1908 Indigenous laws decreed by Zelaya's government, which had made many Indigenous communities disappear.[29]

To this day, land title is important for Veracruceños because it not only deems them to be the rightful owners of the territory, but because it also 'legally demonstrates' that they *are* an 'Indigenous community' according to Nicaraguan law. It is the oldest written record of their presence as an Indigenous people in the region. Although new copies have been legitimately made, the community still zealously keeps the original antique title as one of their most precious and historical documents. In 2001, CCL Arturón Morales illustrated the importance of their land title as it follows:

When people tell me that I am not an Indigenous person because I don't speak an Indigenous language, I tell them that I am an Indigenous person because I was born Indigenous and in an Indigenous territory. If they don't believe me I tell them that we have a document to prove it. Our land title clearly says we are an Indigenous community.[30]

Gow argues that a land title is not a representation of the land of a community primarily because it looks like it, but because its 'standing for' that landscape has the potential to be effected as concrete social action.[31] Given the major importance encoded in the land title, this otherwise inanimate object produced by humans under particular social relations of production, has been attributed life, autonomy, power and dominance, conditions typically associated with commodity fetishism. Gordillo illustrates a similar case of what he calls 'ID-paper fetishism' among the Toba of Argentina. He argues that these people seem to regard legal government documents as valuable and important possessions, while showing critical awareness of the power embedded in modern forms of bureaucracy.[32]

The link between people, land, history and group identity is by no means unique to the Veracruceños. The same relationship between territorial integrity and ethnic identity has been extensively researched elsewhere.[33] Similar relationships between territorial integrity and ethnic identity have been researched elsewhere. For example, White in his study of nationalism and territory found that territoriality plays an essential role in the construction of group identity.[34] According to Saltman (2002) human behaviour is affected by the multiple ways in which people identify with land, topography and natural resources.[35] Saltman found a growing trend towards defining physical space in specific ethnic contexts. In many respects, Veracruceños' preoccupation with their ethnic identity is also grounded on historical attachments to their land. Beyond its irreplaceable role in sustaining life or pragmatic utility, symbolically, their land is regarded as the tangible trace of their history as a distinct people. The construction of an ethnically meaningful past 'is a project that selectively organizes events in a relation of continuity with a contemporary subject, thereby creating an appropriated representation of a life leading up to the present, that is, a life history fashioned in the act of self-definition'.[36]

Veracruceños construct their history by speaking about it; 'in speech history is made'.[37] Past events are made relevant to the present through cultural categories of continuity.[38] In some respects, by consciously promoting the ancestral, historical and traditional values of Indigenous medicine, CCL are reinventing tradition in Veracruz.[39] By overtly evoking the past to reconstruct and validate the present tradition is therefore also altered. Borofsky (1989) argues that very often in the process of being preserved, Indigenous traditions are also being altered.[40] However, in being altered, they are also being preserved because 'the past is being made meaningful to those upholding it in the present'.[41] Borofsky argues that, ironically, [Indigenous people] and anthropologists preserve a past that never was, but they preserve it in a way that is meaningful to present-day audiences. However, this seems to be an inevitable and necessary process because traditional knowledge must continuously adjust to changing circumstances.

Although the historical memory of Veracruceño Indigenous ancestry and land is generally seen as immemorial, the purchasing of their territory in the nineteenth century is regarded as the most immediate historical reference. Purchasing their land seems to have become for many Veracruceos a historical landmark of their culture, identity and territory. Nevertheless, many CCL believe that the cultural boundaries that have historically distinguished group identity on the basis of biological descent and territoriality in Veracruz are gradually becoming indistinguishable in their community. As new cultural elements, such as exogamy, mestizo and global capitalist values, permeate the community, old signifiers of group identity are rendered precarious. Furthermore, for many Veracruceños local territoriality is beginning to lose its binding quality as many indigenous families move outside the legally recognized Indigenous territories. In this context, the need for strengthening 'ethnic boundaries' takes urgency as Indigenous identity in Veracruz.[42] Living among an overwhelming presence of mestizo culture and faced with the social effects of globalization, Veracruceños emphasize their distinct Indigenous identity through a substantial array of cultural practices and strategies. These strategies include the revitalization of their perceived 'Indigenous medicine' as grounded in their historical presence on their land. Although Veracruceños continuously construct their ethnic identity through 'social performances', they conceive their group identity as a fixed essence embedded in a set of primordial attachments accorded to them at birth by the very fact of being born in an Indigenous territory that is both physical and subjective.[43] The subjective meaning of being is seen as objectively grounded in their territory. Most Veracruceños strongly emphasize a qualitative fixity in their ethnicity which they also regard as being historically grounded in the land, from which notions of ancestral spirits, medical configurations, group history and sense of place emerge. Given its irreplaceable role in sustaining life, for many Veracruceños their land is a tangible representation of the historical continuation of their community, and a landmark of their culture and group identity.

> Preserving our territory is preserving our Indigenous identity ... In disunity, we will not be able to claim our rights, protect our land, and keep our culture. Without communal land it will be more difficult to call ourselves Indigenous people.[44]

The symbolic and the concrete

> Originally, the territory our ancestors purchased measured around 50 square kilometers. Several signposts were placed to demarcate the territory. For our people those signposts had great value ... they are symbols of our territorial Indigenous identity... Without a doubt the most memorable relic, even today, is la Piedra Labrada.[45]

La Piedra Labrada is a fancy carved stone brought from Granada, Nicaragua, in the late nineteenth century as an emblem to demarcate the newly purchased Indigenous territory. It is still in its original spot where it was placed almost 150 years ago, right at beginning of the Camarón River. Two other equally important, but less elaborate, stone signposts were also erected around the same time. Their location is south of the Piedra Labrada and over the mountains, passing Rio Grande (formerly called El Tempisque River) and ending in Los Horcones, near the mouth of Guchipilín River. As noted by Maurice Bloch about the Zafimaniry summits in Eastern Madagascar, in Veracruz the carved stones and other long-lasting monoliths can also represent the history of the people.[46] But more importantly, these stone posts represent the achievements of their ancestors who have inscribed themselves on to the seemingly unchanging land. They are specially inscribed in those points where the demarcations of place are less visible and therefore more urgently needed, given the tension between their territory and the ever-growing mestizo one.

After it was initially purchased, the Veracruceño territory remained practically unchanged for almost a century. However, in the mid-1960s a fraudulent new demarcation of their territory took place. Juan Salinas, an individual with no relation to the community and under the protection of the Somoza dictatorship, illegally claimed ownership of over one-sixth of the Veracruz territory. Fortunately for the Veracruceños, during the Sandinista agrarian reform of the 1980s, these usurped lands were confiscated and allocated to a cooperative comprised of people from Veracruz. 'It was because of this government initiative that the lands we had lost in the 1960s were indirectly returned to our community' (CCL Pedro Gonzáles).[47] Nominally both local and national laws still protect the land rights of Veracruceños. Indigenous communal lands cannot be sold, confiscated, taxed, expropriated or subjected to any agrarian reform. Furthermore, Veracruceños' communal laws ensure that every member of the community owns the piece of land where he/she dwells. Movement within the territory is unrestricted; but no one can cut a tree or make major alterations to the landscape without the approval of the monéxico.

In theory, every member of the community has equal access to arable land for subsistence agricultural purposes (41 per cent) and commercial crops (59 per cent). An annual fee of five córdobas (0.50 C$) per acre must be paid to the community's administrators to be granted permission to use the land for subsistence or cash crops. Individual use of communal land only gives people rights to the crops, not to the land itself. In recent years, however, unequal access to the arable land has instigated conflicts among a few families. Some land issues have been communally solved, while others have escalated to occurrences of physical violence and accusations of witchcraft. In fact, social dialectics of power expressed in witchcraft are also essential local ingredients for some degree of social harmony. For Veracruceños witchcraft also operates as a levelling device that enhances group unity by lessening differentials in wealth. Families with more human and economic resources tend to be able to rent more communal land than small families with fewer economic resources. In addition to agricultural usages, communal land in Veracruz is also used for grazing cattle, hunting, gathering and fishing. These activities are free from any form of taxation and community or national regulation. This traditional land tenure regime is an ancient practice in Veracruz and one considered essential for keeping a vibrant Indigenous community in the face of the permanent threat posed by the mestizo culture.

But the value and importance of land for Veracruceños goes beyond the practical benefits they receive from it as the sustainer of life. Veracruceños seem to value and respect their land because they regard it as the mother and ultimate sustainer of both their physical and spiritual existence.

> Our Indigenous territory is, and has been for time immemorial, the base of our material, social and spiritual existence. That is why we refer to our land in general as our motherland, not in the patriotic sense, but in an infinite maternal and transcendent nurturing way. It gives us life; it gives us medicine. We and the land are one. Therefore, we value the land simply because we value ourselves.[48]

The Veracruceños' territory seems to be the single most important feature of the material and cultural patrimony of the community. In January 2002, CCL conservative leader Pedro Gonzáles told me that their Indigenous territory is an essential part of their history, culture, subsistence, and sense of place.

> Our land is a tangible symbol of our Indigenous unity, continuity and pride. It is reference of our history and ethnic identity. We see ourselves as part of the land, and the land as part of us. It is like being one and the same.[49]

As I lived in Veracruz, I became increasingly aware of how Veracruceños speak of their Indigenous territory as both a physical landscape and a conceptual topography of meanings. This particular understanding pervades almost all other spheres of their social, material and ideational life. As will be clear, it is precisely this mode of relating to their landscape that allows Veracruceños' medical experiences to exist in a physical and magical territory in which the presumably discrete demarcations between the objective and the subjective are not clearly defined. Through magical healing and/or medical witchcraft, Veracruceños move in and out of the boundaries between everyday life and a timeless, sacred, but also contemporary order of subjective reality, which they, nevertheless, see as being grounded on the conspicuous objectiveness of their landscape.

Not surprisingly, Veracruceños typically reckon and construct their sense of a distinct Indigenous identity in reference to two main organizing principles, they are: sense of people and place. On one hand, Veracruceños see their Indigenous identity as marked by a Nahua genealogy that extends well into history, and on the other, by primordial ties to a place they call their *territorio Indigena* (Indigenous territory). Whereas '*el pueblo*' refers to all members of the Indigenous community living both in and outside the legally owned Indigenous territory, '*el territorio*' refers to the land that the community legally possesses. One constitutes a political unit, and the other a geographical space. But within these two general categories, they also speak of a non-physical territory as encompassing another form of spatiality. This non-physical territoriality is the subjective space they call their 'Indigenous culture', which is nevertheless conceived as grounded on both the objectivity of their landscape and their historical presence on it. This dialectical relationship between land, culture and history is similar to what Keesing found among the Kwaio of Papua New Guinea, who see their landscape not only as divided by invisible lines into named land tracts and settlement sites, but also as a geography structured by history and meanings.[50] The Veracruceño sense of people and place also seems to reflect the Sauerian (1974) dialectic model where culture is seen as the agent, the natural area as the medium, and cultural space as the end result.

The link between people, land and history in Veracruz is a powerfully unifying conceptual experience. Land is a symbol of ethnic identity for Veracruceños as a people, but keeping it has also been a chronic and severe source of anxiety and tension vis-à-vis the mestizo society and geography. The historic purchasing of their current territory and the subsequent struggles to retain it reveal these tensions and the symbolic importance of territoriality for Veracruceños. In addition to its pragmatic utility, land tenure for Veracruceños is a means for shaping, expressing and preserving their cultural identity. The stories of 'the purchasing of the land' and 'the journey to bring La Piedra Labrada to the community' are often told to children by the elders in Veracruz with such reverence that the stories have somewhat acquired the status of local 'origin myths' of place as the rebirth of a people. As origin myths of place these historical events neatly integrate community social experiences with a wider set of assumptions about group history and identity derived from the contradictions and tensions between their Indigenous position in *alterity* to Nicaraguan mestizos.[51] At the same time, the stories are also reified as the objective realities of place. Both the land and the symbolic markers of the Indigenous territory are tangible and contemporary signifiers of identity and a sense of place. Gordillo, argues that 'places are the result of social contradictions embedded in them' and that therefore, examining these contradictions 'is crucial to dismantle the appearance of places as well-bounded entities, for it reveals, first, the fractures and struggles that make them ongoing, unstable and unfinished historical processes and, second, the relations that integrate them with other geographies'.[52]

A Landscape of Illness, Medicine, Spirits and Evil Forces

In order to speak of, or to distinguish, the city, or a sense of urbanity in general from the rest of the landscape, Veracruceños (and many people in Central America) use the general term 'el campo', literally, the countryside. El campo, however, is further divided into another specific subspace referred to as *el monte*. Although sometimes both terms are used interchangeably, in most contexts *el monte* refers to the more wild, untamed spaces contained within el campo. For instance, the village of Veracruz is situated in *el campo*, but no one is said to live in *el monte*. These two conceptual spaces are usually negotiated by the presence or absence of human dwellings and other symbols of urbanity on the landscape. Sometimes the boundaries dividing these dynamic spaces seem to be indistinguishable. In its practical everyday usage, however, Veracruceños clearly use *el monte* to designate any space of the landscape laying outside the limits of their dwellings, sense of urbanity, or simply beyond human landscape agency. The distinction between *el campo* and *el monte* also constitutes disputed territories in the mind because it implies a partitioned nature that is nevertheless the product of context. Conceptually, *el campo* and *el monte* are mutually exclusive landmarks and places delineated by a culturally structured sense of nature in Veracruz.

During a trip CCL Alfredo López and I took to *la Piedra Labra* in December 2001, amid the overwhelming sound of the howler monkeys (genus *Alouatta* monotypic in subfamily Alouattinae), I was walking with such apprehension that he told me that one should never be afraid of *el monte*, but that nevertheless, one should respect it. 'The trees, rivers, mountains, creeks, bushes, land tracks and animals you see here', he said, 'conceal other forms of life, spiritual life, that can either protect you or harm you'.[53] As I lived in Veracruz, it became increasingly clear to me that the meanings of *el monte* contained within their landscape went beyond its physical appearance. Several Veracruceño healers also told stories that made me aware of how the entire Veracruceño territory was endowed with spiritual powers, attributions and functions that related people in a medical, spiritual and moral sense to their land. The landscape is said to be ruled by its own physical geography as much as it is by powerful spirits permanently dwelling in it. The following quotes best described this notion.

> One day my grandfather lost his great gift for healing because he broke the spiritual rules that had given him the power to heal. Indigenous healing has spiritual rules that one must follow. Regrettably, my grandfather decided to massage an animal after massaging a human. Different spiritual forces rule healing animals and healing humans. One must never treat animals if one is treating humans, and vice versa ... Also there are spiritual rules for gathering medicinal energies from plants and animal. For example, when you want to cut the bark from the mongo tree, you have to make sure you cut it from a part of the tree facing the morning sun. Don't ask me why. These are secret spiritual rules that I was taught as a healer.[54]

> After a birth the placenta has to be burned on coals and buried in the backyard of the house where the birth took place. It has to be there, nowhere else. Those are spiritual laws of the land we have to follow.[55]

Knowing the rules or understanding the particular spiritual grammar of the landscape is a condition that is necessary for effective healing in Veracruz. Having an understanding of the cause of illness is essential for knowing how to treat it. The particular course of action both a healer and patient may take will always depend on the mutual understanding of the place of origin of the illness. 'Physicians know how to treat only common illnesses. Our Indigenous knowledge cures evil and spiritual illnesses because we know its sources, its origin'.[56] In this sense, knowledge about the places, physical, spiritual and otherwise, from which an illness originates, is inversely proportional to having the knowledge for diagnosing and treating an illness. While the sources of some illnesses in Veracruz are regarded as ubiquitous, others are seen as originating in specific landmarks within their landscape. Geographical etiology plays an important role in the classification of illness for Veracruceños. Depending on the place of origin of an illness, a set of identical symptoms can sometimes be caused by different agents. Due to the particular importance placed on the relationship between landmarks and illness, even one illness can, in some instances, have different etiologies. For example one can get a rash by having physical contact with a poisonous plant or by encountering an irritated spirit in a human or animal-like shape near a creek, a waterhole or any landmark (rock or any other geographical features). Furthermore, pathoplasticity or lack of uniformity in the way in which people with the same illness or injury appear to respond to the same or almost identical situations is explained by geographical etiology in Veracruz.

Spatial references to illnesses and healing experiences are also marked by ideas about the proximity or the distance of a place. In this regard, Veracruceños distinguish between local and foreign illnesses. In 2002, CCL Alfredo López declared that outsiders had brought several foreign illnesses to their village. In the excerpt below, López makes a clear reference to a spatial distance between Veracruceño land and other places. Its cultural and geographical distance in addition to its alien origin indicates the foreignness of an illness.

> Illness such as cancer, A.I.D.S., and some others new illnesses in our community are not originally from here. We may suffer from them now because they came from the outside. These maladies are not from this land. People who travel to Costa Rica, Managua and even the United States frequently bring illnesses from those places. These illnesses are foreign illnesses. But, as you know it, it is nothing new. It is always the same story. When the Spanish came to these lands to invade our people, they also brought with them many illnesses. Of course, we were not free of illnesses ourselves. There have always been some illnesses that you can get in this place. That is why you have to know where you go and when to go to certain places here.[57]

Typically, for Veracruceños the Spatial orientation about the origin of an illness is a significant and necessary condition for an effective treatment. It seems that because the healing powers are grounded within the Indigenous territory, the effectiveness of treatment is thus enhanced by the physical proximity to the source. Thus, locality seems to play a significant therapeutic role. Being physically located within the Indigenous territory has an important medical function for Veracruceños. It is a way of reifying their sense of an inherent connectivity thought to exist between place, people and spiritual beings. The following testimony by healer Cipriano M. (an influential leader and healer from Veracruz), well illustrates this point.

> There was a man who was to have surgery. His family came and asked for my opinion. 'We have been told by the physician that if he doesn't undergo surgery, he will die', one of his sisters said to me. 'Noway! Don't waste your money. What they want is to rehearse on patients like your brother,' I told them. 'Do you think you could cure him, then?' they asked me. 'Yes,' I replied. The problem, however, was getting him out of the Rivas hospital. So I told them he had to be brought back to Veracruz for the treatment. If I try to treat him in Rivas, my medicine may not have worked. The healing must take place here in Veracruz so that the spirits can help us. They went back to the hospital and managed to get him out by lying to the hospital staff. They brought him here. 'What's wrong with him?' they asked me. He has an imposed cancer. Someone has sent him this illness through witchcraft. Without undergoing surgery, now the man is healthy again ... the medicinal powers of God and the spirits, who ultimately

do the healing, work better if I treat patients here in the community. El monte is laden with healing powers, some of it comes in plants. That is why people come to see me here. I rarely go out to treat people in Rivas or other places because healing powers seem to be stronger here.[58]

Although in general, Veracruceños believe in the divine origins of illnesses, as did the ancient Nahua people of Nicaragua, their etiological theories can be divided into two main types of illnesses: *enfermedades comúnes* (common or natural illnesses) and *males puestos* (imposed or supernatural illnesses).[59] Common illnesses in Veracruz are typically explained in terms humoural pathology; imbalances caused by exposure to cold air, overeating of 'hot' or 'cold' food, viruses and bacteria, physical or psychological trauma, exposure to poisonous fumes, ingestion of poisonous substances, animal bites, and lack of proper nutrition. *Males puestos* or imposed illnesses on the other hand are part of a personalistic, and sometimes moralistic system where illnesses are caused by the active, purposeful intention of a '*sensate* agent'.[60] Some of these other-than-human persons may be supernatural such as a deity or a god, ghosts, ancestors or any of the many spirits and mystical powers dwelling in their landscape. Although witchcraft is a common diagnosis for some illnesses, misfortunes and even the occasional death, harmful powers ultimately derive from the spirits dwelling in their territory, and in particularly from *el monte*.[61]

The most salient geographical features of *el monte* in Veracruz are rivers, creeks, waterholes, mountains, valleys, a few small grasslands and a jungle laden with many species of plants and wild animals from which healing powers as well as harmful substances can be extracted. For many people in Veracruz, these geographical features constitute a cultural topography of medical meanings where healing powers and illness-causing agents are found. As a whole, *el monte* is regarded as inherently possessing and eradiating a variety of healing, life-giving and harmful energies. In addition to providing people with an everyday subsistence, *el monte* in general can also bring the blissful benefits of health or the dreaded danger of illness and death. Veracruceños typically believe that distinct energies dwelling in various parts of the landscape have naturally occurring powers that can heal or harm people by rewarding or punishing their behaviour. For many Veracruceños, the political economy of moral panic between illness and people's behaviour depends on the benevolence and harmfulness of the other-than-human inhabitants of the land. In fact, the realness of these of other-than-human inhabitants of the land is illustrated by how Veracruceños typically and frequently seek the benevolent protection of these healing agents. Linda Garro, in a different, but related context, claims that to allow for illness and misfortune occurring as a consequence of not living up to one's obligations to other-than-human persons involves an acceptance of the ontological reality of such beings as well as perceiving oneself as dependent on the continuing benevolence of such beings and the necessity to live in a manner that recognizes this dependence.[62]

Although these envisaged energies and sensate agents permanently dwell in the landscape, some of them only manifest themselves at certain times and localities. This is why the healing of some illnesses can only be performed at night time and in especially designated places. For example, the Spirit of the Earth responsible for causing lost soul can only go out at night time, and hence its healing ritual can only take place during the night. These unseen energies can either be personal spirits such as the Spirit of the Earth, or impersonal forces, such as an evil wind, commonly associated with some occurrence of witchcraft.

This particular understanding of the healing and harmful powers naturally occurring in the landscape was also found among the Ancient Nahua people in Nicaragua. They believed that all important landscape features, especially places where clouds would gather to produce rain, were deities in themselves. They also believed that both healing and ailing powers came not only from these sacred places, but also from dreaded places in their landscape, particularly, gloomy creeks, rivers, caves and isolated clearings.[63] In Veracruz many maladies are said to come from mountains, rivers, abandoned or empty roads, and *el monte* in general. Among the most common illnesses people can get from these places are headaches, chest pains, earache, shoulder pains, cramps, muscle spasm, convulsions, paroxysm, madness, shivers and inflammations without any apparent cause. However, some of these illnesses can also be regarded as only symptoms of other maladies. For example, la *perdida del tumal* or soul lost can manifest itself as madness, convulsions, paroxysm or social and personal withdrawal. Although soul lost does not occur very frequently, is one the most dreaded illness in Veracruz caused by spiritual forces found in several places throughout their landscape. When suffering from this illness the Spirit of the Earth allegedly takes one's soul away. To treat it, a healer must supplicate the Spirit of the Earth to return the soul of the patient, in exchange for a better gift that the healer will provide. The following is my English translation of the Spanish healing prayer used to treat soul lost in Nicaragua.

> Earth: Universe of my soul: Where did you pick this person's soul up? Where did you frighten this person? Let this person go ... Give this person to me so that I can take her with me in my arms. Perhaps you too are carrying her in your arms. Let this person free so that I can take her with me ... Don't take this person away ... Let this person go ... I and you will let this person go ... Then, I will visit you ... I will bring you a gift ... but let her go ... You have this person under your armpit ... Don't frighten this person ... Person, raise from wherever you are with your sad gaze. Sit down Universe of my soul ... Give her to me ... Let this person go so that I can hold her under my armpit. Here, I will leave this gift for you ... Seven Thursdays after you let her go, I will leave, but let this person go ... Don't incarcerate her ... You are pulling her hair ... Give her to me ... and I will also give you a gift ... I will give you a more precious offer-

ing than the one you have ... May be you are not able to go in day light ...You only go out at night time ... But because I will give this offering you will be able to go out in daylight ... You may ask me anything you want ... If you want this person rather than a more precious gift, then you will let you have her.[64]

Land in Veracruz is also regarded as a multilayered structure where vertical and horizontal orientations determine the distribution of its benevolent and harmful powers. The topsoil, for example, is endowed with extraordinary healing and life-giving faculties. Its benevolent life manifests itself through crops, flowers, fruits and medicinal plants that grow on the topsoil. The lower layers of the ground, according to local beliefs, are inhabited by the dead and contain destructive telluric forces and demons that can bring illness, misfortune and death. The deeper one penetrates the ground, the more dangerous it becomes. This geological spirituality is also part of ancient Nahua mythology in Nicaragua.[65] Ancient Nahua people referred to the topsoil as *la madre piel de la tierra*, Spanish for the Mother skin of earth. In Veracruz, this conceptual skin is believed to provide additional protective powers for humans. It protects people from the evil forces, and from the occult dwellers of the underground world. The Mother skin of earth impedes the surfacing of underground negative energies, regarded by Veracruceños as the ultimate agents of misfortune, illness and death. Social relations and everyday tensions are seen as only the proximate, not ultimate, causes of illness and misfortune.

Even after death, these occult telluric forces must be dreaded given their harmful nature. Moving vertically on the ground is seen as an invasive action that will always bring an unpleasant encounter with the underground spirits. This explains the custom of making a cross of salt at the bottom of the grave before any one is buried in Veracruz. Deep below the topsoil in the burial place, the body of the deceased is no longer protected by the Mother skin of the earth. The body is then in a vulnerable place, totally exposed to the evil and diabolic unseen powers dwelling in the lower layer of the earth. The cross of salt provides the necessary protection for the buried person. On December 2002, I told Alex Morales, a prominent cultural consultant in Veracruz, that I had noticed how every time someone was buried in the community there was always a cross of salt made at the bottom of the grave.[66] Sensing my inquisitiveness, he replied as follows:

> If we don't put a cruz de sal [cross made of salt] at the bottom of the grave, the devil will come to disrespect the body and could even take it away. This is a way to ensure the dead will rest in peace. The cross of salt provides Christian protection to the body and keeps away the demonic forces that dwell deeper in the ground ... below the topsoil there are evil spirits.[67]

Vertical movement within the land in Veracruz is by all accounts a dangerous enterprise. For instance, after digging a well in the community a blessing ritual must be performed before using it. This is done to ensure that the water coming from out it will be free of the demonic forces dwelling underground. In fact, graveyard soil is generally seen in most of Nicaragua as inherently evil. In November 2001, healers Cipriano M. explained to me how both under and above ground spiritual forces can be manipulated by *brujos* (witches) through witchcraft. According to Cipriano M. *brujos* can magically harness these powers to either free people from the suffering of illness, or make them sick, and bring misfortune and even death upon them. He was particularly concerned with assuring me that he had never done any witchcraft himself, but that as a healer, he had learned how such evil winds were cast. During one of our many interviews, Cipriano M, told me how an evil wind spell was cast using graveyard soil:

> An evil wind can be cast in different ways. I'm going to tell you only about a few of them. Sometimes people use a glass full of soil from the graveyard and another glass full of snake powder to cause an illness or bring misfortune to an individual[68]. This mix of graveyard soil with snake powder can be spread around your house and illness or misfortune comes to you and your family. If, for example, you are building or improving your house, you won't be able to finish it if an envious person places an illness in your house. By spreading this evil mix powder, members of a whole family can get sick or start endlessly fighting amongst themselves. It is the soil what brings disharmony to a household. For example, if you and your wife fight all the time, it's because someone has spread some of this evil soil on your doorstep.[69]

Although not overtly admitted in Veracruz, witchcraft has a well-defined place in Indigenous medicine and in everyday social life. The predominance with which people perceive and express the experiences of illness and healing in terms of the absence or presence of witchcraft reveals how Veracruceños see their social life as embedded in a pervasively medical and magical world. According to many Veracruceños, *brujos* have access to the spirits of apparently inanimate things and plants dwelling in the landscape, usually *el monte*. Although *brujos* can and do gather the powers they use to bring health or sickness to people, elements in the mystical landscape are nevertheless regarded as autonomous. Mist emanating from waterholes, rivers and creeks can also cause several illnesses without having to be manipulated by *brujos*. For instance, a person can fall ill if proper protocol is not followed when using elements and energies found in *el monte*. According to local healers in Veracruz, if a person does not ask permission to drink water from a natural source in *el monte*, she or he may become sick with a variety of physical ailments, ranging from a skin rash to even madness. Furthermore, some of the trees featured in the landscape also have the power to make people ill. Perhaps the most commonly reported one in Veracruz is the Chilamate tree (*Ficus costaricana*). Before one can safely rest in its shade, one should ask for permission to avoid falling ill. Chilamates are seen as having a particular mystical effect on the landscape because its copious foliage usually produces a gloomy atmosphere, but also because it is a sacred tree in ancient Nahua mythology. In November 2001, a key cultural consultant in Veracruz told me that his grandfather had once advised him to show reverence to the Chilamate tree before resting under its shade, and that failing to do so would result in suffering horrible headaches or skin rashes.[70]

Despite the many harms believed to come from *el monte*, in general, however, vegetation in the Veracruceño landscape is seen as inherently benevolent. This is illustrated by following the testimonies of three Veracruceño healers who I interviewed several times between October 2001 and December 2002.

> Here in our garden we have medicinal plants for almost all of the illnesses we treat in our community. I learned how to identify plants because my mother used to tell me about each plant and what their healing properties are. But even if I don't have a particular plant in my garden for an illness, chances are my neighbours have it. Sometimes you can find the medicine in the bush. I also keep oils and fat from animals that we use for healing. Everything we need to treat our illness is here on our land, endowed with abundant healing powers.[71]
>
> Whenever we are sick, we find our medicine in our land, here in this territory. The jungle is laden with medicinal powers. That is why you cannot sell nor buy the herbs and plants that have healing powers. That's how we learned it from our ancestors ... Here in our territory, as you can see, we have plenty of medicinal plants. We have a tree named Quelite Fraile (*Cnidoscolus aconitifolius*), which I also use to treat bones and muscle problems ... It does miracles on broken bones ... These plants are the best anti-inflammatory I know of; and we have it right here on our medicinal land.[72]
>
> We know when a person has been bewitched and know what to do, medically. We know what herbs and roots to use. Physicians are trained to understand pharmaceutical things. They must go to a pharmacy. We go to *el monte*. There we find medicine for our illness.[73]

The description I have given here of the Veracruceño configuration of spatiality is in relation to local concepts and experiences of illness and healing, and hardly reflects the complexity of their entire Indigenous medical system. Beyond my brief and specific account, the Veracruceño Indigenous medical system is ancient, sophisticated and dynamic. It draws upon Nahua mythology, cosmology, cosmogony, epistemology and a historically shaped worldview. Furthermore, since the arrival of the Spanish conquistadors, people have had to imaginatively incorporate new elements, theories and practices into its already existing structures, without losing its ancient Nahua character and essence. Despite its seeming fixity, the Veracruceño medical system is an unfinished and in a constant process of becoming.[74] Its connection to an ancient past is regarded in Veracruz as an essential aspect for both the physical and spiritual survival of a people. And in most recent years, it has been made into a political tool to resist any form of cultural domination through medical and other means.

We have culturally survived and resisted the Spanish invasion, colonial domination and mestizo oppression thanks to our Indigenous medicine. It is and it has been vital for our physical and spiritual survival (Pedro Gonzáles).

Our Indigenous medicine is a way of preserving an autochthonous quality in our health issues and culture. Our ancestors always healed themselves with traditional medicine, and thanks to it, they were able to live healthy lives. Occidental [Western] medicine is relatively new in our community. However, we all know that through medicine and other modern stuff, they [non-Indigenous people] are trying to domesticate us, of taking away our traditions, our Indigenous identity, our culture and our own way of surviving with our own Indigenous medicine.[75]

These testimonies, and a general conscious renewal of Indigenous spiritual medicine in Veracruz, are consistent with a national trend found among many Indigenous communities in Nicaragua. In the last two and a half decades, Indigenous people, particularly in the southwest region of Nicaragua, have been consciously using Indigenous spiritual medicine as a new strategy to reaffirm their collective Nahua identity.[76] Through rhetoric and political action an elite of CCL in Veracruz has been promoting the idea that, beyond its practical medical value, Indigenous spiritual medicine represents an important political and historical tool for demarcating and safeguarding a culturally distinct Indigenous identity.[77] Similar strategies have been developed in, and implemented by, several Indigenous communities throughout Central America. Cultural reinvigoration in Veracruz has been actualized by the revival of an Indigenous spiritual medicine considered historically grounded on a primordial connection to a simultaneously physical and cultural territory.

The temporal process of place making through medical narratives seems to allow people in Veracruz to make an ancient history of spirits relevant to the present. Past events are made relevant to the present through cultural categories of continuity. Place and its inhabitants (human and non-human) provide that relevance. Thus, spiritual medicine is, in a sense, seen as historically timeless and indissoluble, but above all as inherent to their place. The conceptual spatiality of spirits dwelling and manifesting in their physical territory provides a greater sense of reality of their medical beliefs and practices. Healing and harmful spirits grounded on their Indigenous territory are seen as somewhat idiosyncratic to the community and culture. Given the perceived and constant threat posed by the mestizo society, interaction between human and other-than-human beings in Veracruz is constantly redefined through medical idioms that relate people to a particular place, history and identity, but always in 'alterity' to an overwhelming mestizo territory and culture.[78] The historical making and remaking of the Indigenous territory as a distinct political unit in Veracruz is based on its mutual exclusion with the mestizo territory. Although healing and harmful spirits and forces are ubiquitous in most of Nicaragua, Veracruceños seem to regard their particular medical and spiritual experiences as inherent and autochthonous to their Indigenous identity.

Veracruños clearly regard both their Indigenous identity and medicine as ancient, stable, and part of their autochthonous cultural institutions. Nevertheless, in a somewhat broader history of 'Indigenous medicine' in Veracruz is the synthesized articulation of different medical beliefs and practices proceeding from multiple sources. Historically, Veracruceños have been able *to adhere* to the already existing pre-Hispanic herbal wisdom and health practices of other medical traditions.[79] The most prominent historical sources that today constitute Indigenous medicine in Veracruz combine African health practices (including witchcraft); Japanese bioenergetics; allopathic medicine; early Arabic medicine and health practices; Greek humoural medicine; Judeo-Christian religious beliefs, symbols and rituals; medieval and later European witchcraft; and modern beliefs about spiritualism and psychic phenomena.[80] Furthermore, although in Veracruz healers make a nominal distinction between their Indigenous and non-Indigenous medicine, in many respects it is indistinguishable from *curanderismo*. In fact, healers in Veracruz also refer to themselves as *curanderos* and *curanderas*, for female healers. *Curanderismo* is a widespread traditional medical system found among Spanish-speaking people in United States and throughout Latin America.[81] *Curanderismo* and 'Indigenous medicine' in Veracruz share many of the most basic etiological theories, pharmacopoeia, healing procedures, diagnostic techniques, and even sickness categories. One good example is *calor de vista* (literally heat of gaze), or 'evil eye', which is the combination of the classical Mediterranean evil eye with an illness ancient Nahua called *iscucuyalis*, which presents the same symptoms and etiology of evil eye. Friar Bobadilla reported in his chronicle how Indigenous people in Nicaragua believed in a deadly infant illness caused by simply staring at a child.[82] Cosminsky argues that the concept of evil eye, which is 'one of the most widespread folk beliefs concerning illness found in Spanish America', seems to have diffused to the New World from Spain.[83] However, *iscucuyalis* indicates how an Indigenous version of evil eye was already present in the Americas.

This is not to say that Indigenous healing is simply a type of filtered-down medical knowledge, but rather to elucidate the point that contemporary Indigenous medicine in Veracruz is also constituted by medical ideas, which came from other medical systems. This is an important premise because, as Kleinman argues, 'there is no essential medicine, no medicine that is independent of historical context'.[84] Pigg, in reference to the *dhâmi-jhânkris* in Nepal (roughly, shamans and other ritual specialist healers), also argues that it is not possible to recover a pure, authentic Indigenous belief system that is clearly separated from someone else's modern ideas.[85] Due to the eclectic character, Veracruceños' medical practices and ideology inevitably overlap with other medical traditions.

Thus, claiming that traditional healing in Veracruz is a culturally homogeneous social reality could lead to a misapprehension of its ethnographic description.

Conclusion

I began this paper by placing health and illness experiences in the general cultural territory where they are created, suffered and confronted by humans, patients and healers alike. I discussed the multiple relationships Veracruceños have with their Indigenous territory, which they regard as an objective symbol of their ethnic identity, as historical continuation, and as a pragmatic material source of subsistence. The Veracruceño people conceive of their territory as a physical landscape continually being transformed by their own historical agency in opposition to the dominant mestizo society. I contrasted the Veracruceño sense of territoriality as material resources subject to pragmatic negotiations between the need for subjective meanings and the objective requirements for subsistence. Having purchased their land in the nineteenth century illustrates the negotiation of those tensions.

I have demonstrated how, besides having a practical and utilitarian relation to their land as the immediate sustainer of an objective existence, Veracruceños also conceive their territory as a subjective cultural space. The Veracruceños' physical landscape is also constituted by a spiritual geography, where an invisible and complex panorama of spirits, elements and evil forces interact with humans through health and illness idioms. Within this ascribed spiritual ecology, places acquire medical meanings that geographically connect people and spirits to a common history, literally grounded in a particular place. In the complex Veracruceño landscape, geographical features become differentiated not only on the basis of their physical characteristics but also on attributed spiritual qualities. Thus, in this 'morphology of landscape', landmarks are fragmented into meaningful units of medically constituted experiences that coalesce people, spirits and history into a realm of a local 'ecological subjectivity'.[86] In this realm, mutually exclusive meanings are contingently assigned to demarcate subdivisions of the landscape in terms of their healing or harmful spiritual powers, which Veracruceños typically regard as historically timeless and indissoluble.

More important, however, is that in this conceptual territoriality the physical and the spiritual realm are brought together in a single and unifying medical narrative. In this envisaged and amalgamated topography utilitarian and symbolic needs become practical meanings through medical beliefs and actions. Illnesses as embodied experiences on the one hand, and spiritual meanings as healing or illness-causing agents on the other, illustrated this point, i.e. the very materiality of one's body simultaneously exists in both an objective and a mental territory conceived as continuum of events where the boundaries between an objective and subjective world are not neatly defined or even seen as remarkably different and antagonistic. Furthermore, in the ascription of multiple meanings to the landscape, it seems that people, place, medicine and spirits are dialectically fused to a common history and ancestry. Subjective meanings are regarded as reflecting a timeless sense of common history given the relative fixity of the landscape, where ancient symbols bear witness to their historical presence in the land. For Veracruceños, the medical meanings embedded in, and produced by, features in their landscape represent the continuation of a common ancestry precisely because of a perceived common history.

Furthermore, *feeling sick* and *feeling healed* as both subjective and concrete bodily experiences are not regarded by Veracruceños as disconnected from the external physical and grounded world in which they occurred. However, as claimed by Damasio emotions evoked by perceptions of bodily experiences and the external physical world are produced by the dialectic relationship between bodily arousal and cognitive interpretation that create meaning.[87] Thus the ascription of meanings to a simultaneously physical and ideational territory serves as the ultimate metaphor that embodies the intangibility of spirits and their conceptual concreteness as they are manifested in people's perceptions of illness, healing, history and place. Furthermore, by engaging a physical and ideational landscape laden with geographical features containing spiritual meanings, people seem to be ultimately confronting illness and promoting health.

The metaphors of territoriality in Veracruz bring people, spirits, medicine and place within a single narrative of history, which for many Veracruceños is a healing experience in itself. The tensions created by the discontinuity between people and spirits, illness and healing, and Indigenous and mestizo territoriality and culture are (if not entirely alleviated) at least partially mitigated by mystical medical narratives. Medical idioms in Veracruz seem to effectively address past and present suffering by relating people and spirits to a historically produced cultural and physical place that Veracruceños call and believe to be their Indigenous territory, always defined in tension with a mestizo cultural geography.

8 CHRONIC DISEASE IN THE YUKON RIVER BASIN, 1890–1960

Liza Piper

Introduction

In the nineteenth and twentieth centuries, chronic illnesses often chased new-comers out of northern environments. Amongst Anglican missionaries in the Yukon alone there are numerous instances of physical retreat. Reverend W. H. Fry, stationed with his wife on Herschel Island in 1916, left the region abruptly in 1919 as a result of his health. Upon his departure he wrote to his superior, Bishop Stringer, that 'The climate I believe is hard on me and perhaps the absence of fresh foods is not agreeable to my inner man'.[1] Although his health was partly restored upon his return to Ontario – he reported gaining 20 pounds within a few short months – Fry nevertheless died within two years. Rev. Fry's experience on Herschel Island was by no means unique. Robert McDonald arrived in Fort Yukon in 1862. He married Julia Kutug, a Gwich'in woman and raised his family in Fort Yukon and later Fort McPherson. But he eventually left the Yukon due to declining health in 1905 and returned to Winnipeg where he lived out his final years. Bishop Geddes similarly left the Yukon as a result of rheumatism, while Archdeacon Whittaker departed from Whitehorse in 1921 due to his wife's ill-health.[2] Chronic diseases afflicted Native peoples as well but for them northern environments were home, not harsh places to flee for health reasons. Julia McDonald, for instance, stayed in the Yukon after Robert's death, dying in Dawson in 1938. Similarly, as more newcomers moved north in the twentieth century and established families and communities there, leaving the region as a result of ill-health ceased to be the preferred alternative. Instead, newcomer institutions joined with pre-existing indigenous healthcare as ways of caring for those with long-term illness.

Chronic disease has an important role to play in understanding the relations between environments, here understood as the living creatures and non-living features found in a particular place, and human health.[3] More is known about northern epidemics, because of their disproportionate impact upon Native populations and their clear relationships to ecological circumstances.[4] Unlike acute infectious diseases which often manifested as epidemics in Canada's northern environments before the 1960s, chronic diseases had different environmental causes and consequences. As with other infectious diseases, organisms such as the tubercule bacilli were part of northern environments. Their spread was influenced by environmental conditions, including the movements of families and individuals. Yet other chronic diseases arose more directly from environmental factors, such as the presence and dissemination of carcinogens, or from nutritional causes, as with the late-twentieth-century rise of diabetes. The treatment and care of people suffering from chronic illness was also instrumental in defining the physical form and character of health care in the North. This paper focuses on tuberculosis and cancer as chronic diseases that offer insights into relationships between northern places and health.[5] The analysis draws upon a 100-year database of health, population and place built using two major record sets: burial registers from missionaries and hospital registers, such as those available from St Mary's Hospital, as well as smaller record sets including the Dawson City funeral listing from 1879 to 1937.[6] This essay explores the role that a regional environment, the Yukon River basin, played in the early twentieth-century history of two chronic diseases, cancer and tuberculosis and in turn, how bodies affected by these diseases translated environmental circumstance and conditions into new built environments.

Within the large central plateau of the Yukon Territory, ringed by the Mackenzie Mountains to the east and the St Elias range to the south-west, the Yukon River and its tributaries form the dominant drainage basin.[7] The main tributaries of the Yukon include the Pelly, Stewart and Klondike rivers in Canada and the Porcupine, Tanana and Koyukon in Alaska, before the river reaches the Bering Sea.[8] The regional dominance of the Yukon basin lay in its role in weaving the large territorial space together well into the twentieth-century. People moved across an enormous region by means of these waterways; in turn the waterways bound communities and camps together by providing the means for social contact. The longer historical significance of waterways to inland transportation is readily apparent in Aboriginal accounts of living on the land.[9] In turn, the boundaries between indigenous linguistic territories mapped closely to waterways large and small. The continued importance of waterways was evidenced by the role of Native pilots who used inherited and learned local ecological knowledge to guide newcomers along the waterways. Other Yukon historians have emphasized the social bonds tying the Yukon, Alaska and northern British Columbia together. This closeness stemmed in large part from the characteristics of the physical environment. Old Crow, Fort Yukon, Whitehorse, Dawson and Fairbanks were just a few of the communities linked together within the Yukon basin.[10] The northern Yukon was bound as well to the north, via the Peel River – a tributary of the Mackenzie and the main thoroughfare by which travellers crossed from the Yukon to the Mackenzie Delta gaining access to the Arctic coast and Beaufort Sea. To the south, the Inside Passage linked the major panhandle communities, Juneau and Skagway, from which travellers crossed inland to Atlin, British Columbia or on over the Chilkoot Pass to the headwaters of the Yukon River.[11] Before the construction of a highway system and the rise of the car and truck, the rivers provided the major large-scale transportation corridors and in this fashion acted as essential conduits for settlement, commercial exploitation, industrialization and state development. The rivers also provided the means by which people visited friends and family, sent their children to school, sought medical aid or travelled to their hunting and trapping grounds.

Cancer

In the closing decades of the twentieth century and the opening of the twenty-first, there are growing concerns about the roles of environmental toxins in contributing to cancers among northern populations.[12] In some instances these toxins are linked to local or regional industrial activities. In 1960s Point Hope, Alaska, the US federal government introduced radioactive materials into the local environment. The discovery of these contaminants, pointed to connections with increased rates of cancer among the Yu'pik population.[13] Toxins from the oil sands development upstream along the Athabasca River have been linked to blood, colon, bile-duct and liver cancers in the community of Fort Chipewyan. The significance of contaminants in northern environments lie partly in the continued reliance, by northerners in general but northern indigenous peoples in particular, upon 'country' foods – meat, fish and plants that they take from their local and regional environments. Concern about environmental contamination is, however, a post-World War 2 phenomenon and the relatively recent emergence of such concern contributes to a prevailing distinction between healthful traditional environments and lifestyles, versus the unhealthy modern experience. This distinction is rooted in important truths about past wellness as communicated by elders and as is readily apparent from accelerated environmental decline in northern environments after 1950.[14] But the distinction also acts to obscure a longer history of environmental health hazards in the Yukon basin.

Cancer did not appear only in the late twentieth century, and questions about the role of northern environment in shaping susceptibility to and mortality from cancer date at least from Vilhjalmur Stefansson's 1960 publication *Cancer, Disease of Civilization?*[15] Robert Fortuine cites paleopathological evidence of cancer found in skeletal remains from St Lawrence Island and Kachemak Bay.[16] Certainly, by the late nineteenth century, Native and non-Native northerners dealt with cancers, possibly even more often than the written records suggest. Certain deaths described as 'consumption' for example, referred to wasting, prolonged ill-health that may have indicated cancer or tuberculosis or another ailment altogether.[17] One of the earlier reports of cancer from the Yukon can be found in Rev. Robert McDonald's diary. In July 1872, he reported that Dr McKay was en route to the Peel River to see Andrew Flett (a Gwich'in man and Hudson's Bay Company employee) 'who has cancer in the lip'.[18] Cancers of the lip or mouth were common among late nineteenth-century diagnoses, both because they were visible and hence readily identifiable, and because they were tied to the frequent use of chewing tobacco and snuff.[19]

From 1900, cancers began to appear regularly as causes of death in the Yukon River basin. From over 3,600 deaths between 1899 and 1970 in this region, the cause of death was identified in 180 cases as a form of cancer. These included many different kinds of cancer, of which stomach cancer was the most common by far (after the general designation 'cancer' or 'tumour'). In general, cancers of the digestive tract significantly exceeded those of either the respiratory or reproductive systems (sixty-two cases to twenty-three and eleven respectively) as fatal cancers in this period.[20] Brain tumours, lung and oral cancers were the next most prevalent after stomach cancer. The vast majority of cancer deaths were recorded within hospital settings, and to a certain extent the distribution of cancer reproduces the biases of the hospital record, most notably that more non-Native than Native people died in hospital prior to 1950. Nevertheless, some general points can be made regarding those who died of cancer in the Yukon basin before 1970. With the exception of the first decade of the twentieth century, when the number of men and women who died of cancer was close to equal (nine men to ten women), more men died in each decade of cancer than women. Men outnumbered women in the general population in each decade from 1900 to 1950, from a high of 572 men to 100 women in 1901 steadily decreasing to 150 men to 100 women in 1951.[21] Cancers principally killed people between the ages of forty and eighty and they principally killed non-Natives (eighty-nine non-Natives to twelve Natives where such identification was possible). This remained so even after 1921, when the Native portion of the total Yukon population rose again above 30 per cent.[22] An occupation was listed in the records of half (n=90) of the cancer deaths. Within this subset, the majority (45.5 per cent) were miners or prospectors, 10 per cent were housewives, and 6 per cent were hunters and trappers although the group included as a whole nurses, retirees, clerks, barbers, hotel keepers and so forth. Most lived and died in Dawson (although again the bias of the hospital records is at work here) and many, both men and women, were 'pioneers' who had arrived in the Yukon during the first rush at the turn of the century and stayed on.

The proportion of cancer deaths peaked in the 1920s and 30s and were concentrated in this pioneer population in Dawson. It is not surprising to suggest that people who lived for twenty or thirty years in a gold mining district may have been exposed to carcinogens, but it is worth taking a closer look at the local environment to identify direct links. Placer gold mining, as was practiced in the Klondike, was a dangerous activity in general. Mining accidents such as cave-ins and rock slides, and suicides 'by gunshot' were all common causes of death.[23] There were further hazards on the Yukon gold mining frontier. The initial rush and influx of miners caused a boomtown to spring up. The initial townsite growth on low marshy lands in the river valley and unmatched by the provision of appropriate sanitary facilities, brought significant health problems. In the hot summer of 1898, hundreds died of typhoid, dysentery or malaria, with typhoid gaining the greatest notoriety.[24] When Dawson City incorporated in 1901, public health and the provision of appropriate sanitary facilities and inspection was a priority. The town introduced rules regarding the appropriate location of privies, pipes and water closets and forced people to take their water from higher up on both the Yukon and the Klondike rivers. Although these measures did not completely eradicate either typhoid or dysentery, they certainly left the town healthier.[25]

In the late 1930s, the territorial government hired Allan Duncan to work as the medical officer of health for Dawson City. He soon voiced concern about the state of Dawson's water supply. Duncan described how the main water well for the site 'was separated from the Klondyke River by a gravel and sand barrier that seemed to give adequate filtration'.[26] Duncan further observed how, in winter especially, but anytime the well was inadequate for the town's demands, 'Then water was pumped directly from the river into the mains'. Unfortunately, upstream from the pumping station worked three huge dredges, with outhouses suspended over each dredge's stern. Duncan soon realized 'that when the level of water was low in the well, raw sewage was being pumped into the city mains'. Duncan wrote to Comptroller Jeckell and the manager of Dawson Utilities advising them to do something as contaminated water could lead to an epidemic. But his concerns went unheeded on the grounds that 'this had been going on for years and ... nobody had worried before'.[27] Duncan's main concern was an epidemic of typhoid but no such epidemic came to pass.

The other threat to the water supply, as described by Duncan, was industrial contamination. Compared to hard-rock gold mining relatively few chemicals were used in placer mining with the main exception of mercury. Gold will amalgamate (effectively dissolve) in mercury. The mercury can then be boiled off, facilitating the separation and concentration of the gold values from host rocks. Miners and prospectors carried mercury into placer gold fields in ceramic jars and from these jars mercury would have disseminated widely into the Klondike River and creeks near Dawson. When ingested, mercury has many nasty consequences for the human body, including neurological, kidney and respiratory damage, but it is not a major carcinogen. Arsenic, however, is. And the soils and gravels from which gold was extracted within the Yukon basin were heavily laden with arsenic. Studies done in the 1970s showed high arsenic concentrations in stream waters and sediments in the Fairbanks area in Alaska, right in the heart of the Yukon basin. As geologists Wilson and Hawkins observe 'placer and lode-gold mining may increase the arsenic content of the waters by exposing arsenic-containing rocks to surface waters and by increasing the load of arsenic-rich sediments in the streams'.[28] During the 1898 typhoid outbreak, one Reverend Rowe had described to a southern audience that the sickness prevalent at Dawson was from 'the Klondike water, which some think is impregnated with arsenic'.[29] Arsenic of course would not have caused typhoid, but it was a carcinogen, natural in the Dawson environment, disrupted and concentrated by dredge mining especially, and from there directed into the town's water supply.

Treatment options for people with cancer along the Yukon basin varied between those who sought hospital treatment and those who were cared for at home. Native men and women treated at home likely received medicine made from sagebrush (*Artemisia alaskana, A. arctica, A. frigida*), gaillardia (*Gaillardia aristata*), and devilsclub (*Oplopanax horridus*) among other plants.[30] Aboriginal healers would remove tumours and relied upon poultices made from fireweed (*Chamerion angustifolium*) to treat surgical wounds. For at least some of those who died outside of hospitals, we know that they lived with cancer for a 'long duration' before dying.[31] Others, Native and non-Native, were brought to hospitals where the principle treatments were surgical; those seeking radiation therapy had to leave the region.[32] Minor and major surgeries could be performed at the main hospitals. Duncan described removing basal-cell cancers from a trapper's ear and a prospector's eyelid while working in Mayo.[33] Moreover, several of those who died from cancer while at St Mary's Hospital, died during their operations. Nurses and doctors in the hospitals also provided palliative care when neither surgery nor travel for radiation treatment was an option. Indeed, elderly cancer patients were among those requiring considerable care from the Sisters at St Mary's in the late 1920s. Five patients who died at St Mary's Hospital in the 1920s spent more than a year in hospital, in one case an elderly patient spent almost three years under the Sisters' care. On average, cancer patients spent fifty days in hospital, and over 60 per cent spent more than a month. Long-term cancer patients requiring palliative care contributed to the indebtedness of St Mary's Hospital in the 1920s, as the Sisters could not afford to maintain the hospital on their own and many of the community sources of income (such as bazaars or 'minstrel shows') no longer provided the same level of revenue, with the healthy population of Dawson in decline.

The other option for men and women who found themselves diagnosed with cancer was to travel (either permanently or temporarily) to Edmonton, Vancouver or elsewhere to receive radiation treatment. For those with money, or with family outside of the Yukon basin, such a choice was easier than for those who had lived in the Yukon their entire lives or who could not afford the expense of travel.[34] The creation of the Charles Camsell Indian Hospital in 1945, and the agreement that it would serve to treat not only Native northerners, but also Metis and indigent whites from the North, created another alternative for cancer care.[35] Although Camsell was best known as the destination for patients with tuberculosis, there were important similarities in the diagnosis and treatment of both diseases before the introduction of antibiotic therapies. X-rays were the most important diagnostic tool for tuberculosis and they played an important although lesser role in the diagnosis of cancers. By the late 1950s, around '40 percent of patients [at Camsell] were being treated for ailments other than tuberculosis'.[36] One doctor at Camsell, Herb Meltzer, applied his expertise at thoracic surgery to the treatment of lung cancer after the switch to more effective means of tuberculosis control.[37] By 1957 it was moreover the policy of the Northern Administration to accept financial responsibility for the treatment and transportation of cancer patients; the same policy applied to tuberculosis patients at this time.[38]

In the early part of the twentieth century, cancer was a not uncommon cause of death, particularly among the non-Native mining population resident in and around Dawson. Based on the local geology it is highly likely that arsenic in the Yukon River basin, and its uptake through the town's problematic water supply system, contributed to cancer deaths particularly among the elderly 'pioneer' population who had been drinking the water for over twenty years. Such a link between environment and health stands as an important predecessor to late twentieth-century concerns about environmental contaminants and cancer and problematizes the prevailing historiographical divide between past health and present sickness. Equally important was the emergent distinction between treatments available for cancer in the Yukon region, and those available outside. In the Yukon there were indigenous and newcomer, surgical, medicinal and palliative treatments. But radiation treatment, at that time considered most advanced and effective, had to be sought elsewhere. Treatment for cancer was among the more prominent of the early chronic diseases that pushed Yukon residents out of the territory in search of better health.

Tuberculosis

If not native to North America, the disease organism causing tuberculosis had certainly arrived in the North by the end of the eighteenth century.[39] Northern environments were as conducive to the survival and spread of the tubercle bacillus as more temperate latitudes. Fortuine notes for example, that, 'during the Russian era tuberculosis was probably no more common in Alaska than it was among the lower classes in Mother Russia'.[40] Between 1862 and 1970 tuberculosis was the most common cause of death among all Yukon residents, with Native peoples contributing over 76 per cent of the tuberculosis deaths. Entire families were often infected. All different forms of tuberculosis appear amongst the indigenous peoples of the river valleys in the nineteenth century. The most common were pulmonary, tuberculous meningitis and scrofula. The Klondike gold rush brought a vast influx of people to the territory, many of whom were likely already infected with tuberculosis.[41] As well, the larger population, and the concentration of this population in the city of Dawson and along the gold creeks, created more opportunities for the spread of infection. Although the missions and hospital only recorded ten deaths from tuberculosis between 1891 and 1900, this number jumped to seventy-six between 1901 and 1910.

Deaths from tuberculosis on the Canadian side of the Yukon River basin peaked in the 1920s, ten years earlier than cancer deaths, although deaths from tuberculous meningitis peaked later, in the 1930s and 40s. Tuberculous meningitis deaths are important markers of the prevalence of tuberculosis in the population. Where tuberculosis is prevalent in a population, meningitis primarily affects young children. Where tuberculosis is less common, meningitis is more commonly found in adults.[42] Meningitis, as a cause of death, was common in young children in the 1930s and 40s and more common in adults between 1891 and 1930. This evidence, in combination with the documentary record which shows increasing concern with tuberculosis towards mid-century, points to the rising severity of tuberculosis infection in the Yukon population before World War 2. Tuberculosis primarily affected young people with close to 50 per cent of deaths in the Yukon among people under the age of twenty (where age is known). There were also a disproportionate number of women who died of tuberculosis, both relative to the numbers dying of cancer and relative to the population as a whole. The larger proportion of women among those dying of tuberculosis reflects the disproportionate number of Native as compared to non-Native women in the Yukon River basin during this period as well as the higher mortality from tuberculosis among Native peoples.

From the statistical record we gain a very different image of those who died from tuberculosis, compared to those who died from cancer. Cancer was primarily found among older, non-Native men and in particular among miners and prospectors who arrived in Dawson in the late nineteenth century. More often than not, tuberculosis killed young Native and Metis girls, many of whom had spent a portion of their childhood attending a mission or residential school, and most of whom lived in predominantly Native communities. These distinctions illuminate the individuals most likely to die from either of these chronic diseases, but cannot be used to extrapolate the relative health of the communities. As a 1955 study on Fort Yukon noted, in that community and in spite of prevalent tuberculosis infection, infant mortality was low and deaths of women in child-birth uncommon.[43] Native elders throughout this period lived to very old ages – into their nineties or over 100 (or alternatively described as 'very old' or 'aged' upon their death).[44] They were often in excellent health and when they died could only be described as having succumbed to 'old age'. In spite of these indica-tors of good health, deaths of young women from tuberculosis contributed to the decline and slow growth of the Native population between 1901 and 1961.[45]

Caused by an organism that shared northern ecosystems with its human hosts, tuberculosis (unlike cancer) travelled. In particular, the spread of this disease accompanied and followed the movements of other infectious diseases in the early twentieth century. In epidemic outbreaks, underlying tuberculosis infection often weakened individuals and left them vulnerable to infection and less able to resist illness. The reverse was also true, where epidemic outbreaks weakened the ability of individuals to resist infection with tuberculosis or a dor-mant infection would become active.[46] A series of 'flu, whooping cough, measles and dysentery outbreaks in the 1920s and 1930s reached all the major com-munities in the Yukon basin and likely contributed to the peak mortality from tuberculosis in that decade.[47] As late as 1955, public health nurse M. Docherty reported on an outbreak of influenza that affected people in Pelly Crossing, Minto, Carmacks, Whitehorse, Carcross and beyond. In the conclusion of her letter she noted that of the five men and women who had the 'flu first, three had active tuberculosis. She added, 'I think the worst part of the illness is the dragged out cough', illuminating how the effects of one respiratory illness – a persistent cough – contributed to the spread of another.[48]

Between 1890 and 1950, tuberculosis was perceived as a disease with envi-ronmental causes and cures. Such perceptions played a key role in shaping the relations between health and place by characterizing certain environments as harmful or beneficial to a particular disease, and hence in turn influencing state policy about where best to locate medical services for treating disease. The crowded, unsanitary conditions found in burgeoning urban environ-ments and particularly in neighbourhoods with large immigrant populations, were understood to be directly tied to high rates of tuberculosis infection. The late-nineteenth-century 'wilderness cure', popular in the western United States saw open-air spaces and wooded uplands as holding curative powers for those afflicted with tuberculosis.[49] Robert Campbell has described how Alaska's Inside Passage suited elite American needs for curative wilderness.[50] Before the Klond-ike rush, the Alaskan interior along the Yukon River and into the Yukon Territory remained difficult to access and hence little known or thought about in south-ern imaginations. The Klondike discoveries, seen in 1900 as 'by far the most important fact in the history of the North-West', gave the 'North-West a world-wide advertisement of inestimable value'.[51] This advertisement focused on the Yukon's mineral riches. The productivity of the Yukon basin were thus embraced within more widely held notions of northern resource wealth.[52] Neither resource wealth nor the Yukon basin had much to offer consumptive urbanites in southern Canada, however. Authors writing for southern audiences, emphasized the remoteness, hardship and cold of the region.[53] Isabel Shepherd, on her voyage in the Bering Sea in 1889, encountered 'a poor Italian priest, a native of Sicily, who had spent a year on the Yukon, and had been thoroughly frozen out. His health had failed him owing to the rigour of the climate and he had been compelled to leave'.[54] The demands the Yukon climate placed upon the health of southerners was indeed a far more common concern than the potential relief its 'mountain fastnesses' might offer for those in search of sublime and restorative wilderness.[55]

Where Yukon environments entered the wider state and professional discourse around tuberculosis prevalence and treatment, it was as a hazard and obstacle rather than a potential source of relief. By the mid-40s, when people began to recognize the scale of the tuberculosis problem along the Yukon River, they also expressed concern about the lack of facilities suitable to treat the disease. In 1944, the USAAF Base Surgeon at Watson Lake examined a Native hunter, his wife and son and found that they were all 'in a tubercular condition at the early stages'. The report then noted that 'They have returned to their hunting grounds and consequently have not received nor will be able to receive any treatment due to there being no facilities for treatment in their District'.[56] Although not an explicit call for new or improved facilities, the RCMP in this report repeatedly expressed their concern that no assistance, medical or otherwise, could be given to this family. Allan Duncan was more explicit in his calls for improved facilities. He wrote Commissioner Gibben earlier that same year regarding the 'real need for some institution in the Yukon to treat suitable early cases of all types of tuberculosis, particularly pulmonary'. He described families and children infected and dying of tuberculosis and argued that due to inadequate facilities, the hospitals could do little more than admit 'moribund cases with little benefit to anyone'.[57] As late as 1949, William Stewart, a doctor in Whitehorse, wrote to the Commissioner about a family living out at Mile 956. The daughter of this family had been diagnosed with active tuberculosis, 'However, as there was no possibility of hospitalization here [the mother] was advised to take the child home and keep her in bed'. Stewart was particularly concerned 'as there is another child in the family and ... it is impossible to isolate the girl properly at home'.[58] The Yukon environment, to the extent that it was a built and institutional environment as well as a natural environment, lacked the facilities necessary to care for the regional population infected with tuberculosis.

The scale of the problem posed by tuberculosis became abundantly clear as a result of mass surveys conducted between 1947 and 1949. The earliest survey focused upon the 'Indians of the Yukon Territory' and was carried out by the Department of Health and Welfare and the Indian Affairs Branch of the Department of Mines and Resources. The survey started with the communities nearest to the Alaska Highway, Watson Lake, Teslin, Whitehorse, Champagne and Carcross, and reflected the new concern for Native health that arose as a direct consequence of the epidemics of measles, jaundice and meningitis in these communities brought by construction workers and soldiers.[59] The survey moved from the southernmost part of the Yukon basin, up to the settlements along the Yukon River and from there beyond to the northern and eastern parts of the territory. In September, the survey expanded to include non-Natives, particularly the military population in and around Whitehorse.[60] In the following year, 1948, a more comprehensive survey was planned. In addition to x-raying people in the major centres (Whitehorse and Dawson), the Indian Affairs Branch combined with the territorial government to survey the entire (Native and non-Native) population on a 'downriver trip' beginning in June 1948. This survey party included the Indian Agent, a public health nurse, a technician, the doctor from Whitehorse and an RCMP constable. The party hired a boat and pilot and then modified the boat with a temporary dark room aboard for developing x-ray films. Several months passed between taking and interpreting the films. As a result of this time lag, the 1948 survey was declared a failure and a further survey for 1949 was planned.

The differences between the 1948 survey and the 1949 survey revealed the emergent geography of the post-war Yukon as it moved away from the waterways onto the newly constructed roads. From the first, proposals for 1949 suggested that the survey party should travel along the Alaska Highway by car starting in early May, 'with possible side trips by water to cover areas not reached by the highway'. This proposal, coming from Meltzer in Edmonton, was promptly criticized because it did not recognize the very poor conditions along the highway in spring, 'as it is then most subject to flood conditions and road blocks of one sort and another'. Moreover, 'most of the Indians are still in the bush, and the Yukon River in particular is not yet open for navigation'.[61] The seasonal constraints of life in the Yukon basin directly influenced how the tuberculosis survey could be conducted. As well, although those from outside the region thought that a highway-based survey would suffice, local administrators stressed that at the very least the survey should travel again down the Yukon River, if not other rivers as well.[62]

Yet the survey was conducted by the Indian Health Services people and Dr Meltzer from Edmonton, and it conformed to their understanding of how to best reach people in the territory. In the end, the 1949 survey travelled the Alaska Highway by car, and then flew into Dawson and Mayo but did not travel down the river. Joseph Locke, the Chief Sanitary Officer for the Yukon, travelled with the 1949 survey and reported on its work. The method used along the highway was to set up the x-ray unit 'at a central point, where the greatest population was situated, and then all vehicles in the party travelled out to more sparsely settled points and brought the people and returned them from x-ray'. This method involved a lot of driving and long hours of work to reach all the people in the vicinity of the highway. Poor road conditions led vehicles to get frequently stuck, in one instance for five hours in a muskeg bog.[63] In spite of the poor conditions, the survey focused on the highway and roads and omitted the river and its tributaries, revealing the shifting geography towards the highway in this period.

In 1950, as territorial administrators sought out the means and ways to address the high rate of infection in the region, Barry Duncan, the doctor stationed at Dawson wrote to Dr Stone, the Regional Director of Indian Health Services expressing a very different opinion than his brother and predecessor at Dawson, Allan Duncan, about the best future for tuberculosis care. His opinion was further solicited by J. E. Gibben, then Commissioner of the territory and cited by C. K. LeCapelain, a representative of the federal Northern Administration. In each instance, Duncan emphasized first and foremost the problem posed by the Yukon climate, insisting that 'the climate of the Yukon territory is not favourable to quick recovery of active tubercular patients. The long cold and dark winter months have a depressive effect on persons afflicted with this disease'.[64] Elsewhere 'speaking for himself and other medical specialists in the T.B. field', Duncan emphasized the problems from 'the lack of sunlight and dietary deficiencies [in the Yukon] which increased the cost tremendously and retarded the recovery of the patient'.[65] Barry Duncan not only expressed the more widely held concerns about the poor facilities in the Yukon, but was also adamant in his conviction that new facilities should be located outside of the territory. In his tone and justification, Duncan articulated what he saw as an expert and objective view of the Yukon environment relative to more southerly places. He argued, taking a position shared with medical professionals and administrators in the Eastern Arctic at this time, that conditions in the region militated against the effective treatment of TB.[66] He was also, unlike his brother, less concerned with the notion that Yukoners, Native and non-Native, should have access to appropriate facilities at home than that they could and should be directed to specialized and expert medical care available elsewhere. In this regard, Duncan's opinion reinforced the attitude held by the federal government as to the appropriateness of southern institutions for northern medical care. In short order Charles Camsell Indian Hospital went from being a possible destination for tuberculosis patients from the Yukon to being expanded to accommodate their certain influx.[67]

In contrast to cancer, tuberculosis was much more widespread along the Yukon River and its tributaries, affected far greater numbers of people, and had a much more complex relationship with the regional environment. We can see the increased presence and geographic spread of tubercule bacilli in the Yukon basin environment with the rise in childhood deaths from tuberculous meningitis in 1930s and 40s. Even as the human population held steady or declined, the number of tuberculosis organisms sharing this space only increased in the first half of the twentieth century. The surveys in the late 1940s revealed the extent of infection and in turn influenced changes in attitudes about the causes and treatment of this disease. Building upon longer southern cultural perceptions of the Yukon environment as a harsh and unhealthy place, after 1950 the Yukon environment was more particularly perceived, as a result of latitude, climate and food resources, as a hazard to tuberculosis sufferers. This new understanding of the relationship between health and place directly influenced the new policy of removal. Before 1949 there was little emphasis upon travelling to the outside for tuberculosis treatment. While travel to hospitals or clinics in Edmonton, Vancouver and beyond was not uncommon for non-Native Yukoners, the notion that the main facilities for treating Yukoners, Native and non-Native, for the primary illness that afflicted residents of the territory at that time should be located outside of the territory, was a new idea in the late 1940s. Where removal, in the case of cancer treatment, reflected primarily the lack of institutional medical facilities in the Yukon, in the case of tuberculosis this new policy was predicated upon the combined rationale of inadequate facilities and understandings of the Yukon as a physically unhealthy place. The physical form of the new medical services in the post-war period also reflected the changed geography of the Yukon basin following the construction of the Alaska Highway and the new reliance upon mobility of both the sick and their caregivers. Because of the significance of tuberculosis as the dominant healthcare concern in the Yukon in the mid-twentieth century, this disease was primarily responsible for the emergent character of healthcare in this period. We now turn to explore in detail the translation of the relationship between health and place in the Yukon (including state attitudes about each) into new medical infrastructure and policies.

Spaces and Places of Medical Care

Before 1920, the most important steps taken by Canadian government with regards to medical care in the Yukon basin dealt directly with the epidemic outbreaks that were seen as the greatest hazards. With the considerable international traffic generated after 1896 by mining opportunities in the Yukon basin, officials responsible for health in Alaska and the Yukon became concerned with international quarantines to guard against the spread of epidemic disease. Following a smallpox outbreak in 1901, the state tightened its powers of quarantine and frequency of inspection, for the arriving steamships in particular.[68] Quarantines prevented movement across international boundaries, imagined lines in the land, as well as movement between watersheds, very real crossing points between the essential transportation corridors.

Yet beyond establishing the means and policy by which the movements of infected bodies could be controlled, the Canadian state did relatively little in offering institutionalized medical care in the Yukon in the opening decades of the twentieth century. A larger, more complex infrastructure existed in Alaska throughout this period, reflecting the larger total and in particular larger non-Native population. The Army and Navy provided most medical services to the Alaskan population in the late nineteenth century, and continued to play an important role in healthcare even after the introduction of civil government in 1884. From the 1880s there were calls for the creation of hospitals to serve the Native population specifically, and in 1910 the federal Bureau of Education, responsible for Native health, opened its first Native hospital in Juneau. By 1913 a Native hospital in the Yukon basin had opened at Nulato.[69] Across the border in the Yukon Territory, the federal government acted to address the health needs of a growing population by establishing the Whitehorse General Hospital in 1902 as well as providing grants to private hospitals and, after 1905, paying the salaries of the physicians stationed at each of the territory's hospitals.[70]

Religious communities played a much greater role in the provision of institutionalized medical care along the Yukon River and its tributaries. The Sisters of Providence, a Catholic order founded in Montreal in 1843, established a hospital in Nome in 1901 and then moved to Fairbanks on the Yukon River in 1910 where they established St Joseph's Hospital and cared for an average of 300 patients annually. Episcopal missionaries from the 1890s travelled 'along the central Yukon to serve not only the Indian population but also the many miners and prospectors who were lured by the smell of gold'.[71] They established hospitals in mining towns such as Circle City and Rampart, and ran St Stephen's Hospital (renamed Hudson Stuck Memorial Hospital in 1920) in Fort Yukon, founded in 1914. The Klondike rush led to the establishment, by competing religious communities, of two hospitals in Dawson City. In addition to St Mary's established by the Sisters of St Ann, the Presbyterians established the Good Samaritan Hospital in 1898, staffed by the Victorian Order of Nurses.

The need for two hospitals in Dawson City declined along with the population after the peak of the gold rush. In 1918, largely for financial reasons, the directors closed the Good Samaritan Hospital. The government sold the buildings to the Anglicans who transformed the space into St Paul's Hostel, a boarding school for mixed-race children.[72] The children at the hostel attended public school, and when they fell ill they too were taken to St Mary's Hospital.

Yet St Mary's also sharply contracted in its activities and by the late 1920s they saw fewer than 200 patients per year. The Anglicans and Catholics each opened a hospital in Aklavik on the Mackenzie Delta after 1925. Mining companies also funded medical services, in particular the Treadwell Mining Company which funded the hospital in Mayo, established in 1927.

These hospitals best serviced the white mining and settler populations, based as they were in the major settlements. The Native population was served in these centres of institutionalized medical care although there was marked social segregation in the Yukon, and in particular as part of community and economic life along the Dawson-Whitehorse corridor. Downstream from Dawson, for instance, was the Native village of Moosehide. According to Ken Coates 'observers suggest that few Natives remained in the towns [in summer], and that when they did live in the towns, they resided on segregated reserves'.[73] Such segregation also prevailed within medical institutions.[74] The hospital at Mayo consisted of a public ward with eight beds and four private rooms, totalling twelve beds in all. In 1928, there was a proposal to construct a one story addition to the hospital 'to accommodate Indian patients'.[75] Up to that point, Native patients had been kept in a tent on the hospital grounds adjacent to the main building as white patients objected to sharing the public ward. In contrast to Alaska, no Native hospitals were erected in the Yukon Territory. The doctors based at these hospitals did travel to outlying villages. The doctor stationed at Dawson was responsible for a larger zone that covered the area north from Selkirk and included the residents of the nearby village of Moosehide.[76] Doctors also travelled to mission stations and the Carcross residential school to look into the health of the predominantly Native population.[77] The RCMP also continued to play a role in providing certain medical services to the largely Native population living beyond the major settlements.[78]

Most importantly, however, the Native population living at a distance from the hospitals provided for their own health and well-being. We previously examined some of the indigenous treatments available for cancer sufferers in the Yukon basin. Catharine McClellan further elaborated upon the medical treatments used by Southern Tutchone, Tagish and Inland Tlingit during her fieldwork in the southern Yukon in the latter half of the twentieth century. She wrote that 'shamanistic cures are primarily a matter of manipulating power, removing disease objects and recovering souls. Their services are also expensive. For minor ailments, people usually resort to traditional home remedies.'[79] The traditional remedies were widely known across the Yukon basin and, with some local variations, employed similar curative herbs, berries and tree saps. Within each band certain individuals were seen as the most skilled practitioners. Midwives were of particular importance as most Native women continued to give birth in their own communities through the first half of the twentieth century, although some Native women (particularly those who lived near the largest centres) gave birth at St Mary's or one of the other hospitals.[80] The Gwich'in in the northern Yukon basin likewise relied upon their own healers and medicines through much of the twentieth century.[81]

Native peoples and non-Natives who lived at a distance from the major settlements regularly travelled to hospitals or elsewhere to seek out medicine and treatment. In October 1920, a Native woman in her mid-twenties came with her husband and two children under the age of ten from Lansing, over 280 kilometres to the west of Dawson.[82] In 1985, Edward Simon recalled taking his daughter Ida from Fort Selkirk in 1937 'over to Mayo with dogteam to hospital. We stay there two months. Doctor said no hope ... I will fly back and leave my wife ... airplane ... will bring them back here'.[83] For those who lived in the northern Yukon basin, around Old Crow in particular, trips west to Alaska for treatment were as common as trips south to Dawson. Archie Linklater, a Scotsman who married Catherine Netro, who was Ninsyag and Vuntut Gwich'in, kept a diary from 1903 until his death in 1941. He and his family frequently travelled to Fort Yukon or Dawson for medical treatment (although from the diary it would seem that all the children were born at home).[84] Frank Foster, an English trapper who lived around Old Crow, reported upon friends and family in hospitals in Fort Yukon, Fairbanks and Dawson in the 1940s.[85] Likewise, those stationed at distant mission or police posts reported visitors in search of medicine. Relocations in search of medical treatment also occurred between the three hospitals. A 1938 letter from the Controller of the Yukon Territory to the *Dawson News* noted that 'many patients are brought from the Whitehorse and Mayo Districts, [to St Mary's Hospital] who cannot be accommodated in the Hospitals at Whitehorse and Mayo'.[86]

Thus, throughout the twentieth century, access to medical care and even institutionalized medical care within the Yukon basin involved considerable mobility. This movement followed the main transportation corridors: The couple that travelled from Lansing most certainly came the direct route, along the Stewart and Yukon rivers. Similarly, Old Crow was not only closer to Fort Yukon than Dawson, but the two communities were directly joined along the Porcupine River. As the significance of certain transportation corridors shifted, so too did their role as routes for those seeking medical treatment. Julie Cruikshank has noted that, in time, the government encouraged families to move to the highway to avoid the costs of medical flights to isolated bush camps and villages and because the state itself had turned away from the rivers as the main highways within the territory.[87] The move to the highways was not just a government initiative. With more private vehicles and more traffic along the highway, more residents turned to the road for travel; easily hitchhiking to larger centres if they did not own a car themselves.[88] The war dramatically changed the Yukon basin and the provision of healthcare services. Construction of the Alaska Highway, in addition to its role in a series of epidemics in the 1940s, more generally reconfigured the medical geography of the territory in a way that reinforced the new government policies of relocation.

These new state policies and practices with respect to the provision of medical services in the Yukon were more complicated than simply directing patients and doctors to travel via the new road network. Foremost, the state dramatically expanded its role in healthcare during this period. From 1944 onwards, it was the stated policy of the Northern Administration that the government would assume responsibility for hospitalization of northern residents 'rather than to delegate this responsibility to the missions, especially where there is no religious denomination already providing service in the field'.[89] During the war, this responsibility meant that the Department looked to acquire surplus equipment and buildings from the US Army.[90] It also signalled a marked departure from previous policy, and one which was not in keeping with the feelings of the churches and missions who continued to see themselves playing a significant role in northern health (and spiritual) care. It was later in 1944 that J. L. Coudert, OMI and Bishop of Whitehorse, wrote to T. A. Crerar, Minister of Mines and Resources in Ottawa repeating the interest held by the Catholic Church in establishing a hospital in the Watson Lake area. The Minister had already refused the request, using the excuse that it would require the Department to approve a 'similar institution' for the Anglicans.[91] There was some truth to this concern, as denominational competition had led to the erection of two hospitals in Aklavik, a persistent irritant to funding-conscious northern administrators. As well, it was a general post-war northern health priority to limit 'duplication and uneconomical use of the limited facilities available'.[92] What the minister left unstated, however, was the fact that even if new hospitals were to be built, it was the government that would build them; a policy that was in keeping with developments in southern Canada where increasingly the state, rather than private citizens or institutions, were seen to be responsible for healthcare.[93]

A chance event in January 1950 facilitated the government's aggressive new role in providing for the health needs of Yukon basin residents. The tuberculosis surveys revealed the extent and magnitude of tuberculosis infection and the fact that it was the major public health concern. The primary response of the government to the extent of infection was to ensure that the active cases received immediate treatment and isolation from the general population so as to curtail the further spread of the disease.[94] In this regard, the policy of isolation followed in the tradition of the state exercising control over the movement of people that had manifested in the first government health policies in the North in response to epidemics. Isolation did not necessarily mean removal from the territory altogether. As noted earlier, there were strong advocates in the 1940s for the construction of suitable facilities in the territory. In the late 1940s, the

Sisters of St Ann and the local hospital board planned the construction of a new thirty-three bed wing to be used for tuberculosis patients, or for infectious disease cases in the event of an epidemic. A 'very complete diagnostic laboratory' was to be added to the wing primarily to deal with typhoid and tuberculosis, and further funding was sought from the federal government to purchase necessary x-ray equipment.[95] The expansion was entirely for the purpose of treating specific regional health needs, as the existing hospital sufficed to deal with the population of Dawson and nearby villages.[96] One doctor in Dawson in 1949, H. A. Proctor, was guarded in his support for the expansion as he wrote to P. E. Moore in Ottawa how 'Conceivably more tuberculous patients could be accommodated at Dawson but supplies are expensive and the staff does not have any special qualifications'.[97] The Sisters, by contrast, used the high cost of salaries, fuel and provisions as part of their justification to ask for more funding.[98]

In their September 1949 request for funding, the Sisters asked for money for a new x-ray unit and for improvements and repairs, but the majority of money sought was for the 'rewiring of the original hospital building (built in 1906) which has become a fire hazard; An electric booster pump to provide sufficient pressure in case of fire; [and a] fire hose & chemical extinguishers'. The need for these upgrades became tragically apparent when, on 10 January 1950, a fire started as a result of unattended candles in the chapel inside the hospital. The fire destroyed the hospital. The elderly Sister Mary Gedeon died from asphyxiation. Otherwise all the patients and some of the hospital equipment were successfully evacuated. Within a week, twelve tubercular patients were sent by Canadian Pacific Airways plane to Whitehorse, followed by three further patients who were evacuated by RCAF plane to Charles Camsell in Edmonton. The burning of St Mary's Hospital was a tragedy for the community and the Sisters, who not only lost one of their number, but also had to rebuild their institution from scratch. For the federal government, however the burning of St Mary's was an opportunity. The Sisters could not afford to rebuild on their own, they required considerable financial assistance which the territorial government could not provide.[99] The federal government, building upon their own policy preference to wrest control of healthcare away from the churches and with advice from Barry Duncan among others that the Yukon was not the appropriate location for specialized tuberculosis care, could better implement their plan now that the major institutional alternative in the Yukon had been destroyed.

By the 1950s, the state, in the guise of both the territorial and federal governments, had almost entirely assumed responsibility for healthcare. In lieu of constructing major new territorial institutions to deal with tuberculosis or other chronic illnesses, the state focused upon relocating the sick to southern facilities. Charles Camsell Hospital in Edmonton became the principle destination. Camsell administrators had initially insisted that only those patients 'requiring chest surgery or other special treatment should be sent out', with those only requiring bed rest remaining in the territorial hospitals.[100] Yet even this smaller category greatly exceeded the facilities in the territory after 1950. The administration upon 'realizing the increasing seriousness of the tuberculosis situation in the Territory, and the necessity of finding a long term solution to this problem', turned to provincial sanatoria to find beds for Yukon residents.[101] The peak in outside treatment came in the 1950s when at least fifty-two 'Indians' from the Yukon were being treated in Charles Camsell alone. By the late 1950s and early 1960s this number had been cut in half. In 1965, ten 'Indian' patients were treated at Camsell, and a further twelve 'white status' patients (therefore either Metis or non-Native) were treated at either Camsell, the Baker Memorial Sanatorium in Calgary, or the Aberhart Memorial Sanatorium in Edmonton. By the late 1950s and 1960s, moreover, patients at Camsell included not just people with tuberculosis, but also cancer as noted earlier, as well as polio, heart disease, mental retardation, epilepsy and one child who was blind and deaf.[102]

In opting for relocation rather than the creation of regional institutions, the government had to make this new system work for those who lived at a distance from the major communities where medical and transportation services now concentrated. RCMP officers continued to act in an emergency capacity, contacting the local doctor or ferrying sick people to the nearest hospital or nursing station as necessary.[103] Policies and practices regarding such intervention by police officers were formalized in the 1950s. In 1965, the territorial government also agreed to pay any costs in excess of $50 one way or $100 return fare for emergency medical transportation from isolated communities.[104] The cornerstone of the new medical infrastructure was the creation of a public health service, ideally staffed by five public health nurses.[105] Each nurse was assigned to a particular district that matched closely to the physical geography of the territory: one was based in Whitehorse; a second along the Carmacks-Haines Road as well as the northern half of the Alaska Highway; a third was directed to cover the region from Whitehorse down to Lower Post, BC including working with the Native population in northern BC and taking charter flights to Telegraph Creek and Ross River; a fourth was to work in the Mayo and Keno area and down to the north side of the Yukon River at Carmacks; the fifth and final was responsible for Dawson, the Dawson Road down to Stewart River Crossing and the area around Dawson.[106] The public health nurses performed combined medical, social and educational services. They visited homes and schools, provided vaccinations and tests, delivered babies and treated venereal diseases.[107] They also consistently complained about being underfunded and understaffed and therefore unable to fully care for the health needs of the population they served.

The new state services continued some of the pre-war practices that had characterized healthcare in the Yukon basin. Most notably, territorial officials, healthcare practitioners and non-Native community leaders agreed that Native and non-Native patients should continue to be treated separately and that

'Indian patients, and the tubercular ones in particular, should be taken care of in a separate institution'.[108] Such segregation, given the scarcity of facilities, was not always possible. At the Camsell Hospital, the principal outside destination for TB patients, 'white patients [were] mixed with natives'.[109] Where Native peoples stayed in the Yukon they typically shared institutions with non-Natives, but were subject to second-rate treatment. In 1953 there were reports that Native peoples at the Whitehorse General Hospital were given substandard accommodation resulting in crowding and patients being put into the corridors.[110] 'First rate' provincial sanatoria in Minette, Manitoba and Fort Qu'Appelle Saskatchewan appealed to policymakers because they segregated Native and non-Native patients. Segregation, moreover, calmed some of the objections non-Native Yukoners themselves held against being sent south for treatment.[111]

The amount of opposition to relocation led the territorial government to empower itself with the Yukon Health Ordinance to isolate patients if necessary. Some people further proposed regulations that would enable the Health Authorities to remove individuals to sanatoria against their will. Such drastic measures were generally seen as counterproductive by tuberculosis experts who insisted that 'Cheerful co-operation seems to be part of the cure'.[112] Cheerful was rather a lot to ask of people being removed from their existing social support networks. The most common objections against medical relocation were shared by Native and non-Native people. They did not want to be removed so far from their home and family. Even when they sought out hospital treatment, parents did not want their children removed from their care indefinitely. Lydia Elias, a Gwich'in elder from Tsiigehtchic (in the western Subarctic but outside the Yukon basin), recalled being informed that her child had tuberculosis,

> We're going to admit your child to the hospital they told me ... It was spring and it was warm and the snow was thawing fast. I told the hospital exactly where my camp was ... I wanted to find out about my son and the illness he had. I want some explanation so I ask Knut Lang to talk to the doctor and he said the person sitting right there is a doctor you can ask him. And so I ask him. I did not know he was taking care of my son too so I ask him about my son and he said he will be not coming home soon. He is a very sick child.[113]

Many of the Native children, removed from their families for extended periods, found it difficult to readjust to homelife upon their discharge from hospital.[114] Many of those sent south for treatment never recovered. They died and were buried far from home.[115]

Conclusions

This essay presents two very different examples of chronic diseases in the Yukon River basin as opportunities to explore the relationships between health and northern places in the early twentieth century. The first example, cancer, was historically not understood as an environmentally-contingent illness. However, given the prevalence of cancers among the pioneer population of Dawson coupled with the known character of that town's water supply in this period, these cancers can be tied to arsenic found in the local environment. By contrast tuberculosis infection was historically perceived as closely linked to environmental conditions. These perceptions exaggerated the significance of regional environments in creating the TB epidemic and encouraged a policy of relocating those sick with tuberculosis to southern medical institutions. In both instances, place not only profoundly influenced the character and spread of these diseases, including the increased prevalence of tubercule bacilli in the Yukon environment in the 1930s and 40s, but also shaped responses to them.

The broader character of institutionalized health care that emerged in the mid-twentieth century must be understood as rooted in specific understandings of both health and place (evidenced in the examples of tuberculosis and cancer), and further shaped by independent factors. Among the independent factors, the most significant was the federal government's desire to transfer responsibility for medical care in the North away from the churches and under its own auspices. During the period when missionaries provided the majority of medical services, with the assistance of government-funded doctors, they reached people in the most efficient fashion: via the network of waterways. The rise of state healthcare coincided with the geographical shift that accompanied the construction of the Alaska Highway, and the peak of tuberculosis infection and concern in the territory. This convergence dramatically reshaped the places of medical care within a decade. By 1950, the government had replaced missionaries with public health nurses. It relocated Native and non-Native patients with serious and chronic diseases to southern institutions for treatment and rehabilitation. It formally recognized, through transport policies and its own practices, the centrality of mobility to the provision of healthcare across this space. But it also chose particular paths, between major settlements and southern cities, and along the developing network of highways and roads, that reinforced a new geography in which the Yukon basin itself retreated as a dominant physical feature to be replaced by a new built environment.

Acknowledgements

I thank the Gwich'in Social and Cultural Institute for granting me access to their unpublished interview transcripts with Gwich'in elders as part of the research for this project. I also thank the Social Sciences and Humanities Research Council of Canada and the Killam Trusts for financial support in researching and writing this article.

9 'AN IDEAL HOME FOR THE CONSUMPTIVE: PLACE, RACE AND TUBERCULOSIS IN THE CANADIAN WEST'

Maureen Lux

In 1895 a group of prominent Calgary citizens extolled the advantages of their city as a site for a national tuberculosis sanatorium. The city, they boasted, was the 'Denver of Canada' and an ideal home for consumptives. Area physicians outlined the specific medical advantages of the region's climate, geography and elevation. Far removed from the congestion and foul air of Europe and eastern Canada the consumptive would benefit from the salubrious prairie west's clear bracing air and endless sunshine. Needless to say the national sanatorium was ultimately established in Ontario. The Calgarians were not, however, eager to attract all consumptives. The region's Aboriginal people, increasingly exposed to infection and to the repressive policies of the state, came to be seen as fundamentally deficient in their reaction to the disease. The Indian reserves served to isolate and contain both their disease and their poverty. Fifty years later, in 1945, hundreds of Edmonton residents publicly and loudly objected to the federal government's plans to establish a sanatorium in their city for Aboriginal people. They demanded that the government establish the sanatorium somewhere – anywhere – else. A spatial analysis of the shifting cultural and medical understandings of the disease, from consumption as a condition of the delicate and wealthy to tuberculosis as an infectious disease of the poor and the Aboriginal, highlights the roles of race and class in the construction of disease and its treatment.

Looking at region or place as a category of analysis somewhat akin to gender, class and race, is particularly helpful in understanding the intersections of colonialism and health that came to define relationships with Aboriginal people. Connections to particular landscapes were fundamental to many Aboriginal peoples' sense of identity. Even the most nomadic groups consistently returned to the same sites every year.[1] Aboriginal creation stories are often characterized by particular landmarks as sites where the people were created and continue to live. According to Stoney oral history, for instance, that nation had always inhabited and hunted in the region that came to be known as southern Alberta, bounded on the west by the Rocky Mountains, on the east by the foothills and onto the prairies, and the south past the international border.[2] They shared their space with other Aboriginal groups, at times peacefully, at times not. But identity, livelihood, and spirituality were intimately connected to landscape. Considering place also yields insights into how colonialism came to affect Aboriginal peoples' health in particular ways. The places that sustained Aboriginal well-being, both physical and spiritual, were quickly appropriated by nineteenth-century newcomers. One might talk about the 'colonization of health' where the mountains, wildlife and grasslands all became part of a larger nation-building project that sought to create a liberal, rational order by suppressing the Aboriginal order.[3]

The search for health by the wealthy was made possible by the same processes that created the conditions for Aboriginal ill-health. Place and space were reconfigured to exclude and isolate Aboriginal people on Indian reserves, thereby creating racial hierarchies defined by illness – although Aboriginal people themselves would not passively accept this classification.[4] A regional focus also highlights how at the turn of the twentieth century the rising authority of Euro-medicine and its practitioners owed much to the increasing public fear of tuberculosis.[5] Physicians as social elites and 'men of science' played an important role in colonizing the region as a haven for the weary and consumptive upper classes. At the same time, a spatial analysis also allows us to examine in Foucauldian terms specific sites of 'disciplination', the sanatorium, the Indian reserve and residential school, whereby administrative and bureaucratic authority was consolidated.[6] Ultimately the discourse of humanitarian concern and dispassionate medical expertise served to isolate and exclude Aboriginal people in service of the public's health.[7]

The meaning of disease is not constant over time. As Katherine Ott argues, it changes under the influence of cultural constructions, personal experience and medical doctrine.[8] The current medical understanding of tuberculosis, an affliction of the immigrant, the AIDS patient and the desperately poor, bears scant resemblance to what was known as 'consumption' a century earlier. Despite Robert Koch's 1882 identification of the tubercle bacillus and its ability to spread infection, the 'consumptive' was not considered to be a threat to the public's health, at least not until after 1900 as the illness became increasingly associated with the poor.[9] Tuberculosis today is understood as an infectious disease caused by *Mycobacterium tuberculosis*. Spread through droplet infection, it most commonly affects the lungs but also can involve almost any organ of the body. Symptoms include fatigue, lethargy, weight loss and night sweats that progress to coughing, chest pain, coughing up of sputum and blood, and shortness of breath. But until the disease reaches an advanced stage, many experience only mild respiratory symptoms similar to the common cold. Unlike other infectious diseases however, tuberculosis has a variable incubation period. Certain factors, especially the quality of nutrition and crowding, determine whether the disease develops.[10] This marks a major change from the turn of the twentieth century, when tuberculosis and its treatment were believed to be governed by climate and individual susceptibility to disease. Indeed, consumption and tuberculosis were often understood as separate conditions. It was in this space opened by shifting understandings of disease that local physicians vigorously promoted Calgary and central Alberta generally as an ideal home for the consumptive.[11]

The boundaries on maps that created the political region of Alberta, the lines that 'opened the west' to Euro-Canadian settlers, attempted to redefine the landscape away from Aboriginal uses and conceptions of the land to harness it to the great project of building the young dominion through investment and development. In 1870 the newly formed Canadian government bought Rupert's Land (the Hudson's Bay Company Territories) in the western interior, including southern Alberta, and subsequently began negotiations for land cession with the region's Aboriginal peoples.[12] The language of Treaty Seven signed in 1877 with the Siksika (Blackfoot), Piikani (Peigan), Kainai (Blood), Tsuu T'ina (Sarcee), and Nakoda (Stoney) stated that the people agreed to 'cede, release, surrender, and yield up to the Government ... all their rights, titles, and privileges whatsoever' to 130,000 square kilometres of southern Alberta in return for annuities, seed or cattle, teachers and reserves.[13] The treaty also promised that Aboriginal people retained the right to 'pursue their vocations of hunting throughout the tract' albeit 'subject to such regulations as may, from time to time, be made by the Government of the country'.[14] Elders see the treaty very differently. They maintain that its text does not reflect the 'true spirit and intent' of the negotiations at Blackfoot Crossing in 1877. The Elders contend that land surrender was never discussed; they had agreed to keep the peace and share the land with the newcomers.[15] Moreover, they understood that their right to hunt, trap and fish was absolute, although the treaty text restricts that right.[16]

Treaties created the relationship between the federal government and Aboriginal people of southern Alberta, but the department of Indian Affairs and the 1876 *Indian Act* determined the nature of those ties. The sweeping powers of the *Indian Act* presumed to regulate most every detail of Aboriginal peoples' lives and marked them as wards of the state, separate in law from the growing (after 1880s) settler population. This legal status was premised on the absence of rational citizenship for the Aboriginal and the inability to acquire it without fundamental changes to their social, cultural and political selves. For nearly a century government policy, whether Liberal or Conservative, sought to protect, civilize, and assimilate Aboriginal people.[17] This policy, truly remarkable for its consistency, supposed that Aboriginal people could not be considered true individuals in the classical liberal model that was hegemonic in Canada since the mid-nineteenth century.[18] It was also predicated on assumptions completely alien to the Aboriginal world view. Theirs was a world where people were but one part of the larger circle of life; with property relations where the group shared possession, and where the value of goods was realized by giving them away. These views stood in stark contrast to the white, liberal view of the individual as those whose body and mind were theirs alone. Efforts to assimilate the Aboriginal people to a Christian, capitalist and liberal norm focussed on missionary education and reserve agriculture.

Reserve lands were apportioned on the basis of 640 acres per family of five, and although reserve lands were to be chosen by chiefs, the location of the Stoney reserve west of Calgary at Morleyville, for instance, was determined by the local missionary, while their familiar hunting and camping grounds were not reserved.[19] As far as the government was concerned the treaties were land surrenders and reserves were intended to provide a land base for the 'civilizing' pursuit of agriculture, regardless of the suitability of the climate, the land, or the wishes of the people. Indian reserve boundaries became the spatial expression of that colonial relationship, what Cole Harris calls the 'primal line on the land … that facilitated and constrained all others'.[20] The surveyors' lines that created the region also created Indian reserves where the acres were meticulously counted out and everything else was for the newcomers. And although the treaties promised freedom of movement throughout the ceded territories, after 1885 reserve boundaries became increasingly confining.[21] The 'internal frontier', the lines between Aboriginal and white drawn on the landscape created a space that came to be defined by race.[22] Reserve boundaries were never absolute of course, and the frontier was tended assiduously by Indian agents and the North West Mounted Police (NWMP). The reserves increasingly became islands of exclusion through the legal and extralegal restrictions on the people's economic and personal freedom. In the decades after the treaties were signed the colonizing constructs whereby Aboriginal people were dispossessed of their lands and livelihood also became the means to relegate them to the lowest socioeconomic rungs of western society.

The destruction of the bison herds which had sustained many of the Aboriginal people of southern Alberta was surprisingly sudden and by 1880 the last of the herds had disappeared.[23] The Blood and Blackfoot were far more dependent on the bison than the Stoney and Tsuu T'ina who continued to hunt in the eastern slopes of the Rocky Mountains.[24] Nevertheless, the collapse of the bison herds aided the government's efforts to move the Treaty Seven people onto reserves. And by 1880 a cattle-grazing industry was firmly established on the grasslands that had once sustained the bison.[25] Wealthy and politically powerful elites prospered under favourable federal legislation that allowed white ranchers to lease 100,000 acres for up to twenty-one years at an annual cost of one cent per acre. The NWMP provided unprecedented protection for the herds, while leaders of the 'cattle kingdom' attended fancy balls, polo matches and fox hunts.[26] Like other Aboriginal people of the Canadian west in this era, the people of southern Alberta descended into hunger and disease as their source of clothing, food and housing disappeared.[27] Government-issue rations were intentionally miserly not only to spare the federal treasury, but also to cultivate habits of industry and enterprise among the Aboriginal people. Prime Minister John A. Macdonald told the House of Commons in 1882 that the government would not let the people die of starvation, but added that his officials in the department of Indian Affairs 'are doing all they can, by refusing food until the Indians are on the verge of starvation, to reduce the expense'.[28] Treaty-making and the establishment of the 'cattle kingdom' served to anchor the region to the newly formed state; the dispossession and impoverishment of the region's Aboriginal people was inextricably linked to that process.

The Stoney and Tsuu T'ina, among other Aboriginal groups, continued to hunt in the eastern slopes of the Rockies, despite attempts to have them confined to reserves.[29] For the Stoney people, the mountains provided much that the people needed, from elk, deer and moose, to herbs and plants for food and medicine, to spiritual sanctuary for vision quests. As elder John Snow explained, 'These mountains are our temples, our sanctuaries, and our resting places. They are a place of hope, a place of vision, a place of refuge, a very special and holy place where the Great Spirit speaks with us. Therefore, these mountains are our sacred places'.[30] But after the mid-1880s the transcontinental Canadian Pacific Railway (CPR) sliced through both their reserve and hunting territory, bringing significant environmental change such as wildfires sparked by the engines. Its trains also brought settlers, physicians, sportsmen and health-seekers. This unwelcome change was accompanied by a change to the Indian Act in 1886 to empower the superintendent general of Indian Affairs to declare that Aboriginal people were subject to provincial and territorial game laws.[31] And in 1887 Aboriginal people were forbidden to hunt in their traditional territory in the newly created Rocky Mountains (Banff) Park. The park, originally twenty-six square kilometres and intended to protect the Cave and Basin Hot Springs, was enlarged to 673 square kilometres in 1887; in 1902 it was further expanded to abut the Stoney reserve and included most of their hunting territory. The CPR, the foremost lobbyist for the creation of the park, limited and controlled access in the interests of wealthy tourists and health seekers.[32] As Theodore Binnema and Melanie Niemi argue, Aboriginal people were excluded from national parks both in the interests of sport hunting, tourism and also to promote Aboriginal 'civilization' by denying them access to wildlife and forcing them into agricultural pursuits.[33] But for the

Stoney the mountains, their 'sacred places', provided not only food and clothing, but also the plant and animal remedies used by their healers. The mineral hot springs, their 'sacred waters', were fundamental to maintaining health and curing illness. Chief John Snow described their importance: 'A person would journey to the sacred waters at the direction of a medicine man or woman and use them with suitable preparation and prayer'.[34] The colonization of the region and its resources in the interests of the CPR, wealthy health-seekers, settlers and the Canadian state also effectively colonized health by limiting Aboriginal access to the restorative properties of the mineral hot springs, the physical and spiritual connection with the lands and the wildlife.

The beauty of Banff National Park and the soothing hot springs were very quickly put to use in the commodification of health when in 1886 Dr Robert G. Brett established a private sanitarium in the park.[35] After graduating from Victoria College medical school in Toronto, Brett headed west with his brother-in-law Dr N. J. Lindsay and in 1883 they arrived in Calgary to become the town's second and third physicians. Brett contracted with the CPR to provide medical services for its construction crews, and spent considerable time at Siding 29 (Banff) assessing the commercial potential of the Cave and Basin Hot Springs.[36] With financial backing from the CPR Brett leased six acres and access to the hot springs for $115 annually for forty-two years, at the end of which the lease was renewable in perpetuity.[37] The Brett Sanitarium had fifty hotel beds, forty invalid beds, tennis courts, and a cricket team.[38] It evoked the elegance and luxury of European mountain spas and advertised its thoroughly modern appointments to the tourist or invalid. Brett boasted of the 'remarkable salubrity of the atmosphere and favorable climatic conditions ... the lightness of the air, its extreme purity and dryness, the almost entire absence of clouds, the long periods of brilliant sunny days'. He promised treatment for 'consumption, chronic affections of the bronchial tubes and pleura and different forms of asthma'. The climate also recommended itself to 'persons in whom the hereditary taint of consumption is known to exist, or in whom its beginnings are suspected rather than diagnosed, as well as those already afflicted'. Moreover, the 'wonderful curative properties' of the mineral waters were prescribed for the 'treatment of enlarged glands, scrofulous tumors, open sores and skin diseases'. In short, there seemed few ailments that could not be treated at the Brett Sanitarium from malarial poisoning, anaemia and neuralgia, to complaints of the kidneys and liver, and overwork. In a fine bit of medical hucksterism the buildings and trees near the mineral springs were adorned with crutches and canes that were apparently abandoned by the newly cured. Health-seekers found comfortable rooms, well-furnished tables, attentive servants and skilful medical advisors, while the rivers 'abound with fish and the forests with game'. The CPR provided special rates for visitors to the Hot Springs.[39] The following year the CPR opened its grand Banff

Springs Hotel to cater to its wealthiest passengers. By 1888 more than 5,000 visitors had used the baths at the Cave and Basin, and Brett's establishment had earned an international reputation.[40] As a loyal Conservative and friend of both the federal government and the powerful CPR monopoly, Brett won access for his medical enterprise to the natural assets of the National Park, and the railway happily accommodated by delivering wealthy patients. The region's reputation as especially restorative, something long understood by Aboriginal people, was reconstructed as a destination for the white health-seeker.

Yet as tourists increasingly flocked to the springs to cure their real and imaginary ailments, at the same time all the Aboriginal groups in southern Alberta experienced a steady deterioration in their health in the decades after the treaty was signed. With the destruction of the bison economy, exclusion from their hunting grounds, and few other resources at their disposal Aboriginal peoples were increasingly impoverished and isolated on reserves. Calgary, less than 12 kilometres north and east of the Tsuu T'ina reserve, provided an early market for reserve produce and Aboriginal labour. But as settlement increased, so did white resentment against Aboriginal competition in the market. Meanwhile, the permit system which prevented Aboriginal people from selling reserve produce without permission from the agent, and the pass system that prevented their movement off reserve without a pass from the agent, further limited their economic opportunities.[41] By the 1890s, for example, relations between the Tsuu T'ina and the growing settler population were becoming strained, and it became an easy matter for the Indian agent to call upon the NWMP to have the people returned to their reserve.[42] Editorials in local newspapers called for stricter patrolling of the reserve boundaries, and that Aboriginal people should be confined to reserves because they hindered progress and development.[43] One Calgary paper decried the presence of Tsuu T'ina people in the city as, 'worthless Indians who were too lazy to work but were around town pilfering and breeding disease'.[44] In striking contrast to the restrictions on the people's economic and personal mobility, non-Aboriginal settlers had relatively easy access to reserve lands. The Priddis Road, a public thoroughfare, ran through the Tsuu T'ina reserve.[45] And the Stoney reserve was bisected by the CPR mainline, giving wealthy health-seekers and tourists access to Aboriginal artifacts and crafts.

These one-way lines of communication also eased the spread of disease as the consumptive flocked to Banff to take the cure. Throughout the region the restrictions on mobility and access to resources led to precipitous declines in reserve populations. On the Stoney reserve crude death rates exceeded birth rates in six of the ten years after 1884.[46] The Tsuu T'ina population fell 29 per cent in the five years after 1890; population losses slowed, but did not stop until after 1930.[47] Dr N. J. Lindsay, contracted by the department of Indian Affairs to treat Aboriginal people of the region, reported in 1895 that he found (in order of prevalence) scrofula, phthisis, sore eyes, syphilis, rheumatism and pneumonia and that 'poverty induces scrofula and numerous diseases resulting in death'.[48] But it was infant and child mortality, the most sensitive indicators of the overall health status of a community, rather than disease *per se* that accounted for the precipitous population losses. On the Stoney reserve for instance, in five of the ten years after 1884 the average child mortality rate surpassed the birth rate; for every child born, at least one and often two children died.[49] Dr Lindsay prescribed cod liver oil 'together with plenty of nourishing food, comfortable clothing, physical labour or exercise in the open air in good weather, and roomy dwellings for winter, well ventilated'.[50] In short, improved living conditions. Given the state of poverty on the reserve, that prescription was well out of reach for most.

Meanwhile, civic leaders in Calgary, politicians, physicians and the board of trade began agitating for a 'dominion sanatorium' to be established in their city. They hoped to attract the attention of the wealthy Toronto publisher William J. Gage who had in 1894 offered $25,000 to establish a home for consumptives. Gage toured British and continental spas and returned to Canada convinced that a 'national sanatorium' was necessary. What he had in mind was an institution supported by public funds and private subscription that would stem the flow of 'hundreds of our young men' who left Canada each year for Europe and the United States in search of health and strength.[51] In 1895 Calgary city council took to heart Gage's public pronouncements that Calgary might offer the same advantages to the consumptive as Denver, Colorado, and that the CPR might win new customers by providing special rates to transport patients to Calgary. The Calgary group did not intend to compete for patients with the Brett Sanitarium, but instead hoped to attract a class of consumptives who were not quite suitable for Banff. Indeed, Dr Brett was one of the ten physicians who attested to the Calgary's medical advantages in the promotional pamphlet, *Calgary the Denver of Canada*. City council resolved that since,

> very many consumptives have been restored to health without special treatment through coming to Calgary to reside; that the air, the water, the sunshine, and general conditions of Calgary are equal, if not superior to those at Denver … and believing that the lives of many, otherwise doomed to an early grave, would be saved if they had the advantages of being treated in an institution specially conducted for their benefit at Calgary.[52]

What is of interest is not so much the fate of the first sanatorium; Gage and the wealthy Massey family built the Muskoka Cottage Hospital in the lake country north of Toronto in 1897. Instead, it is the efforts of the Calgary group, especially the physicians, to entice consumptives to the region that provides insight into the medical and popular understanding of the disease.

As the group enthusiastically portrayed it, Calgary offered magnificent views of the Rockies; it boasted electric lights, waterworks, good shopping, churches, schools, two 'substantial hospitals', and an opera house for its slightly more than 3,000 inhabitants. Residents were 'of a superior class, many of them being highly cultured, intelligent people, and parties coming here to find health, can also find homes and enjoy all the advantages of good society'.[53] After charting the social and practical advantages of the region, including attractions for the sport hunter and angler, the Calgary boosters outlined the specific medical advantages for the consumptive. The region, according to the ten area physicians, was free of 'endemic' disease, including typhoid and malaria. The altitude, at between three and four thousand feet above sea-level, was 'admitted by the highest authorities to be the most desirable to attain, and is the one best adapted to afford relief to consumptives in the various stages of the disease'. Elevation was thought to stimulate circulation and respiration allowing the 'aseptic character of the atmosphere' to be drawn deeply into the lungs. Calgary's long hours of sunshine and dry climate created an atmosphere that was especially remarkable for producing a 'buoyancy and elasticity' that allowed 'candidates for consumption, who have had a bad family history, or been subjected to severe depressing influences ... [to] throw off and apparently outgrow their weakness and tendency to fall into a tuberculous condition'.[54]

It was this construction of place as inherently beneficial and restorative that Calgary's physicians and civic leaders had hoped would attract the publicly-financed 'national sanatorium'. Those with 'incipient consumption' and sufficient means were invited to come to Calgary for the cure, as well as to take advantage of the region's abundant lands and economic opportunities. Stirring testimonials from the apparently cured were a large part of the promotional pamphlet. The first, and most 'important', testimonial was from a clergyman of the Church of England (and therefore presumably trustworthy) who had suffered from tuberculosis for three years after an attack of pneumonia in London, England in 1892. He travelled to European and American spas in search of the cure before settling in Calgary where, in just seven and half months, he gained eighteen pounds, his cough abated, his appetite improved, and he was able to return to work. Another 'incipient consumptive' removed to Calgary from Ontario after her specialist 'gave the case up as absolutely hopeless;' her sister had died of consumption, and she herself had always been extremely delicate. But, once in Calgary she quickly gained thirty pounds and her cough disappeared; in a short time she was to all 'practical purposes cured and had never enjoyed better health'. Her husband supposed that her rapid improvement was also somehow due to horseback riding, but that the climate was the 'main factor'. Others claimed that they tried Colorado Springs, but their condition only improved once they settled in Calgary.[55] The testimonials made clear that Calgary's climate and elevation worked marvellous cures. What is less evident was the need for a sanatorium given the region's natural medicinal benefits, but presumably the institution might provide the individual care, healthy diet and medical expertise to hasten the climate's good effects.

The board of trade's brochure was of course intended to entice investment and settlers to the city, and the area's resident physicians hoped to draw prospective patients to the city of slightly more than 3,000 disappointingly healthy citizens. Trading on the proximity to Banff's mountain resorts and the natural assets of the National Park, the Calgary boosters endeavoured to attract the invalid trade away from the American destinations of choice, Denver, New Mexico, West Texas and California.[56] It was challenging to build a medical practice in southern Alberta in the late nineteenth century and few physicians had Brett's close connections to the National Park. Dr J. D. Lafferty, who initiated the bid for the national sanatorium, had, like Brett, moved west with railway construction and used his association with the CPR to engage in real estate speculation. He served as Calgary's mayor in 1890, and operated a string of banks across the southern prairies, although the Canadian chartered banks forced him out of the business by the early 1890s.[57] As a Liberal in a profoundly Conservative region Lafferty had to wait until his party was returned to power in Ottawa in order to benefit from government patronage, especially department of Indian Affairs work. Medical entrepreneurship and the notion of a climatic cure for 'incipient consumption' constructed a powerful image of the region as an attractive home for settlers and health seekers. Physicians were selling the region and health at a time when fears of tuberculosis far outstripped medical remedies. And while they lost the national sanatorium, as they waited for patients they were able to access public funds through medical contracts with the NWMP and the department of Indian Affairs, as well as private contracts with the railway and mining companies in southern Alberta.[58] Brett and Lafferty were also actively involved in limiting and defining who could practise medicine in the west, forming the North West Territories Medical Council in 1889, and the Alberta Medical Association in 1906. In 1915 Brett was named the province's second lieutenant governor. Building successful practices and building the west were one and the same.

The Muskoka Cottage Sanatorium, as noted, was eventually opened with thirty beds in 1897 by William Gage in the lake country north of Toronto. It was financed by wealthy donors and its middle and upper class patients. The Sanatorium, in the climate of southern Ontario lacked the elevation and mountain air of the Rockies, but was fashioned after E. L. Trudeau's Adirondack Cottage Sanitarium which opened in 1884 in rural New York and popularized the approach that consumption might be averted or cured by building resistance through a regimented environment and a return to nature. Physicians as patients, including Trudeau himself, were among the earliest and most committed converts to the sanatorium cure.[59] It was a very class- and race-based notion of both disease and cure. As Katherine Ott argues, other classes and races were excluded from participation in a disease that 'resulted in refinement of the body and ennoblement of the soul'.[60] In retrospect, Koch's detection of the tubercle bacillus appears integral to an understanding of the disease, but at the time it did little to explain why, if the germ was ubiquitous, some became ill and others did not. There were two categories that might explain the 'exciting causes': internal or individual behaviors, and external or environmental causes. It appeared certain that other factors, age, gender, class, race, moral failings or personal disposition, were to account for the disease. Medical discourse framed this apparent ambiguity by the metaphor of 'seed and soil'; the seed of tubercle bacillus was necessary for illness to develop, but individual disposition, a receptive soil, was also necessary.

The sanatorium cure hoped to address both individual and environmental causes through the moral regulation of conduct and thought, and by exposure to a bracing climate. An early patient at Muskoka Cottage Sanatorium in 1900 recalled (fifty-three years later) that the 'cure' consisted of twenty-four hours of fresh air and six feedings per day consisting of plenty of milk and raw eggs. Rest was not emphasized. Instead he joined other male patients on long daily walks, rowing and fishing on the lake, and tennis on the lawn. These things, he explained, 'kept the emotions controlled as well as the muscles properly exercised'. Several times a week, and always on Sunday, they walked the nearly five kilometres to Gravenhurst to tramp around the town, and then 'hustle back to be on time for the next luncheon or meal'. [61] Stanley's recollections evoke the picture of young, homosocial health and vitality, not disease. Since there was no nursing care at Muskoka, patients helped each other 'In fact it was a bit of real happiness for one fellow to be able to help another. The intimate association of one man with the others around him in entertaining one another, in extending help to one another ... all combined to create a fellowship that was indispensable ... and one of the outstanding treasures of my life'.[62] It seems clear that Stanley suffered from what was termed 'incipient consumption' at a time when it was possible to feel 'a little bit consumptive'.[63] As treatment at Muskoka and the Brett Sanitarium made clear, only the white middle and upper classes suffered from the disease that could be cured at these institutions.

In the first decades of the twentieth century, however, the understanding of tuberculosis and its treatment was changing. A clearer understanding of the disease as infectious and more closely associated with the poor meant that the invalid trade was no longer welcome in Alberta. In 1907 concerned citizens petitioned the legislature to prevent the consumptive from descending on the region. They wanted the province to search out all cases of tuberculosis, to require the ill to report to the Board of Health, to restrict the tubercular from entering the province, or failing that, that they be denied lodging in hotels, boarding houses and private homes.[64] As tuberculosis increasingly became a public health concern optimistic voluntary and government agencies worked to break the grip of the 'white plague' through education and sanatorium treatment. But it was the continuing ambiguity in etiology and diagnosis that created the space for medical and bureaucratic discourse to solidify their prescriptions for social order and public health.[65]

Tuberculosis on reserves was seen as different. The 'seed' of tuberculosis was the same, but the 'soil', Aboriginal people, were seen as especially prone to fall into illness and spread disease from reserve to town. The longstanding policy of the department of Indian Affairs to assimilate Aboriginal people focused on agriculture and especially giving their children Christian education in residential schools, what historian Ian McKay called 'Christian/liberal manufactories of individuals, pre-eminent laboratories of liberalism, [where] First Nations children were 'forced to be free', in the very particular liberal sense of 'free', even at the cost of their lives'.[66] But by 1907 the 'civilizing and christianizing' mission appeared to falter when the horrendous physical condition of the schools was brought to the public's attention. Dr. Peter H. Bryce, former secretary of Ontario's Board of Health and actively involved in the anti-tuberculosis societies in Canada and the United States, was appointed in 1904 as chief medical officer of the department of Indian Affairs. His report on the church-run and government-owned schools found an 'intimate relationship between the health of the pupils while in the schools and that of their early death subsequent to discharge'.[67] The schools were overcrowded and the children undernourished. Although he did not examine the children, he claimed that in all cases tuberculosis was considered the cause of death. The government's per capita grants to the churches were never adequate to feed and clothe the children well *and* maintain the institutions, so more children were enrolled, they were put to work, and their health suffered as a result.[68] Bryce's recommendation that the government take over full management of the schools was rejected.

The following year, 1908, J. D. Lafferty, former Calgary booster and now the department's medical officer in southern Alberta, inspected the region's schools and found on both the Stoney and Tsuu T'ina reserve schools that 100 per cent of the children were ill with tuberculosis. According to Lafferty the children were disposed to the disease because they possessed little resistance due to the change from the outdoor life to school.[69] The next year Bryce joined Lafferty in yet another school inspection which had now become the weapon of choice in the public health movement. Eschewing the accepted methods of diagnosis (tuberculin testing, Roentgen rays with a fluorescent screen and sputum examination) as too time-consuming and expensive, they instead noted temperature, pulse, respiration, the condition of the nose, throat and chest, and general appearance. Although it is impossible at this distance to know what the physicians saw, Aboriginal bodies would have been perceived as very different from the 'normal' white body. Nevertheless, Bryce reported that the children were exposed to tuberculosis in their homes and that all children awaiting admission to school showed signs of the illness. He suggested that each student should be considered an 'individual case of probable tuberculosis' and that government establish a sanatorium using the 'Frimley method'. The Brompton Sanatorium in Frimley, England developed a cost-effective treatment that stressed graduated exercise, strict discipline and manual labour. The historian Linda Bryder suggests that this 'pick-axe cure' was similar to labour colonies for the unemployed.[70] Bryce's recommendations were again rejected by the department of Indian Affairs which was under intense pressure from the Christian churches to leave the educational system essentially unchanged, although there were efforts to build open-air dormitories, to provide a minimum diet, and increase per capita grants to cover the added expense.[71]

Bryce consistently noted in his annual reports to the department that tuberculosis on reserves could be alleviated with better housing and sanitation, as well as quarantining the sick. He did wonder how it was that Aboriginal people who lived an outdoor life, such as the Stoney and Tsuu T'ina in the shadow of the Rockies and its clean mountain air, suffered so terribly from tuberculosis. As he noted, the climate in southern Alberta was the most salubrious on the prairies 'in a district famous, and properly so, as a health resort for the white consumptive'.[72] Rather than question the climatic theories of the day, Bryce provided a popular racial explanation that Aboriginal people were moving through a difficult stage of civilization; a tendency to tuberculosis was a marker of their social and cultural inferiority. Social Darwinism suggested that the white (probably British) race had, through natural selection, risen to a position of superiority. Aboriginal people were considered to be moving (however slowly) towards civilization, and their poor health was evidence of racial weakness and natural stage in the evolutionary process. Bryce noted that there were two Aboriginal groups who suffered least from tuberculosis; those who remained in their 'natural state' and far removed from society; and those who had undergone an 'advance in general intelligence of how to live, through the valuable admixture of white blood with its inherited qualities'.[73] That Bryce's prescription for health, assimilation through 'white blood', bore a strong resemblance to long-standing departmental policy of complete assimilation is perhaps not surprising given his role as departmental employee. What is rather more notable was how Bryce as tuberculosis expert manipulated 'scientific' understandings of disease to produce racial explanations that left climatic theory intact.

By the 1920s tuberculosis rates in Canada were steadily falling and had been declining well before active measures were taken to control it.[74] Enthusiastic voluntary anti-tuberculosis associations were established across the west in the early decades of the century, and their fundraising efforts were focused almost exclusively on the goal of establishing a local modern sanatorium. Enthusiasm was not enough however, and it was only the federal government's healthy per diem payments for the treatment of World War I veterans that allowed sanatoria in the west to become financially secure.[75] These provincial sanatoria of the 1920s and 30s were hybrid institutions that developed from nineteenth-century notions of 'consumption' as a wasting disease that required rest and feeding, as well as from the belief that tuberculosis could be controlled by the removal of the infected from home and society. The institutions had much in common with the early health resorts, from an architecture that evoked the chalet style, to locations in the bucolic countryside, and an emphasis on open-air treatment. Although chest surgery was becoming increasingly popular in tuberculosis treatment, moral regulation of thought and behaviour continued to play a significant role in the cure. Dr R. G. Ferguson, medical superintendent of Saskatchewan's Fort Qu'Appelle sanatorium and national tuberculosis expert, advised his non-Aboriginal patients in 1920 '... "the cure" is not a bottle of medicine, nor a surgical operation, but an Idea: a way of life, to apply to every moment of the day, every activity ... part of the cure is the development of a spirit of faithful endeavour, helpfulness, earnestness, good humour, kindliness and forbearance.'[76] The newly-established provincial sanatoria were public institutions intended to manage a disease that was increasingly seen as a public health threat associated with the poor and the working classes.[77] As Ferguson's advice to patients makes clear, the sanatorium cure relied on spatial isolation where the tubercular might cultivate modern attitudes and behaviours of the responsible, hygienic self.

Aboriginal people, however, because of their race were deemed incapable of this sort of self-regulation and, with few exceptions, were explicitly excluded from sanatorium treatment, ostensibly because their care was the responsibility of the federal government.[78] Sanatorium directors, represented by the Canadian Tuberculosis Association (CTA), exerted considerable pressure on the state to deal with the 'Indian problem'. The group noted with pride that white tuberculosis rates were declining, but drew attention to apparent unchecked tuberculosis on reserves. A western sanatorium director characterized the reserves as a 'menace ... to the health of ordinary citizens' and urged the federal government to 'remove from the doorstep of the provinces the anomaly of conditions of uncontrolled nuisance and menace that the Federal government is responsible for, but is doing little or nothing about'. Isolation on reserves was no longer adequate because they 'never were water-tight or disease-tight compartments, and in these days of easy travel are becoming less and less so'. Disease 'leaked' into non-Aboriginal communities through work, and through handling of berries and handcrafts.[79] As the medical and scientific authority on tuberculosis, the CTA began agitating for separate government-funded facilities to treat Aboriginal people citing the 'growing anxiety among the white population living adjacent to certain Indian bands ... and the leaders of certain bands of Indians publicly agitating for increased facilities for diagnosis and treatment'.[80]

Institutional care for Aboriginal people in southern Alberta, before the 1940s, was confined to mission hospitals on reserves.[81] These charity hospitals, managed and funded according to the imperatives of Christian stewardship and government subsidies, were associated with the schools to treat sick children; students might then remain on the school rolls and stay eligible for per capita funding. It was also hoped that the civilizing mission of the hospital might eventually touch the parents as well. By 1921 the long-neglected Anglican-run Tsuu T'ina reserve school was converted into a hospital of sorts with Dr. F. T. Murray appointed in the dual role as physician and Indian agent.[82] As noted, the childrens' chronically desperate condition had already been identified in school inspections in 1907, 1908, and 1909, when it was reported that every child in the school suffered from tuberculosis.[83] Yet another medical inspection in 1920 drew attention to one particular child 'curled in a bed that is filthy in a room that is untidy ... both sides of her neck and chest are swollen and five foul ulcers are discovered when we lift the bandages'.[84] And another medical inspection the following year found similar conditions: dirty floors and windows, and the bed linen 'stained with blood and puss [*sic*] marks old and recent'[85] The boarding school was subsequently termed a 'hospital' and the whole reserve considered a 'hospital area'.[86] Sleeping porches were added to the school and an assistant nurse was hired, but other than Murray's presence as physician, there was little to indicate that the school had become a hospital. By 1932 with only a 'practical nurse' and a cook in attendance it was judged 'scarcely a hospital'.[87] The opportunity for more than custodial care was severely limited by the extreme poverty of the reserve generally. For example, x-ray examination was impossible because the reserve remained without electrical power until 1937, although the nearby city of Calgary had enjoyed it since at least the 1890s.[88] But the conversion of the missionary school to government-funded 'hospital' was more than merely the discursive practice of institution-naming; it also indicated an increasing concern that the racial boundaries of reserve and disease be more vigilantly monitored.

The focus of efforts in the school/hospital continued to be to confine and isolate the children from their own families, and to isolate the reserve from the wider Alberta community. Elder Helen Megunis who attended the school in the 1920s recalled,

> ... [my] early experiences was being lonely and afraid....To me the feeling was we were here we have lived an isolated life, after I became a young girl in my teens were still isolated, there was no TVs, phone, electricity, plumbing, newspapers. It was strange visiting Calgary during the stampede was our only contact with alien people of Calgary. To me when I think of growing up I was living in a cocoon afraid to explore outside the safety of my reserve [*sic*].[89]

The continued isolation of the reserve that literally adjoined the burgeoning city of Calgary was made possible through formal and informal restrictions on the people's movements, always enforced by the Mounted Police. The rationale for isolation had certainly shifted from ostensible efforts to 'protect' the Aboriginal people from unscrupulous whites, to efforts to contain disease on the reserve and thereby safeguard the Canadian public's health. The Tsuu T'ina experience was not representative of all schools, but the differences were quantitative not qualitative.[90] The expedient of confining the ill and dying to reserve schools or mission hospitals rather than admitting them to local hospitals was dictated by the department's concerns for economy. But there were larger issues that influenced the form and place of medical treatment for Aboriginal people in the Canadian west.

Sanatorium directors, through the CTA, continued to call for racially-segregated care for Aboriginal people. At their annual meeting in 1935 the CTA devoted a session to 'Indian tuberculosis' and sent a 'strong resolution to the prime minister and minister of health, pointing out the menace of uncontrolled tuberculosis on Indian reserves to the surrounding white population, and suggesting that more active measures be taken'.[91] It goes without saying that the association never considered whether to expand provincial sanatoria to accommodate Aboriginal patients. Racially-segregated hospital care had become 'normal' and was taken for granted. The modernizing hospital after the 1920s began to attract patients who demanded, and would pay for, the benefits that medicine seemed to promise. Relatively safe and effective surgery, the availability of professional nursing, technological innovations such as x-ray, and doctors intent on preserving medical authority over health, all combined to transform the hospital from a social to a medical institution.[92] Medical care for the poor was increasingly separate from, and to a certain extent dependent upon, the fees charged to paying patients, thereby creating a system of hospitals segregated by class.[93] But it also created hospitals segregated by race. Racially-segregated wards were prevalent even in community hospitals that relied on department of Indian Affairs funds for their financial survival. After all, keeping Aboriginal people apart was vital to attracting paying patients.[94] Yielding to pressure from the CTA to provide care, and recognizing that it could not rely on provincial sanatoria, in 1936 the federal government opened the Fort Qu'Appelle Indian hospital in southern Saskatchewan, across the lake from Ferguson's Fort Qu'Appelle sanatorium. In 1939 the Dynevor Indian hospital was opened outside of Winnipeg in a former residential school, and in 1941 the Coqualeetza residential school in British Columbia was converted into an Indian hospital. These facilities also signalled a shift from the kind of patriarchal charity that characterized the missionary management of reserves, to a medically expert management through institutional confinement.

In early 1945 the Advisory Committee on Indian Tuberculosis (essentially the management committee of the CTA) was established by Order-in-Council and recommended that the government establish a large 'Indian hospital' in

Edmonton.[95] The site, a recently acquired American military headquarters, was transferred to the newly-established department of National Health and Welfare. It seemed a radical departure from longstanding policies to isolate Aboriginal people from the larger community. Edmonton citizens agreed. A large delegation representing twenty-two different organizations petitioned the mayor to protest the government's plans. They objected to the buildings' being used to accommodate 'tubercular Indians' in a residential neighbourhood, and pressed for the site to be used instead either to hospitalize returned veterans, or to convert its buildings into housing for veterans. The mayor pressed federal ministers to locate the hospital somewhere else.[96] The Edmonton *Bulletin* claimed that veterans 'who fought the Empire's battles huddle in dark, ill-ventilated basements' for a lack of housing in the city.[97] Other veterans groups petitioned the prime minister to use the buildings to accommodate tubercular veterans who were entitled to hospitalization.[98] The minister responded by assuring veterans that they did indeed have priority in government planning. But he also explained the desirability of the hospital in a discourse that acknowledged public concerns over the 'dangers' posed by Aboriginal people. First, to address the need for racial segregation, 'A section of the institution will be used for the ordinary hospitalization of Indians, and thus relieve the public wards of the Edmonton hospitals from treating Indians in these institutions ... This, undoubtedly, is better for the Indians and for the general public'. Second, to address the need for isolation, 'The Indian patients will be kept within the institution and from a public health viewpoint it would seem much more desirable to have these people under treatment than to have tuberculous Indians wandering about the streets of Edmonton and other Alberta cities and towns spreading the disease'.[99]

Agitation continued however. A mass protest meeting on 25 November 1945, attended by 300 citizens and deemed a 'riot' by the press, demanded that the buildings be given over to veterans to ease the housing shortage in Edmonton; or if the buildings must be used as a sanatorium, they should at least be reserved for veterans. Mayor Harry Ainley's telegram to the minister made the point: 'There would be no objection to the buildings being turned over for a hospital for veterans, and we understand there is an urgent need for accommodation for tubercular veterans in this province'.[100] An undercover RCMP officer in attendance, keeping a watchful eye on the volatile combination of disgruntled veterans and the Communist Labour-Progressive Party's involvement in the protest, noted that the speeches criticized the government 'sharply'.[101] The city attempted unsuccessfully to block the government's plans by claiming the hospital violated zoning by-laws. A petition from more than 300 residents of the hospital's Westmount neighbourhood claimed that the Indian hospital would affect their property values, although they were willing to accept a veteran's hospital. The minister assured the neighbours that 'Every effort will be made to see that neither staff nor patients, nor hospital visitors cause any nuisance in the community'.[102] The minister's promise of 150, and then 200, jobs for Edmonton citizens went some way to calming the protest.

In 1946 Canada's head of state, Governor General Field Marshall Viscount Alexander of Tunis, officially opened the 500-bed Charles Camsell Indian Hospital in Edmonton.[103] It was high state drama intended as a very obvious display of modern and effective health care for Aboriginal people by the flagship of the welfare state, the department of National Health and Welfare. As the Edmonton protesters were told, it was necessary to isolate and segregate Aboriginal people who were increasingly seen as 'dangerous' not just because of their supposed proclivity to disease, but precisely because they were seen as lacking the liberal values of individualism, as rational, self-governing citizens. It was necessary to make a very public demonstration of the state's commitment to protect all Canadians by segregating those who threatened the public's health and security. Confinement on reserves was not enough. The Edmonton site recommended itself because it was economical; a 'borrowed building' already owned by the state. Edmonton was also the geographic centre of the province with access to Aboriginal people in the north and south, but more importantly it was central to the experts who would endeavour to normalize health, behaviour and thought.[104] And it was a mass project. Dr Percy Moore, director of Indian Health Services, boasted that in the 1950s more than 90 per cent of the Aboriginal population was x-rayed 'at one point I had nearly half of them in hospitals'.[105] Alberta had indeed become an ideal home for the consumptive.

The Tsuu T'ina and the Stoney, along with other Aboriginal peoples, consistently protested that their health status was a symptom of the larger social, economic and political policies that colonized their lands and attempted to undermine their communities. Government policy, however, worked to repress Aboriginal conceptions of health, land-use and livelihood in order to fashion rational, liberal citizens; that their health deteriorated was variously seen as either cause or consequence of their unreformed selves. A spatial analysis of the changing meaning of tuberculosis underscores how the construction of health and its maintenance were culturally produced and served to inscribe racial and class difference. Lines of segregation and isolation, drawn on the landscape, tended by the power of the state, and rationalized in the language of medical humanitarianism were not a negation of Canada's liberal democratic values, but integral to the formation of the welfare state.

Acknowledgements

I would like to thank CIHR and Associated Medical Services for the research funds for this study. I would also like to thank the editors and especially my colleague David Schimmelpenninck van der Oye for his valuable comments.

10 SERBIAN LANDSCAPES OF DREAMTIME AND HEALING: CLEAR STREAMS, STONES OF PROPHESY, ST SAVA'S RIBS, AND THE WOODEN CITY OF OZ

Marko Živković

After Milošević's fall in 2000, and the assassination of the Prime Minister Zoran Djindjić in 2003, the Serbian political scene has been characterized by the struggle of contending political groups to legitimate their visions of Serbian identity. One common method is to entrench these visions in political rituals situated at particular dates and places. As anchors for collective memory and narratives of national origin, both the calendar of official holidays, and the map of 'famous historical places' become battlegrounds for contesting agendas.

On the other hand, widespread concerns with pollution and purity, alternative healing methods, and various 'energies' – long associated in anthropological literature with anxieties over social boundaries or intrusions of global capitalism – tend to be anchored in the places purportedly endowed with special energies – the 'places of power'.

By 'places of power' I mean named places that have become widely shared symbolic tokens in a particular polity because they accumulated many and varied layers of meaning. For instance, such places of renown or 'power' tend to act as 'pegs' or 'anchors' not only in the 'national geography of the mind', but also in the 'social frameworks of memory' on very intimate, personal and familial scales. In short, we need places to hang our life memories on, and the powers that be always seek to insert their ideology through these locations on which we drape our memories. The memories of my generation, for instance, would hang on the streets and schools named after heroes of socialism, or on the school excursions to famous battlefields of the WWII Partisan struggle. New generations are hanging their intimate memories on different pegs.

This density of (often contradictory) meanings makes such places not just effective tokens in political debates but also sites of rituals, commemorations, pilgrimages sacred and secular, and other politically effective performances. Altogether, I consider 'places of power' to be among the most crucial battlegrounds for contesting agendas in times of radical social, economic and ideological change.

Paying attention to shifts in how places are named and used should help illuminate shifts in ideologies. My focus here, however, will be to see whether thinking with places helps us understand something about links between places, social/political changes and notions of health/healing.

A very romantic passage from an essay on dreaming will, I think, be a good starting point. The whole of Greece even today, concludes Carl Alfred Meier in his essay on 'The Dream in Ancient Greece and Its Use in Temple Cures (Incubation)', is imbued with myth.

> ... looking at the map you will realize it is the geography of the human soul ... Spread over the peninsula and its islands are hundreds of places each of which has its special myth, its cult and cult-legends, and sanctuaries, each of which would take care of one or another of the most basic problems of human life in the most varied, complete, beautiful, and healing way. If you had been in need of help in those days, you would have known exactly where to go to find enacted for you the appropriate archetype.[1]

So Greek landscape serves as a 'mythological grid' – a classificatory system on which dream interpretation and healing are based. Every disturbance you experience can be inserted into a proper place. What is healing in rituals is an insertion into, and alignment with such comprehensive symbolic maps of the universe. Ritual effects a mutual mapping of domains onto each other. Body with its illness, on the one hand, and heavens, the world of sacred animals or, what I am particularly interested in here, the dreamtime landscape of a nation, on the other, thus get ritually mapped onto each other. Once correspondences are established, manipulation on one of these levels could bring about change on others – typically both the patient and the immediate group afflicted are re-aligned with the mythological grid and thereby healed according to the classical anthropological explanation for the efficacy of rituals.[2]

If that's the case, and if the list of ailments and its appropriate cures does tend to get encoded in, or anchored in topography, then perhaps one could reconstruct a Serbian map of healing analogous to Meier's Ancient Greece, and read from it about major sources of anxiety following a long tradition in anthropological theory that relates such widespread concerns with healing and harmful energies to anxieties about the social boundaries,[3] or intrusions of capitalism and commodity fetishism.[4] I am still far away from constructing such a map and reading from it the current anxieties of Serbian society. What I will offer here instead is my first preliminary attempt to 'think with places' in Serbia in the hope that this will be the first step towards a more comprehensive 'reading'.

In the summer of 2007 I made three trips to 'places of power' in Serbia accompanied with a minimal film crew as an initial foray into what should become a larger project that will include the making of a documentary. For this first fieldtrip I settled on the Zlatibor region. The second was to Niš, and the third to Eastern Serbia. I will focus only on the first trip here and see how fruitful it is to take 'places of power' as tools of analysis.

Family of Clear Streams: EcoDreams and Catastrophe

I have been vaguely aware of the Family of Clear Streams (*Porodica bistrih potoka*) for years. I knew it had to do with some combination of communal living, ecological activism and artistic colony. It turned out that my soundman's wife was friendly with someone who lived there and needed a ride, and besides the place was very conveniently on our way to Zlatibor. So this was our first stop.

We stop first at the local village store and buy some oil and sugar since I heard that this is a customary gift brought by visitors. We follow the unpaved road to the foot of the mountain. Up the steep wooded slope we climb and emerge into a clearing with several peasant-style buildings. The sun is setting and the grassy hill above the buildings is golden. Grass is being cut. We are welcomed heartily by Boža Mandić, the founder and the soul of the Family. We are treated to a simple and very tasty meal of boiled rice, white cheese and tomatoes. Wooden bowl and wooden spoons. Racing with the setting sun we set up the camera and the microphone, and Boža immediately launches into his animated presentation of the place, walks, jumps, gesticulates expansively. He is a writer and very much involved in theatre, obviously a person of considerable histrionic talents.

Over and over again Boža emphasizes simplicity of living, openness and hospitality, and doing away with material possessions. He often jokes, he tells us, that he is 'one of the richest people in Europe without a dime in my pockets'.[5] 'And when they ask me how I came to these riches', he says, 'I tell them – by not charging anyone anything'. Boža emphasizes sharing and mutuality, and a 'narrative warmth' for the 'young people who come here because they need to talk it out'. 'We engage here', he says, 'with nature, art and humble economy. We are a paradigm showing it's possible to live without profits, markets, money ... All that's important are soul, love and embrace'. The basis of their economy: 'all we have we want to share; all we need we'll somehow get'. Inside the oldest house he shows many rustic objects, such as roughly hewn wooden ladles and crude earthen bowls, all brought by others, he hastens to say. And in another room, objects on the wall are hard to discern in the twilight. They are art pieces made of cow dung, wood, stone and wool to be put on exhibition called 'Art toward Freedom' at the Belgrade National Museum.

Boža started The Family of Clear Streams in 1977 when he moved there with his wife and infant daughter from the city of Novi Sad. 'Some 30,000 people passed through in the last 30 years', he says, 'and this place has passed through many stages – a commune, an intensive commune, a family. I live here alone with Jelena and of course, with people who come'. This will last a long time, he says, 'and that's primarily because I feel so great here. And who wouldn't feel splendid here in the mud, in the wood and stone, with plants and winds, with trees, with the spring?'

Then he walks to one of the houses and jumps on the porch fence made of rough logs. 'They are all crooked', he says, 'just like my art – this is my auto-portrait. And I am coming to resemble my own art more and more. I came here as a writer who protects nature and now I am more and more a writer who nature protects'.

The last house he shows us is made of wood – 'with axe only, no nails just by fitting planks together'. 'This is an old principle of living in Serbia, ' he says. And then he senses that he's embarked on a certain dangerous track. The houses are obviously made in a Serbian peasant style. Serbia is mentioned for the first time. He hastens to add: 'I must say I belong to this local culture. We recently talk a lot about "ecological patriotism". I am not a nationalist, on the contrary, I am plan-etaristically [*sic*] oriented, but it is really nice that where you live you like what you live – which means I like the beech [*bukva*], the hornbeam [*grab*], the oak [*hrast*], I like my ditch [*jendek*], my stream'. Then he turns to the wooden house and remarks that it 'almost resembles [Wilhelm] Reich's boxes – where people come to feel very good'.

And finally, jumping on a roughly hewn wooden podium that serves as their summer stage, with beautiful grassy hill, trees and a vine framing him, he launches into his last oration on the importance of returning to the 'purity of beginningness' (quoting Emil Cioran) of going back to roots ('I believe in roots, in the rhyzomatic culture') so as to start a new civilization again not beguiled with speed, gigantism, materiality, destruction and alienation as ours is. At first, he says, 'when I came here, I wrote exalted panegyrics to nature. Now, as the twenty-first century is 'getting more and more entrenched in the 'pessimistic code' – fetishes, plastics, alienation', his texts are increasingly turning to critique. His last book is titled 'The Plastic Mind', and it is a warning to the twenty-first century to 'return to soil, trees, and ants'. 'And if humankind does not possess consciousness, at least it might have the instinct to stop on the brink of the abyss, just as an individual instinctively stops before the chasm', he says bodily enacting the teetering at the edge of his wooden podium. If humankind doesn't stop of its own accord, the Nature will stop it with a cataclysm'. There is no war that Nature does not win', Boža says.

A lover of smallness and of roots, practitioner of 'wildism' (*divljizam*) in art who makes sculptures out of cow dung, wood, stone and wool, and plays sponta-neous, physical theatre based on energy and rhythm – this is how Boža presents himself. People come and bring salt, sugar, oil. Peasants teach the urban family how to recognize plants, milk the cow, till the soil. Alienated youth, holy fools, artists and famous film makers visit, stay, move on. Stories and simple food are exchanged. The Family of Clear Streams is a symbol in Serbia, Boža says, 'of the return from city to nature'.

The three clear streams that gave name to the Family are now polluted by the Austrian company that has bought the nearby stone quarry and Boža has lost his environmental campaign against it. He exudes optimism and hope before us but there is no telling what part of it is an outward show. For my purposes, it suffices that the Family has indeed accumulated some fame, and does offer perhaps the longest-lasting and successful example of an experiment in return to nature, simplicity and communitarian sharing in Serbia.

The Family presents the visage of a distinctly rural character, a peasant arcadia Serbian style and Boža is aware that his houses resemble ethnological museums. The family had to get along with the peasants around them, and it was from these peasants that they learned their simple economics. Their dwellings and utensils are local, thus peasant and recognizably Serbian, and yet Boža is at pains to distance himself from certain associations such places would bring in today's Serbia where tokens of romanticized peasantry are a major ingredient in the mainstream celebration of ethnos and national ideology. Ecological philosophy of his type, with its localism, tends to exhibit affinities, willy-nilly, with the celebrations of the ethnic, just as hippy communes in the US and elsewhere tended to imitate the romanticized eco-wise Natives. Boža is swift-footed. His localism, he says, is not nationalistic chauvinism but planetarian eco-patriotism.

In Serbia, as in many other places, idealized countryside and peasant lifestyle are identified with health, while cities, with their speed, crowding and pollution, are suspected of being fundamentally diseased. Clear springs, clean air, 'natural food', and simple physical labour are all longingly exalted by the urbanites as the right way to live. In simple rural virtues lies salvation for the jangled nerves and bad digestions of urbanites, as a widespread fantasy would have it.

Family of Clear Streams definitely lends itself to this popular rural utopia of healthy living, but with a difference. What is often implied in the popular idyll in Serbia as well as in many other places, is that the village life is fundamentally the right, pristine, way the nation should live. The healing power of the countryside then resides not just in ethnically neutral pure water and air, but also in the 'naturally Serbian' way of life epitomized by peasants. Urbanites are then 'poisoned' not just by car exhaust and shocking city rhythms, but also, implicitly or explicitly, by foreign influences that the cities of peripheral nations who typically receive their modernity from the Western Core are the first to incorporate and then disseminate to the countryside. Flight to the last remnants of the still unspoiled countryside is then also an imaginary retreat into what is most 'ours'.

Boža, however, refuses to endorse the healing power of ethnic identity. The healing force of his wooden house is not in the traditional Serbian way it was built, but in the Reichian Orgone energy it accumulates.

Boža proudly reiterates that nobody is charged for anything at the Family of Clear Streams, but at another rural utopia, Kusturica's Drvengrad on Mokra Gora, guests are charged for everything, even just to look around if they are not staying.

After we finish filming we sit before the summer stage in the approaching dusk and talk for a while. It is already dark when we leave for Mokra Gora.

Drvengrad: Kusturica's WoodTown of Oz

Drvengrad (Woodtown) perches on top of Mokra Gora in the Zlatibor region. It grew around the stage set for Kusturica's 2004 movie *Life is a Miracle* (*Život je čudo*) and is now a fully functional combination of a theme park and upscale bungalow accommodation framed as a complete if miniature city. There is a main street, a pastry shop, a library, a hi-tech movie theatre, a restaurant and a bar, an art gallery and a bookstore. There is even a jail with prisoners painted on the doors behind the painted bars. Pavements are all made of log sections that used to be railway ties, and nearly everything is made of wood. The main street, lined with colourful polka-dotted flower pots, is visually dominated by a small, sharply pointed wooden church of St Sava that glows golden in the sunset. In front of the church is parked a Trabant *limousine* prepared for the wedding party. One restaurant offers the traditional Serbian rustic fare, the bar serves pizzas and other cosmopolitan food, while the pastry shop specializes in Bosnian delights (the Turkish art of sweets). All serve fruit juices so thick they often have to be forced by vigorous shaking out of bottles shaped exactly as the old Yugoslav *Vitasok* juice bottles. The juices tend to induce a kind of fruit ecstasy combined with Yugonostalgia.

Drvengrad is a rich combination. Besides Kusturica's international fame, and well-known patronage of Prime Minister Koštunica, it combines the ethno and eco with magic realism. Its all-pervasive wood is a diacritic of ethnic peasant essence, as opposed, for instance, to cobblestone (*kaldrma*) as a diacritic of Ottoman urbanity, stone as Roman legacy, or asphalt as modern urbanity (see Spasić 2006). It sports a tiny St. Sava church but also a host of socialist nostalgia markers such as Che Guevara and Tito images, or the Trabant limo. And it is bursting with little winks. Kusturica's self indulgence is playful and often exaggerated right to the point of self-parody. The Yugo and socialist nostalgia shimmers undecidably between seriousness and irony, markers of rustic ethnicity are subtly mocked through magic realism and quasi naïve painting mannerisms, and so on. And yet, all of this could be taken quite literally as an open-air ethno-village, a genre recognized in Serbia (and we will visit its other incarnations later).

The eco part is straightforward. The juices are phenomenal, the food excellent and Zlatibor has been enjoying the fame of the premier Serbian 'air spa' (*vazdušna banja*) for a long time. Kusturica's internationally acclaimed magic realism Balkan-style, is, in a sense, crafted precisely to mediate between the ethno-local and Metropolitan Cosmopolitanism. Drvengrad enacts this mediation beautifully. It is cutely, endearingly local and ethno, but one senses that it would be quite commonplace to be passed by Maradona, Iggy Pop, or some other International Celebrity on the main street (they are all Kusturica's personal friends). Drvengrad thus beautifully performs a favourite utopia – we are cosmopolitans (not backward provincials) unfazed by the greatest celebrities from the Wide World (*iz belog sveta*) beating their path to our doors (because we are fascinating, of course) without us being corrupted by that Wide World, and without us giving up on being fully ourselves, utterly and authentically unique.

Finally, that Kusturica changed his Muslim first name Emir into the ur-Serbian Nemanja (the founder of the Nemanjići dynasty no less!) could be mocked (and is, sometimes quite viciously), but St Sava Church could not be. All else around it offers itself to ironic, parodic, or undecidably shimmering readings, but St Sava Church pierces as a golden arrow this melee of the carnivalesque. St Sava and Serbian Orthodoxy are an Axis Mundi of the Serbian Planet, and wherever they are put, they establish the 'vertical' of Serbian spirituality. There is no joking there!

For us, Drvengrad was a base of operations, and our main excursion was to the nearby village of Kremna – the home to the most famous Tarabići Prophecy, and, as it turned out, a great rival to Drvengrad.

Kremna – The Serbian Delphi: Illiterate Peasant Prophets, Scheming Priests, EthnoTheologians, and Saints of Serbodoxy, with Air Spa, Healing Waters, and Clairvoyant Stones Thrown in ...

I have known of Kremna Prophecy and Tarabić family for a long time but I cannot recall since when. What was lodged in my mind was that this was *the* Serbian prophecy, the equivalent of Nostradamus, that it was of nineteenth-century provenance, and that during the socialist era it was surrounded with a kind of hush-hush awe reserved for things deeply Serbian that 'they' (communist authorities) didn't want you to talk about.

Dragan Pjević, an engineer from Kremna is the main promoter of the village and the Prophecy. He established the tourist agency 'Kremnaturist', built what is now the third 'Memorial Home' (*Spomen dom*) since the previous ones were torched to the ground, and published a book on Kremna Prophecy.[6] He welcomes the steady traffic of guests and lectures on the prophets and the village.

The inside of the Memorial Home is filled with newspaper clippings, photos and maps pinned to the walls that relate to Kremna, and there is a table where his daughter, a student of tourism, sells Kremna souvenirs. In blistering heat he graciously gave us his lecture in several installments. The first two at the Memorial Home, one at the grave of the prophets, and one at the spring, allegedly with healing and mystical properties, that happens to be on his land. Later, we were treated to his home-brewed plum brandy in his yard.

According to the legend, Dragan lectures, the Kremna valley was created when 'a celestial body entered the earth's womb here leaving the limestone (*kremen*) with miraculous properties that gave the name to the village'. This stone emits 'biogenic' radiation that brings health, longevity and special mental powers. Kremna had produced the most intellectuals in Serbia relative to its population, but most importantly, there is something in the place itself that stimulates clairvoyance since Tarabić family are just the most famous, but as Dragan never tires in pointing out, by no means the only prophets the village has produced. The Kremna Prophecy is mostly concerned with Serbian rulers and the country's destiny. Rulers who listened to Kremna prophets did well, while those who ignored them all fared badly, Dragan points out.

Kremna is notoriously difficult to photograph from the air, and its miraculous stones have been pilfered by various Westerners who tried examining them in their labs. Dragan is not quite sure whether to encourage people to take Kremna stones home or leave them where they are 'so as not to diminish the power of the place itself'.[7] Pjević sells them embedded in various little trinkets, keychains, etc., and I bought quite a bunch as a way to thank him for his hospitality and willingness to sweat in the sun for our camera.

The story of the Prophecies, it turns out, is quite convoluted. The popularly accepted outline that Dragan endorses (with a few peculiar twists) runs more or less like this: Miloš Tarabić (1809–54) and his nephew Mitar (1829–99) were illiterate peasants who told their prophecies to the Kremna priest Zaharije Zaharić (1834–1918) who wrote them down. The original manuscript has never been found and it is believed that, conserved in a jarful of oil it had been buried in the foundations of Zaharije's friend's house. In 1915, the theologian Radovan Kazimirović talked to Zaharije and published the only 'authentic' Kremna Prophecy first in the *Niški Glasnik* in 1915, and later as a part of his ethnological study on the 'Mysterious Phenomena among our People' (*Tajanstvene pojave u našem narodu*) published in Belgrade in 1941.[8] In 1982, Golubović and Malenković published another Kremna Prophecy with new, hitherto unknown Tarabići prophesies (Malenković as Zaharije's grandson being supposedly privy to unpublished family lore), but suspicious because of its communist tinkering. Finally, Dragan himself, upon becoming the president of the village municipality in 2000 as a candidate of the opposition (DOS), builds the tombstone to Miloš

Tarabić in 2002 (the sanctification ceremony of which is attend by auspicious atmospheric phenomena) and starts promoting the prophecy. He claims that he was the one who invited Vojislav Koštunica to come to Kremna on the eve of the September 2000 elections when the opposition won and ousted Milošević.[9]

The latest instalment of prophesies comes from the prominent Serbian immunologist Dr Todor Jovanović who has talked with Miloš Tarabić in his dreams, on the astral plane, and published the new prophecies in the magazine *Twilight Zone* (*Zona sumraka*) Aug 20, 2002 issue. He has apparently also talked with Nikola Tesla, Mileva Marić (Einstein's wife), Milutin Milanković, and Mihailo Pupin (all Serbian scientists of some world fame). Dragan Pjević fully endorses this new prophecy, and reports it in his book, as well as in his lectures. Most interestingly, this latest instalment of the prophecy foretells that Serbia will become a kind of Noah's Ark, the last refuge from an ecological catastrophe in the future. But it is actually the Kremna region that is the true safe haven according to Miloš Tarabić as channelled by Jovan Todorović, and in turn adapted by Dragan Pjević. This is where one should go in case of war, for in Kremna, Mokra Gora, and Bioska, 'there are springs and lots of healthy water. People born there have strength, are not tired, not decayed. Others can go there too to rejuvenate themselves, and many will suddenly be attracted there because there are vibrations and the power circulating through you all the way to the center of the earth ... these are perfect places for healing... because the plants are more healing there than in other places. Nothing can destroy this area because the mountains are placed in a certain way. These are the places for salvation'.[10]

Voja Antonić made a thorough study of the Prophecies and concluded that most of them were actually retrodated – published after the events they predicted. Those prophecies that were published before the events were mostly wrong, and the rest is so vague as to be interpretable in any which way.[11]

I wish to very sketchily enumerate a few further ingredients of the Kremna syndrome. For one, there is a St Sava token there. Pjević asks himself at the beginning of his book – what is the secret of Kremna's power? 'Why do we find the footprints of the "God-Man" (Bogočoveka) people call the "footprints of St. Sava"? Why did the prophets live here? Was it because of the God or stones? Both are present in this valley for millions of years'.[12] He further relates Kremna to the Nemanjić dynasty when he mentions that they had their villas there. He also mentions that later Ottomans had their villas too, and even Tito.

Finally, he points out that the Kremna municipality map uncannily resembles both the map of Serbia and that of former Yugoslavia rotated 90 degrees – thus showing itself a fractal replica and microcosm of the nation as a whole. This is for him yet another sign that Kremna is fatefully connected to the destiny of the country of which it is a part, the fact that rulers of that country, if they are wise and concerned about the country and their own destiny should heed.

Scientific adviser of the Geographical Institute of the Serbian Academy of Arts and Sciences, Dr Radovan Ršumović, is extensively cited in Pjević's book. Ršumović says that Kremna is a sacred, cultic place of the Serbian people, 'a great luminent (*svetlosna*) cathedral of Orthodoxy built not by man but by God himself'. Kremna is the Serbian Mecca, the Hilandar in Serbia (Hilandar is the Serbian monastery on Mt Atos), and all Serbs should at least once in their life-time make a true pilgrimage there. This should not be just a perfunctory visit. The pilgrims should spend at least a day and night in Kremna, follow in the footsteps of the Prophets, bow to their graves, and experience the nature of the place as intimately as possible.[13] Under the influence of healing and spiritual energies they will then get attuned to 'evangelist laws' (*jevandjeljskim zakonima*) and experience enlightenment. All troubles should fall from the pilgrim because he will enter in the new luminent era full of positive energies. This is the era after the Third World War when our fatherland will 'again be free, larger and more powerful than ever before'.[14]

In an aside that I found particularly interesting, moreover, and that returns us to dream practices and Mayer's quote about the ancient Greek landscape of the soul, Dragan also mentioned that people will sometimes have Tarabići prophets appear in their dreams and command them to come to Kremna. He advises them all to first go visit a village nun who is adept at interpreting such dreams, and who will then direct pilgrims to what particular ritual acts they need to perform. It seems then that we are witnessing an incipient 'visitational dream' tradition arising around the Kremna prophets.[15]

Another interesting addition to the Kremna literature is a little book by one of the more publicly prominent psychiatrists in Serbia, Dr Petar Bokun (2002). He writes with the authority of a scientist, yet after reading the book one is not at all sure whether he endorses or deconstructs the prophecy. The book is incoherent to the point of inducing nausea (in those of us addicted to consistency in thinking), but here I want to mention just a few interesting points Bokun mentions.

His main thesis is that the prophecy was the priest Zaharije's fabrication rather than the product of illiterate Tarabić peasants. This is his 'demystification' part, but he actually celebrates Zaharije for being a genius of psychological war-fare, a precocious Serbian master of propaganda, perhaps a sort of Nikola Tesla of PsyOps – all for the greater good of his nation.

The famous clarity and swiftness of mind supposedly exhibited by the Kremna villagers, Bokun speculates, may be owed to their position on the borders – 'of Byzantium and Hungary, Austria and Turkey, Serbia and Bosnia ... an eternal place of breakdown between the East and the West'.[16] Being a borderguard fosters alertness and mental acuity. Moreover, due to all this border traffic between civi-lizations passing through Kremna, the Kremanci are cosmopolitans, wise in the ways of the wider world, rather than illiterate and ignorant provincial peasants.

The Serbian scene has been crowded by psychiatrists acting as prophets, interpreters of the national psyche and character, and even political leaders during the Milošević era (1988–2000). The first leader of Croatian Serbs, Jovan Rašković was a psychiatrist, and so was, infamously, the leader of Bosnian Serbs, Dr Radovan Karadžić. At the time this text was being written in the Summer of 2008, moreover, Radovan Karadžić made news worldwide when he was arrested in Belgrade and extradited to the International Criminal Tribunal for the former Yugoslavia in The Hague. What was fascinating was that Karadžić, sporting a long white beard and topknot, had successfully posed as an alternative medicine healer in Belgrade for years under the false name of Dragan David Dabić. A published poet and author of one children's book, a psychiatrist and apparently successful and charismatic alternative healer, and yet responsible for massive crimes against humanity in Bosnia 1992–5 (with the killing of approximately eight thousand Muslim males at Srebrenica as the most egregious), Karadžić is a hieroglyph of recent post-Yugoslav history that I will not even attempt to decipher here. It suffices to note, however, that his successful cover attests to the relative 'normalcy' of alternative medicine in the former Yugoslavia.

Other prominent psychiatrists in Serbia at the same period were Jovan Marić,[17] Dragan Kecmanović,[18] Vladeta Jerotić, and Bokun himself. It is interesting also to note the profiles of those who have recently written about Kremna: Pjević is an engineer, Ršumović is a geologist – a scientific expert on soil and stone (of our land). Psychiatrists are experts on the collective psyche, or national character (which is rooted in our soil/rock). Todorović is an immunologist and inventor of *Todoxin* – a very popular (and expensive) poultice reputed to boost immunity, and cure not just herpes, but even AIDS. He is an expert in the perils and pollutions threatening the body, and in ways of strengthening its internal defences, while prophecies he receives in his dreams from Tesla, Tarabić's, Pupin, and other illustrious Serbs could be seen as a sort of '*Todoxin*' for the National Body.

To sum up. Kremna is the Serbian Delphi (Bokun mentions that Delphi is on the same altitude as Kremna), a place of celestial impact, miraculous stone, clean air, healing clear water and extraordinarily potent plants. It is a Noah's Ark for Serbs from all the world where they will find the only safe refuge after the Ecological Catastrophe of World War 3. Kremna is a microcosm of the country of which it is a part, and fatefully linked to its rulers throughout history. Those rulers who listen to Kremanci will prosper and bring prosperity to the country; those who don't are doomed. Nemanjići built their villas there, and St Sava left his footprints. Kremna is a natural, open-air cathedral and an Orthodox Temple, a Serbian Mecca and Hilandar in Serbia that all Serbs should make a pilgrimage to at least once in their lifetime. Zaharije is an autochtonous genius of psychological warfare in the best interests of Serbdom. Kremna is the centre of Serbdom and home to peasant-cosmopolitans of unusual mental powers. And it is the Orthodox Church that is deeply involved in all this. There is Zaharije, a priest of no small influence in Serbia of his time, followed by the pivotal Kremna prophecy disseminator, the ethno-theologian Kazimirović, and last, but by no means the least, Kazimirović's classmate and good friend who wrote the Introduction to his 1941 book – who turns out to be none other than the 77th Saint of the Serbian Orthodox Church, St Nikolaj Velimirović of Serbia.

In a contest for the most essentially, archetypally Serbian village, Kremna would be a contender, especially if your notion of Serbdom geographically encompasses the Bosnian Serbs as well as Serbia proper. In Serbia proper, a village that represented the Serbian heartland would perhaps be a stronger one, but if the 'Western Serb lands' are both literally and symbolically limestone, and the heartland is mud, then Kremna could be seen as a good mediator between the wild highlander's stone and lowlander's soft soil. Surely, a place that combined Delphi, Hilandar (or Mecca), Noah's Ark and St Sava's footsteps with quick-witted borderguard peasant-cosmopolitans, mastermind priests, stone, air and water that bring health, longevity and clairvoyance, must be a contender indeed.

Let me now quickly finish recounting our first trip because we visited two more places that offer good points of comparison to the Family of Clear Streams, Drvengrad and Kremna.

First we paid a visit to Sirogojno, the home of well-known homespun raw wool sweaters with folkloric motifs – a good example of socialist ethno-enterprise. We visited the 'Old Village' there – an ethnological museum in the open that combines meticulously reconstructed peasant households of the Zlatibor type with tasty and well-appointed bungalows in the same rural style. This is indeed an ethno-village constructed according to the strictest criteria of ethnological science. There is a great deal of attention to detail and a painstaking effort to use the actual buildings taken from nearby villages rather than build new models. I visited the village in 1995 when it was still quite new, and it looked as well kept in 2007 as it was then. It was quiet and there were a few guests mulling around. The sweaters were being sold in a double row of about a dozen or so stalls on top of the hill. There was a church there as well, but the town itself seemed very much to be like it was in socialist times.

And finally, we passed through Zlatibor itself. I was warned repeatedly but still got shocked by how the place has changed. It was a favourite resort way back then when I visited as a young boy, but instead of one hotel (Palisad) there is now a huge, densely packed summer villa-city stretching as far as you could see, and a town made of cafes and boutiques of a density and acreage not to be seen in Belgrade itself. My quest has been to find the 'Tower of Milić of Machva' – an exotic local attraction in the old days. I remember it being quite a walk through empty fields to get there. It was a wooden house built in an exaggerated and eccentric 'ethno' style, uninhabited even then in the 1970s but somehow enchanting. Elsewhere I showed how Milić, the Mad Painter, channelled and scrambled together the Byzantine Great Tradition, Serbs as the Most Ancient People and the Peasant Volksgeist (Ethno).[19] His style was a mix of Salvador Dali, Pieter Brueghel, Hieronymus Bosch and local naïve painters, and he mixed peasants, icons and Lepenski Vir figurines with his trademark flying logs. He was a major proponent of Serbs as the Most Ancient people theories in the 1990s, and a self-styled high priest of a more populist version of that neo-Byzantinism mixed with the Balkan magic realism that Milorad Pavić of the *Khazar Diction-ary* fame represented at the more elite/intellectual end of the spectrum.

We found the Tower, still abandoned (the family is in estate dispute after his death) with buildings added to the old wooden one I remember, but this time densely surrounded by summer villas. It was very hard to find, and nobody seemed to pay attention to it. *Sic transit gloria mundi*. And yet, I felt that this was the germ out of which the Splendid Wooden Town of Oz has sprung, that this one house was the seed, and Milić of Machva Kusturica's forerunner and spiritual father. For here too, you could see a self-indulgent (Balkan Dali-esque) self-exoticizing play on the ethno theme, the antics of a Balkan Barbarogenius, a shimmering undecidability between irony and seriousness. Milić's was a search for the autochthony of autochthonies, a movement of turning inside and digging into soil and depths of time in search of that archetypal, pristine essence that makes us most truly ourselves. Kusturica adds Gypsies and their ambiguity as a trope that has long made them so useful for Serbs as a mode of self-display/self-criticism.[20] He has taken over Milić's mantle but made it a cosmopolitan brand. I couldn't resist the feeling that there was a genetic connection between Milić's abandoned tower and Drvengrad, just a few miles away, and that the logs that pave the streets of Drvengrad were the flying logs taken from Milić's paintings and cut into sections.

Eco, Ethno, and St Sava as Aboriginal Ancestor

So how far can we go thinking with these places? The Family of Clear Streams is about the eco. The houses are rural, but this ethno aspect is assimilated to a 'planetaristic' ideology of local eco-patriotism. Boža loves his beech, hornbeam and oak trees not because they are Serbian, but because they are local *nature*. He comes from a milieu of 1960s artistic experimentation in Tito's Yugoslavia, heady times that produced extraordinary achievements. I am sure that his refer-ence to Wilhelm Reich's Orgone Accumulators comes easily to someone who belonged to the same circle as Dušan Makavejev of *William Reich: Mysteries of the Organism* fame. No St Sava here, and no Orthodoxy.

Drvengrad and Sirogojno Old Village are mediated by Milić's abandoned Tower. Old Village is a scientific reconstruction of peasant homesteads, a serious

Ethnological Museum in the Open. No mixing of genres here, and no St Sava or Orthodoxy either. Kusturica's Drvengrad is Milić's tongue-in-cheek self-exoticizing made Cosmopolitan – Serbian bizarreness for the International Jetset.

Kremna is in competition with Drvengrad. The competition is obviously for tourist revenue, but it involves political patronage including that of Premier Koštunica himself. There is convoluted local politics and economics that meshes with the current Serbian neo-feudal capitalism at play here that needs to be seriously taken into account.

Eco and *ethno* seem to have an elective affinity in the dream logic of Serbian places of power. What is authentically *ethno* is by definition pristine, unspoilt (by modernity, industry, civilization, culture) thus close to nature, hale, whole, healthy, and wholesome. What is *ethno* is by definition also *eco*. And what is *eco*, since it is close to pure nature, is also *ethno* since the local almost inadvertently takes on some hues of *ethno* (from the way houses are built to the images of animal husbandry and community with local peasant neighbours). A retreat from the City to the Nature, as in the very clear example of the Clear Stream Family, happens concretely to be a return to village, thus the peasant way of life is idealized as gift economy and ecologically pristine.

Eco and *ethno* also share the logic of what Marilyn Ivy (1995) writing of Japan calls the receding remainders of modernity. Since modernity comes from foreign places (see Greenfeld 1992) and spreads outward from the local urban centres (Belgrade, Tokyo) erasing its opposite, the traditional/autochtonous in the process, the remnants of autochthony/tradition, that is, the 'true' national identity, can only be found in ever receding (vanishing) places.[21] In that sense, the provincial, the remote, the marginal, and peripheral become the locus of the authentic. In Japan and in Serbia this could be the literal remote – far away from the Centre (Belgrade, Tokyo) or remote vertically – i.e. mountains as the refugee of the authentic. In Japan and in Serbia this dynamic is very much evident in tourist discourses.

Eco and *ethno*, however, seem to be very significantly mediated and legitimated in present day Serbia by perhaps the most powerful ideological force – the Serbian Orthodox Church. The Church has emerged as the central clearing house and legitimator of beliefs and practices of place in Serbia. Through it are channeled all kinds of 'pagan' and New Age beliefs, and it anoints historical as well as natural sites as uniquely Serbian and worthy of respect, worship or healing pilgrimages.

I prefer, however, to give a special name to this aspect of Serbian Orthodoxy insofar as it acts as a legitimator of a particular Serbian ideology (or imaginary or dreamworld) I am concerned with here. I propose to call it 'Srboslavlje' (lit. SerbWorship) rather than 'Pravoslavlje' (the usual word for Serbian Orthodoxy, lit. RightWorship), for what I am talking about has really little to do with Christianity as a universal religion but rather with Ethno Self-Worship. The God of Serbodoxy is Serbian, and St Sava is his avatar, in fact, his only Son and Serbo-Christ himself.

Both Kremna and Drvengrad, players for higher stakes than the relatively marginalized Family of Clear Streams and Sirogojno Old Village, are claiming the most powerful patronage of all – that of St Sava and Serbodoxy.

The Kremna prophecy has been channelled (some say invented) by priests, EthnoTheologians, and sanctioned even by Nikolaj Velimirović himself, the most recently consecrated saint of the Serbian Orthodox Church. Emir Kusturica converted to Orthodoxy, changed his name into Nemanja and stuck the pointed church of St Sava in the dead centre of Drvengrad as his unassailable flag and ideological anchor – something that cleanses him of all his taints (one can think of Turkish, Gypsy and Cosmopolitan taints to start with).

Historians of religion have examined the extensive St Sava folklore as a syncretic amalgam of old pagan legends about peripatetic gods, origin of lakes, springs and other local topographic markers, and popular Christian cults of miraculously curative springs near monasteries, healing tombs and relics, and so on.[22] The St Sava cult is a huge topic and needs much research. But I trust my instinct of heeding the words of the living saint of Serbian Poetry, Matija Bećković in this case, as in all matters of the Serbian Dreamworld, for he is perhaps its most powerful mouthpiece. And I will go straight to what Matija has to say about St Sava.

> The whole of Serbian soil is adorned with Sava's name, from the Sava field by the Hilandar – all the way through river Sava, Savine, Savince, Savovo, Savovska, Savovac, Savino selo – to Sava's spring on top of Mt Durmitor. Following Sava's footsteps, on Sava's soil, it is possible to travel from Sava's monastery to Sava's monastery. The Serbian soil is the visible hagiography of St Sava. *Serbian geography is the objectified biography of St Sava.*
>
> In this soil Sava's footsteps, foothills, mountains, springs, rocks, chairs, dining tables [*trpeze*], dwelling places forever remain. Eternalized are his stone sandals [*opanci*], imprints of his bedding [*postelja*], his walking stick and the water gourd. Sava's ribs remain imprinted so as to be visible on whole regions for all time. *This is the longest rib our man has ever had and from it we are all chiseled out* [*To je najduže rebro koje je imao naš covek i od njega smo svi istesani*].[23]

As a mythic ancestor, St Sava has left his imprints all over Serbian soil – in fact, 'Serbian geography is objectified biography of St Sava'. Those familiar with classical anthropological writings on Australian Aborigines and their relationship to their landscape will recognize the almost identical pattern that Bećković lays down here in his poetic exaltation, without the benefit, I am pretty sure, of having any acquaintance with this literature.[24]

But one doesn't have to be immersed in Bećković's national metaphysics in order to seek some sort of healing in particular places that dot the Serbian landscape conceived in some manner vaguely akin to 'dreamtime' of Australian Aborigines or Apache Places of Wisdom as analysed by Basso.[25] Drvengrad attracts not only with Kusturica's charisma and Western recognition, but also as an 'air spa' – a place where one can combine the goodness of *eco* and *ethno* and at the same time accrue health benefits. The Family of Clear Streams has over years attracted variously disturbed people and offered them 'narrative warmth', clean air, simple food, and even Reichian 'orgone accumulators' produced by old local housebuilding craft.

Zlatibor has long been known as a prime 'air spa' offering plentiful health benefits. New places of renown also tend to covet the 'air spa' designation. It is my hypothesis that places that have accumulated some sort of renown, be it historical, national or natural, will also tend to 'attract' (or claim for themselves) other kinds of power, most notably, some sort of healing power. It is as if other kinds of renown or notoriety become healing in themselves. One doesn't need to stray too far from classical Durkheimian insights here. Nations are our social bodies charged with collective force. If they tend, as they do, to get objectified as national landscape (among other things), then this social body, conceived analogously to human body, could have nodes or loci of concentrated power (daoist meridians and acupuncture points) objectified as particular named places. Pilgrimages to such places and ritual acts performed there (even under the guise of tourism) could then effect changes in the physical body by operating on the social body as an 'expressive-iconic model'.[26]

As a final illustration, I offer the strange case of Najdan's circles. A local dowser, Najdan Rakić discovered a healing circle about 3m in diameter in the village of Mala Krsna near Smederevo in 1999. It is located in a private yard and is regularly visited by people seeking remedy for various illnesses by standing within the circle for ten to twenty minutes on two consecutive days followed by another session after thirteen days. Claims about miraculous cures have spread widely through word of mouth and have been publicized in the popular press. It is interesting that other places appeared subsequently that claim to have Najdan's circles. When we were in Kremna we met a couple from Zrenjanin (in Vojvodina) who were visiting with their teenage daughter. They gave me contact phone numbers for Najdan's relatives who could tell me more (Najdan himself having died a couple of years previous). Our host, Dragan Pjević, the curator and promoter of the Kremna prophecy, then promptly claimed that Najdan's circles have been positively identified in Kremna as well, and that they might be even more powerful than the original ones. Whatever the truth of this, the logic makes sense – there is nothing surprising about such a powerful place as Kremna also boasting the positive, healing energies of Najdan circles. Mala Krsna, and the private yard of housewife Jelka Petrović have very little going for them in terms of rich histori-cal, mystical, national or natural associations.[27] I wouldn't be surprised if Najdan circles eventually migrate to more prominent places such as Kremna (especially if the process is helped along by such relentless promoters as Pjević).

Places emerge from comparison with other places. When places are compared you learn a lot about values of those who do the comparing – what emerges is a (wavering, ambiguous) image of good lives and good people, good communities. What can also emerge from a controlled comparison of places are the implicit and unsystematic, and yet culturally specific popular 'theories' of health, illness and healing. What studying places and practices associated with them might fur-ther reveal is how these 'theories' relate to notions of community, and of group history and identity for which places tend to be important anchors or 'pegs'.

NOTES

Introduction

1. A. Young, 'The Anthropologies of Illness and Sickness', *Annual Review of Anthropology*, 11 (1982), pp. 257–85.

2. See for example, C. Briggs and C. Mantini-Briggs, *Stories in the Time of Cholera: Racial Profiling During a Medical Nightmare* (Berkeley, CA: University of California Press, 2003), for an excellent and current example.

3. N. Adelson, 'The Embodiment of Inequity: Health Disparities in Aboriginal Canada', *Canadian Journal of Public Health* 96, Supp. 2 (2005), pp. S45–S61 provides a comprehensive argument supporting this position in Canada.

4. Valliantos's chapter (this volume) draws on this tradition in locating women's bodies in resource-poor spaces and subsequently as spaces in their own right. Das and Das (V. Das and R. K. Das, 'How the Body Speaks': Illness and the Lifeworld among the Urban Poor', in J. Bieh, B. Good and A. Kleinman (eds) *Subjectivitiy: Ethnographic Investigation.* Berkeley: University of California Press, 2007, pp. 66–97), have likewise brought attention to how subjectivities and illness experience are enmeshed in the mass habitations of urban slums. Finally, Ramphela (M. Ramphela, *A Bed Called Home: Life in the Migrant Labour Hostels of Cape Town* (Cape Town: New Africa Books, 1993), addresses the minimalist space of the 'bed-hold' in the constitution of migrant workers in South African townships.

5. E. S. Casey, 'How to Get from Space to Place in a Farly Short Stretch of Time', in S. Feld and K. H. Basso (eds) *Senses of Place* (Sante Fe, CA: School of American Research, 1986), p. 46.

6. N. Lovell, 'Introduction',in *Locality and Belonging.* London: Routledge, 1998, pp. 1–24. K. Basso, '"Speaking with Names": Language and Landscape among the Western Apache', *Cultural Anthropology*, 3:2 (1988), pp. 99–130. J. P. Brosius, 'Analyses and Interventions: Anthropological Engagements with Environmentalism', *Current Anthropology*, 40:3 (1999), pp. 277–309.

7. Sahlins begins *Islands of History* (Chicago, IL: University of Chicago Press, 1985) 'History is culturally ordered, differently so in different societies, according to meaningful schemes of things. The converse is also true: cultural schemes are historically ordered, since to a greater of lesser extent the meanings are revalued as they are practically enacted. The synthesis of these contraries unfolds in the creative action of the historic subjects, the people concerned', p. vii.

8. In particular see: A. Baker, *Geography and History: Bridging the Divide* (Cambridge: Cambridge University Press, 2003); C. Harris, *Making Native Space: Colonialism,*

Resistance, and Reserves in British Columbia (Vancouver: University of British Columbia Press, 2002); A. K. Knowles (ed.), *Placing History: How Maps, Spatial Data, and GIS are Changing Historical Scholarship* (Redlands, California: ESRI, 2008); C. Philo, *A Geographical History of Institutional Provision for the Insane from Medieval Times to the 1860s in England and Wales: The Space Reserved for Insanity* (Lewiston and Queenston: Edwin Mellen Press, 2004); and D. Livingstone, *Putting Science in its Place: Geographies of Scientific Knowledge* (Chicago, IL: University of Chicago Press, 2003).

9.   See for example: J. Reinarz (ed.) *Medicine and Society in the Midlands, 1750–1950* (Midland History Occasional Publications, 2007); and special volume with 7 articles and three reviews: P. Twohig (ed.), 'Written on the Landscape: Health and Regionalism in Canada', in *Journal of Canadian Studies*, 41:3 (2007).

10. D. N. Livingstone, *Putting Science in its Place: Geographies of Scientific Knowledge* (Chicago, IL: University of Chicago Press, 2003).

11. A. Kleinman, V. Das and M. Lock *Social Suffering* (Berkeley, CA: University of California Press, 1997). V. Das, *Remaking a World: Violence, Social Suffering, and Recovery* (Berkeley, CA: University of California Press, 2001).

12. M. Jackson, *Minima Ethnographica: Intersubjectivity and the Anthropological Project* (Chicago, IL: University of Chicago Press, 1998).

13. N. Scheper-Hughes and M. Lock. 'The Mindful Body: A Prolegomenon to Future Work in Medical Anthropology', *Medical Anthropology Quarterly*, new series, 1 (1987), p. 21.

1 Vallianatos, 'Placing Maternal Health in India'

1.   Maternal mortality was reported as 440 deaths per 100,000 live births in 1995, but has increased to 540 deaths by the early twenty-first century (UNDP 2007, 2008). Female literacy (aged fifteen and above) was 44.5 per cent in 1999, versus a male literacy rate of 67.8 per cent (UNDP 2001). This has increased slightly, to a literacy rate of 47.8 per cent for women and 73.4 per cent for men (UNDP 2007). Over 30 million women are said to be 'missing' in India, due to gender biases leading to premature death (including female feticide). The outcome is evident in unbalanced sex ratios favoring men (Sen 1992, 2003). A. K. Sen, 'Missing women', *British Medical Journal*, 304 (1992), pp. 586–7; A. K. Sen, 'Missing women – revisited', *British Medical Journal*, 327 (2003), pp. 1297–8.

2.   M. Lock, 1993, *Encounters with Aging: Mythologies of Menopause in Japan and North America* (Berkeley, CA: University of California Press, 1993).

3.   E. S. Casey, 'How to get from Space to Place in a Fairly Short Stretch of Time', in S. Feld and K. H. Basso (eds), *Senses of Place* (Santa Fe, NM: School of American Research, 1996), pp. 13–52; M. C. Rodman, 'Empowering Place: Multilocality and Multivocality', in S. M. Low and D. Lawrence-Zúñiga (eds), *The Anthropology of Space and Place* (1992; Malden, MA: Blackwell Publishing, 2003), pp. 204–23.

4.   Casey, 'How to get from Space to Place', pp. 13–52; T. Csordas, *Embodiment and Experience* (Cambridge: Cambridge University Press. 1994); M. Richardson, 'Being-in-the-Market versus Being-in-the-Plaza: Material Culture and the Construction of Social Reality in Spanish America', in Low and Lawrence-Zúñiga (eds), *The Anthropology of Space and Place*, pp. 74–91.

5.   K. H. Basso, 'Wisdom Sits in Places: Notes on a Western Apache Landscape', in Feld and Basso (eds), *Senses of Place* (Santa Fe, NM: School of American Research, 1996), pp. 53–90; S. M. Low and D. Lawrence-Zúñiga, 'Locating Culture', in Low and Lawrence-

Zúñiga (eds), *The Anthropology of Space and Place* (Malden, MA: Blackwell Publishing, 2003), pp. 1–47; Rodman, 'Empowering Place', pp. 204–23.

6. H. J. Nast and S. Pile, 'Introduction: MakingPlacesBodies', in H. J. Nast and S. Pile (eds), *Places Through the Body* (London: Routledge. 1998), pp. 1–19.

7. Rodman, 'Empowering Place', pp. 204–23.

8. Consult H. Vallianatos, *Poor and Pregnant in New Delhi, India* (International Institute for Qualitative Methodology Series. Walnut Creek, CA: Left Coast Press, 2007).

9. A. Bose, *India's Billion Plus People: 2001 Census Highlights, Methodology and Media Coverage* (New Delhi: B.R. Publishing Corporation, 2001).

10. GNCTD (Government of the National Capital Territory of Delhi), 2002, Economic Survey of Delhi, 2001–2.

11. World Bank, *Attacking Poverty: World Development Report 2000/2001* (New York: Oxford University Press, 2001).

12. See A. Ali, 'Nutrition', in A. Mukhopadhyay (ed.), *State of India's Health* (New Delhi: Voluntary Health Association of India, 1992), pp. 1–50; R. Balakrishnan (ed.), *The Hidden Assembly Line: Gender Dynamics of Subcontracted Work in a Global Economy* (West Hartford, CT: Kumarian Press, 2002); L. Benería and S. Feldman, *Unequal Burden: Economic Crisis, Persistent Poverty and Women's Work* (Boulder, CO: Westview Press, 1992); C. D. Deere, H. Safa, and P. Antrobus, 'Impact of the Economic Crisis on Poor Women and their Households', in N. Visvanathan, L. Duggan, L. Nisonoff and N. Wiegersma (eds.), *The Women, Gender & Development Reader* (London: Zed Books, 1997), pp. 267–7; T. Manuh, 'Ghana: Women in the Public and Informal Sectors under the Economic Recovery Programme', in N. Visvanathan, L. Duggan, L. Nisonoff and N. Wiegersma (eds), *The Women, Gender & Development Reader* (London: Zed Books, 1997), pp. 277–84; F. Meer (ed.), *Poverty in the 1990's: The Responses of Urban Women* (Tours: UNESCO and ISSC, 1994); K. Staudt, *Policy, Politics & Gender* (West Hartford, CT: Kumarian Press, 1998); M. Swaminathan, *Weakening Welfare: The Public Distribution of Food in India* (New Delhi: LeftWord Books, 2000); UNDP (United Nations Development Programme), *Human Development Report* (New York: Oxford University Press, 1995).

13. See Vallianatos, *Poor and Pregnant* for a more in-depth description.

14. P. Berman and P. Dave, 'Financing Health Care', in A. Mukhopadhyay (ed.), *State of India's Health* (New Delhi: Voluntary Health Association of India, 1992), pp. 341–9; A. Mukhopadhyay, 'Health Systems and Services', in A. Mukhopadhyay (ed.), *State of India's Health* (New Delhi: Voluntary Health Association of India, 1992), pp. 53–85.

15. A. Islam and M. Z. Tahir, 'Health Sector Reform in South Asia: New Challenges and Constraints', *Health Policy*, 60 (2002), pp. 151–69.

16. A. Mukhopadhyay (ed.), *Report of the Independent Commission of Health in India* (New Delhi: Voluntary Health Association of India, 1997).

17. Ibid.; B. C. Purohit, 'Private Initiatives and Policy Options: Recent Health System Experience in India', *Health Policy and Planning*, 16 (2001), pp. 87–97.

18. I. Qadeer, 'Health Care Systems in Transition III: India, Part I. The Indian experience', *Journal of Public Health Medicine*, 22 (2000), pp. 25–32.

19. World Bank, *Attacking Poverty*.

20. Mukhopadhyay, *Report*.

21. *Ibid.*

22. Purohit, 'Private Initiatives'.

23. Ali, 'Nutrition'; Mukhopadhyay (ed.), *Report*; Swaminathan, *Weakening Welfare*.

24. B. Kang and A. Pillai, 'Starved of Logic', *Outlook*, 41 (2001), pp. 22–8; B. K. Taimni, *Food Security in the 21 Century* (Delhi: Konark Publishers PVT Ltd, 2001).

25. In 2001, US$1 was approximately equal to Rs. See Taimni, *Food Security*, p. 45.

26. R. Radhakrishna and K. Subbarao, *India's Public Distribution System: A National and International Perspective* (Washington, DC: World Bank, 1997).

27. Swaminathan, *Weakening Welfare*.

28. GNCTD, 2002.

29. See J. C. Bhatia & J. Cleland, 'Health-Care Seeking and Expenditure by Young Indian Mothers in the Public and Private Sectors', *Health Policy and Planning*, 16 (2001), pp. 55–61; V. R. Kutty, 'Historical Analysis of the Development of Health Care Facilities in Kerala State, India', *Health Policy and Planning*, 15 (2000), pp. 103–9.

30. Vallianatos, *Poor and Pregnant*.

31. GOI (Government of India), *Annual Report 2000–2001* (New Delhi: Department of Health, Ministry of Health & Family Welfare, 2001); K. Mitra and K. Basu, 'Health problems and practices of slum women in Delhi', *South Asian Anthropologist*, 19 (1998), pp. 37–43; R. Nagarajan, in 'Delhi's government hospital: Have a baby, get abuses for free', *Hindustan Times* (Retrieved 20 June 2003, from http://www.hindustantimes.com, 3 November 2002); Vallianatos, *Poor and Pregnant*.

32. GNCTD, 2002.

33. Vallianatos, *Poor and Pregnant*.

34. Ibid.

35. Ibid.

36. See A. M. Basu, 'Is Discrimination in Food Really Necessary for Explaining Sex Differentials in Childhood Mortality?', *Population Studies*, 43 (1989), pp. 193–210; J. Caldwell and P. Caldwell, 'Patriarchy, gender, and family discrimination, and the role of women', in L. C. Chen, A. Kleinman and N.C. Ware (eds), *Health and Social Change in International Perspective* (Boston, MA: Harvard University Press, 1994), pp.339–71; B. Harriss, 'The Intrafamily Distribution of Hunger in South Asia', in J. Drèze, A. Sen and A. Hussain (eds), *The Political Economy of Hunger: Selected Essays* (Oxford: Clarendon Press, 1995), pp. 224–97; D. Jacobson and S. S. Wadley, *Women in India: Two Perspectives* (New Delhi: Manohar, 1995); D. Kandiyoti, 'Gender, Power and Contestation: "Rethinking Bargaining with Patriarchy"', in C. Jackson and R. Pearson (eds), *Feminist Visions of Development: Gender Analysis and Policy* (London: Routledge, 1998), pp. 135–51; D. G. Mandelbaum, *Women's Seclusion and Men's Honor: Sex Roles in North India, Bangladesh, and Pakistan* (Tucson, AZ: University of Arizona Press, 1988); B. D. Miller, *The Endangered Sex: Neglect of Female Children in Rural North India* (1981; Delhi: Oxford University Press, 1981); G. Santow, 'Social Roles and Physical Health: the Case of Female Disadvantage in Poor Countries', *Social Science and Medicine*, 40 (1995), pp. 147–61.

37. Nast, 'Introduction: MakingPlacesBodies', pp. 1–19.

38. Consult S. Derné, *Culture in Action: Family Life, Emotion, and Male Dominance in Banaras, India* (Albany, NY: State University of New York Press, 1995); S. K. Khanna, '*Shahri* Jat and *Dehati Jatni*: the Indian Peasant Community in Transition', *Contemporary South Asia*, 10 (2001), pp. 37–53; M. N. Srinivas, *Village, Caste, Gender and Method: Essays of Indian Social Anthropology* (Delhi: Oxford University Press, 1998).

39. P. Kolenda, *Regional Differences in Family Structure in India* (Jaipur: Rawat Publications, 1987).

40. See S. K. Khanna, 'Traditions and reproductive technology in an urbanizing North Indian village', *Social Science and Medicine*, 44 (1997), pp. 171–80; Mandelbaum, *Women's Seclusion*; Jacobson & Wadley, *Women In India*.

41. See G. Eichinger Ferro-Luzzi, 'Food Avoidances of Pregnant Women in Tamilnad', in J. R. K. Robson (ed.), *Food, Ecology and Culture: Readings in the Anthropology of Dietary Practices* (New York: Gordon and Breach Science Publishers, 1980), pp. 101–8; I. Hutter, *Being Pregnant in Rural South India: Nutrition of Women and Well-being of Children* (Amsterdam: PDOD Publications/Thesis Publishers, 1994); P. Jeffery, R. Jeffery and A. Lyon, *Labour Pains and Labour Power: Women and Childbearing in India* (London: Zed Books Ltd, 1989); M. Nichter & M. Nichter, 'The Ethnophysiology and Folk Dietetics of Pregnancy: A Case Study from South India', in M. Nichter and M. Nichter (eds), *Anthropology and International Health: Asian Case Studies* (Amsterdam: Gordon and Breach Publishers, 1996), pp. 35–69; M. Rao, 'Food Beliefs of Rural Women during the Reproductive Years in Dharwad, India', *Ecology of Food and Nutrition*, 16 (1985), pp. 93–103.

42. Eichinger Ferro-Luzzi, 'Food Avoidances'; Hutter, *Being Pregnant*; Jeffery, *Labour Pains*; Nichter, 'The Ethnophysiology'; Rao, 'Food Beliefs', Vallianatos, *Poor and Pregnant*.

43. Vallianatos, *Poor and Pregnant*.

44. This is not to neglect the range of relationships that mother- and daughter-in-laws do have. While the hierarchy remains, the everyday practices demonstrating this hierarchy were quite variable, from friendly, equitable relations to contentious, troubled relationships. It was interesting to me though, to hear many daughter-in-laws admitting that when they became mother-in-laws, their behaviours would not be so distinctive from what they themselves had experienced. In other words, many expected to repeat histories of family hierarchies.

45. Vallianatos, *Poor and Pregnant*.

46. A type of rice-based dish that may include vegetables, lentils or meat. Among the study participants, because of the economic situation, this dish was simple, containing a few cheaper vegetables or lentils.

47. Mung beans (*Vigna radiata*) that have been dehusked and split, with a flat, yellow appearance.

48. Nichter, 'The Ethnophysiology'.

49. S.C. Babu, S. Thirumaran and T.C. Mahanam, 'Agricultural Productivity, Seasonality and Gender Bias in Rural Nutrition: Empirical Evidence from South India', *Social Science and Medicine*, 37 (1993), pp. 1313–19; A. M. Basu, 'The Status of Women and the Quality of Life among the Poor', *Cambridge Journal of Economics*, 16 (1992), pp. 249–67; M. Chatterjee and J. Lambert, 'Women and Nutrition: Reflections from India and Pakistan', *Food and Nutrition Bulletin*, 11 (1989), pp. 13–28; Harriss, 'The Intrafamily'; Kandiyoti, 'Gender'; Miller, *The Endangered*; Santow, 'Social Roles'.

50. Vallianatos, *Poor and Pregnant*.

51. GNCTD, 2002.

52. B. Bogin and R. Keep, 'Eight Thousand Years of Economic and Political History in Latin America Revealed by Anthropometry', *Annals of Human Biology*, 26 (1999), pp. 333–51; J. M. Tanner, 'Growth as a Measure of Nutritional and Hygienic Status of a Population', *Hormone Research*, 38 (suppl 1) (1992), pp. 106–15.

53. (Vallianatos 2007; WHO 1995) Vallianatos, *Poor and Pregnant*.

54. IOM (Institute of Medicine), *Nutrition During Pregnancy. Part I, Weight Gain; Part II, Nutrient Supplements*, Committee on Nutritional Status During Pregnancy and Lactation, Food and Nutrition Board (Washington, DC: National Academy Press, 1990); Vallianatos, *Poor and Pregnant*;

55. Vallianatos, *Poor and Pregnant*.

56. Consult ibid.

2 Reinarz, 'Putting Medicine in its Place'

1. S. Ward, 'On Shifting Ground: Changing Formulations of Place in Anthropology', *Australian Journal of Anthropology*, 14:1 (2003), pp. 80–97; P. Levitt and M. Waters (eds), *The Changing Face of Home: The Transnational Lives of the Second Generation* (New York: Russell Sage Foundation, 2002); C. Gallaher, C. T. Dahlman, M. Gilmartin, A. Mountz, P. Shirlow, *Key Concepts in Political Geography* (London: Sage, 2009), pp. 291–92.

2. Ward, 'On Shifting Ground', p. 92.

3. T. Cresswell, *Place: a Short Introduction* (Oxford: Blackwell Publishing, 2004), p. 1.

4. Ibid.

5. Ibid.

6. Ibid., p. 12.

7. S. Shapin, 'Placing the View from Nowhere: Historical and Sociological Problems in the Location of Science', *Transactions of the Institute of British Geographers*, 23 (1998), pp. 5–12; D. Livingstone, *Putting Science in its Place: Geographies of Scientific Knowledge* (Chicago, IL: University of Chicago Press, 2003).

8. N. Rupke, 'Introduction: Historical Geographies of Science', in Rupke (ed.), *Medical Geography in Historical Perspective* (London: Wellcome Trust, 2000), p. 9.

9. Livingstone, *Putting Science in its Place*.

10. Ibid., p. 11.

11. M. Dettelbach, 'Humboltian Science', in N. Jardine, J. Secord and E. Spary (eds), *Cultures of Natural History* (Cambridge: Cambridge University Press, 1996), p. 298.

12. E. Ackernecht, *Medicine at the Paris Hospital, 1794–1848* (Baltimore, MD: Johns Hopkins Press, 1967); S. Lawrence, *Charitable Knowledge: Hospital Pupils and Practitioners in Eighteenth-Century London* (Cambridge: Cambridge University Press, 1996); J. Reinarz, *Medicine and Society in the Midlands, 1750–1950* (Birmingham: Midland History Society, 2007).

13. E. Jenner, *An Inquiry into the Causes and Effects of the Variolae Vaccinae: a Disease Discovered in some of the Western Counties of England, Particularly Gloucestershire, and known by the Name of the Cow Pox* (London, 1798).

14. H. A. Waldron, 'James Hardy and the Devonshire Colic', *Medical History*, 13 (1969), pp. 74–81; S. Q. Saikat, J. Carter, A. Mehra, B. Smith and A. Stewart, 'Goitre and Environmental Iodine Deficiency in the UK – Derbyshire: A Review', *Environmental Geochemistry and Health*, 26 (2004), pp. 395–401.

15. Riley, *The Eighteenth-Century Campaign to Avoid Disease*, p. 87, p. 104.

16. J.H. Warner, 'The Idea of Southern Medical Distinctiveness: Medical Knowledge and Practice in the Old South', in J.W. Leavitt and R. L. Numbers (eds), Sickness & Health in America: Readings in the History of Medicine and Public Health. (Madison, WI: University of Wisconsin Press, 1985), p. 88.

17. Ibid., p. 61.

18. Inkster and J. Morrell, *Metropolis and Province: Science and British Culture, 1780–1850* (Philadelphia, PA: University of Pennsylvania Press, 1983).

19. Ibid.; Naylor, 'Introduction', p. 6.

20. H. Marland, *Medicine and Society in Wakefield and Huddersfield, 1780–1870* (Cambridge: Cambridge University Press, 1989); J. V. Pickstone, *Medicine and Industrial Society: A History of Hospital Development in Manchester and its Region, 1752–1946* (Manchester: Manchester University Press, 1985).

21. The regional studies of Scottish medicine are far too numerous to list. For Welsh medicine, see A. Borsay (ed.), *Medicine in Wales: 1800–2000: Public Service or Private*

Commodity? (Cardiff: University of Wales Press, 2003); P. Michael and C. Webster (eds), *Health and Society in Wales, 1800–2000* (Cardiff: University of Wales Press, 2006); A. Roberts, *The Welsh National School of Medicine: The Cardiff Years, 1893–1931* (Chicago, IL: University of Chicago Press, 2009).

22. See, for example, J. Lane, 'A Provincial Surgeon and his Obstetric Practice: Thomas W. Jones of Henley-in-Arden, 1764–1846', *Medical History*, 31:3 (1987), pp. 333–48.
23. J. Lane, *A Social History of Medicine: Health, Healing and Disease in England, 1750–1950* (London: Routledge, 2001).
24. Cresswell, *Place*, pp. 26, 97.
25. E. Hopkins, *Birmingham: The Making of the Second City, 1850–1939* (Stroud: Tempus, 2001), p. 12.
26. E. Hopkins, *The Rise of the Manufacturing Town: Birmingham and the Industrial Revolution* (Stroud: Sutton Publishing, 1998), p. 5.
27. Lane, *A Social History of Medicine*, p. 23.
28. J. Reinarz, *The Birth of a Provincial Hospital: The Early Years of the General Hospital, Birmingham, 1765–90* (Stratford: The Dugdale Society, 2003), pp. 3–13.
29. Cresswell, *Place*, pp. 15–51.
30. J. Reinarz, 'The Transformation of Medical Education in Eighteenth Century England: International Developments and the West Midlands', *History of Education* (2008), pp. 558–9.
31. Tomlinson, *Medical Miscellany*, p. v.
32. Ibid., pp. 203–4.
33. University of Birmingham Special Collections (UBSC), Birmingham Dispensary, Annual Report, 1840.
34. Tomlinson, *Medical Miscellany*, p. 89.
35. J. Darwall, *De Morbis Artificum*. Edinburgh, 1821.
36. J. Darwall, 'Observations on the Medical Topography of Birmingham, and the Health of Inhabitants', *Midland Medical and Surgical Register*, 2 (1830), p. 111.
37. J. Darwall, 'Introductory Lecture to a Course of Lectures on Botany, Delivered at the Birmingham School of Medicine and Surgery', *Midland Medical and Surgical Register*, 1 (1828–9), pp. 118–30.
38. UBSC, Birmingham Dispensary, Annual Report, 1840.
39. Riley, *The Eighteenth-Century Campaign to Avoid Disease*, p. 10.
40. J. T. J. Morrison, *William Sands Cox*, pp. 98–9.
41. D. Livingstone, *Putting Science in its Place: Geographies of Scientific Knowledge* (Chicago, IL: University of Chicago Press, 2003), p. 3.
42. Ibid.
43. L. Wilkinson and A. Hardy, *Prevention and Cure: The London School of Medicine and Tropic Hygiene* (London: Kegan Paul, 2000); J. Reinarz, *Health Care in Birmingham: The Birmingham Teaching Hospitals, 1779–1939* (Woodbridge, 2009), pp. 227–30.
44. Morrison, *William Sands Cox*, pp. 20–1.
45. Wilson, 'Conflict, Consensus and Charity: Politics and the Provincial Voluntary Hospitals in the Eighteenth Century', *English Historical Review* (1996), p. 602.
46. *Aris's Gazette*, 18 November 1765.
47. Hopkins, *The Rise of the Manufacturing Town*, pp. 28–30, 78–9.
48. Reinarz, *The Birth of a Provincial Hospital*, pp. 7–8.
49. The casualty service that evolved as a result of the Manchester Ship Canal project is less unfamiliar territory, see R. Cooter, *Surgery and Society in Peace and War* (London: Macmillan, 1993), pp. 100–3.

50. BCLA, General Hospital, Birmingham, Register of inpatient admissions, 1803–23, HC/GH/4/2/ .
51. BCLA, General Hospital, Annual Reports, 1803–6, MS 1921/414.
52. BCLA, Registers for medical and surgical inpatient admissions and discharges, August 1839–June 1848; July 1848–June 1858, HC/GH/4/2/13–14; 26; 33.
53. BCLA, General Hospital, Birmingham, General Committee Minute Book, 1766–84.
54. BCLA, General Hospital, Birmingham, Annual Reports, 1860, 1870, 1880, 1890, 1900, GHB 417–23; J. Reinarz, 'Charitable Bodies: The Funding of Birmingham's Voluntary Hospitals in the Nineteenth Century', in M. Gorsky and S. Sheard (eds), *Financing Medicine: The British Experience since 1750* (London: Routledge, 2006), p. 43.
55. Birmingham Central Library, Local Studies (BCLLS), Birmingham Eye Hospital, Annual Report, 1884.
56. BCLLS, Queen's Hospital, Annual Report, 1848.
57. M. Gorsky and J. Mohan with T. Willis, *Mutualism and Health Care: British Hospital Contributory Schemes in the Twentieth Century* (Manchester: Manchester University Press, 2006), pp. 18–27.
58. *Birmingham Daily Post*, 17 March 1873.
59. Gorsky and Moran, *Mutualism and Health Care*, p. 37.
60. J. L. Bronstein, *Caught in the Machinery: Workplace Accidents and Injured Workers in Nineteenth-Century Britain* (Stanford, CA: Stanford University Press, 2007).
61. BCLLS, Birmingham Skin Hospital, Annual Reports, 1882–1900.
62. Census 1881; 1891.
63. R. Waterhouse, *Children in Hospital: A Hundred Years of Child Care in Birmingham* (London: Hutchinson, 1962), pp. 32–4.
64. BCLA, Birmingham Children's Hospital, Annual Report, 1862–1900, HC/BCH/1/14/1–7.
65. BCLA, Birmingham Children's Hospital, Medical Committee Minutes, 1861–8, HC/BCH/1/4/1.
66. BCLA, Children's Hospital, Annual Report, 1862–1900, HC/BCH/1/14/1–7.
67. E.M.R. Lomax, *Small and Special: The Development of Hospitals for Children in Victorian Britain* (London: Wellcome Institute for the History of Medicine, 1996), pp. 94, 182–3.
68. J. Woodward, *To Do the Sick No Harm: A Study of the British Voluntary Hospital System to 1875* (London: Routledge, 1974), pp. 127–37.
69. BCLA, Birmingham Children's Hospital, Medical Committee Minutes, 1861-8, HC/BCH/1/4/1.
70. C.A. Vince and J. T. Bunce, *History of the Corporation of Birmingham, 1885–99* (Birmingham: Cornish Brothers, 1902), pp. 108–13.
71. D. Guthrie, *The Royal Edinburgh Hospital for Sick Children, 1860–1960* (Edinburgh: E. & S. Livingstone Ltd, 1960), pp. 10–11.
72. Lomax, *Small and Special*, pp. 94, 180–90.
73. Thanks to Graham Mooney for assistance with this graph.
74. Lomax, *Small and Special*, p. 126.
75. Ibid., p. 94.
76. P. Harvey, *Up the Hill to Western Bank: A History of the Children's Hospital, Sheffield, 1876–1976* (Sheffield: J.W. Northend, 1976), pp. 55.
77. Naylor, 'Introduction', p. 10.

3 Mullally, 'Finding Place in *The Big-Little World of Doc Pritham*'

1. D. C. Wilson, *The Big-Little World of Doc Pritham* (New York: McGraw-Hill, 1971), front and back matter.
2. Ibid.
3. I have examined this in greater detail elsewhere in 'Canadian Medical Life-Writing and the Historical Imagination: Unpacking a Cape Breton Country Doctor's Black Bag', E. Heaman, A. Li and S. McKellar (eds), *Essays in Honour of Michael Bliss: Figuring the Social* (Toronto: University of Toronto Press, 2008), pp. 435–69.
4. M. Rutherdale, 'Nursing in the North and Writing for the South: The Work and Travels of Amy Wilson', in M. Rutherdale (ed.), *Caregiving on the Periphery* (Montreal and Kingston: McGill-Queen's University Press, 2010), pp. 158–80.
5. J. W. Leavitt, '"A Worrying Profession": The Domestic Environment of Medical Practice in Nineteenth-Century America', *Bulletin of the History of Medicine*, 69 (1995), pp. 1–29.
6. An early call for greater attention to regional frameworks in the history of medicine is C. E. Rosenberg and J. Golden (eds) *Framing Disease: Studies in Cultural History* (New Brunswick, NJ: Rutgers University Press, 1992). See especially pp. xiii–xxvi. Peter Twohig has noted a recent resurgence of interest in regional and local studies in Canadian health history as well. P. Twohig, 'Health and Region in Canada', *Journal of Canadian Studies*, 41:3 (2007): 5–17.
7. This literature developed from John Harley Warner, 'The Idea of Southern Medical Distinctiveness: Medical Knowledge and Practice in the Old South', in J. W. Leavitt and R. L. Numbers (eds), *Sickness and Health in America: Readings in the History of Medicine and Public Health*, 2nd edn (University of Wisconsin Press, 1985), pp. 53–70. Recent works include Sandra Barney's treatment of the particular way medical authority became gendered in Appalachia in *Authorized to Heal: Gender, Class, and the Transformation of Medicine in Central Appalachia, 1880–1930* (Chapel Hill, NC: University of North Carolina Press, 2000) and regional medical 'orthodoxies' derived from professional cultures and traditions of practice are likewise explored in S. Stowe, *Doctoring the South: Southern Physicians and Everyday Medicine in the Mid-Nineteenth Century* (Chapel Hill, NC: University of North Carolina Press, 2004).
8. He worked for the local railroads offering medical service and first aid in return for free use of the rails in his medical calls. Pritham also seems to have been a regular physician to the employees of the larger pulp and paper companies in northern Maine. On the occasion of his fifty-year anniversary in medical practice in 1956, he was honoured by the Great Northern Paper Company. A program for the event is kept in see Folio 8, Box 2073, Dorothy Clarke Wilson Collection, Fogler Library, University of Maine, Orono, ME [hereafter referred to as DCW Collection].
9. D. C. Wilson, *The Big-Little World of Doc Pritham*, pp. 24–5.
10. The medical school at Bowdoin would not survive the Flexnerian reforms, but when Pritham was a student, the curriculum required the last two years combining lectures and clinical rotation at the Maine General Hospital in Portland. Subjects for advanced classes included internal medicine, surgery, *materia medica*, therapeutics and obstetrics. His most absorbing interest was in surgery, although his training only allowed him to observe live cases. The biography recalls '[s]tudents were required to add bandages and dressings and perform operations on the cadavers under the supervision of instructors.'Ibid., pp. 37–8.

11. Pritham's practical experience as Externe House Office inspired his medical school thesis on 'Labour Abnormalus'.This was his only post-graduate training. Ibid., pp. 38–41.
12. Ibid., pp. 63–5.
13. Ibid., dust jacket.
14. Ibid., preface.
15. Ibid.
16. Ibid.
17. She later wrote, 'Even then the fabric of my future career as a biblical writer was being woven'. D. C. Wilson, *Twelve Who Cared: My Adventures with Christian Courage* (Chappaqua: Christian Herald Books, 1977) 12.
18. The only other man featured in her biographical works is Dr Paul Brand, a physician who pioneered a novel surgical approach to the treatment of leprosy. Ibid.
19. Ibid.
20. Ibid.
21. Dorothy Clarke Wilson, Personal Interview, 21 June 1999.
22. He makes special mention of a 'Voice of America' interview in his first telegram to Wilson over which he expressed regret. Telegram from Dr. F. Pritham to Dorothy Clarke Wilson, 18 March 1969. Folio 51, Box 2072, DCW Collection.
23. Wilson, *Twelve Who Cared*, p. 199.
24. Telegram from Dr. F. Pritham to Dorothy Clarke Wilson, 21 March 1969. Folio 51, Box 2072, DCW Collection. In an act of unspoken sarcastic retaliation, Wilson scrawled 'obvious burst of emotion ' to herself over his message.
25. The doctor supplied 'names of persons, descriptions of places, of horses, boats, cars, snowmobiles, lumber wagons, weather conditions, numbers of miles traveled, cases treated, operations', Wilson, *Twelve Who Cared*, pp. 203–4.
26. Dorothy Clarke Wilson, Personal Interview, 21 June 1999. She reiterates the importance of this source in her memoir. Wilson, *Twelve Who Cared*, p. 201.
27. Ibid., p. 208.
28. By all accounts, the doctor was just over five feet tall.
29. Ibid.
30. Sadie Pritham, for instance, found many of the journalists disrespectful. She remembered one particularly unlikable writer who landed unexpectedly one day demanding Pritham drop everything for the surprise interview. When his wife suggested he wait until the doctor was finished his work and talk to her in the meantime, he blustered, 'I've come to talk with a *real man!*' Ibid., p. 211.
31. Letter. Howard Pritham, Sr to Dorothy Clarke Wilson, 21 January 1970. Folio 54, Box 2072, DCW Collection.
32. Letter. Howard Pritham, Jr to Dorothy Clarke Wilson, 8 October 1970. Folio 54, Box 2072, DCW Collection.
33. Interview. Dorothy Clarke Wilson. Orono, ME. 21 June 1999.
34. When he decided to cooperate with Wilson's biographical project, the first avenue of research he suggested was a paper he had published twenty years before, in commemoration of the Maine Medical Association's 100 anniversary talk and to mark his own fiftieth year in practice. Telegram from F. J. Pritham, M D. to Dorothy Clark Wilson, 21 March 1969. Folio 51, Box 2072, DCW Collection.
35. Wilson, *Twelve Who Cared*, p. 209.
36. Letter from Dorothy Clarke Wilson to Dr. Fred and Sadie Pritham, 15 December 1969. Folio 51, Box 2072, DCW Collection.
37. Wilson, *Big-Little World*, pp. 209–12.

38. [promotional materials].
39. A. Elden, 'Maine's Most Remarkable Country Doctor often Risks His Life Saving Others', *Portland Sunday Telegram/Portland Daily Herald*, 6 May 1928: D1. Folio 45, Box 2072, DCW Collection.
40. Ibid.
41. Fred Pritham, 'North Country Doctor', *Portland Sunday Telegram*, 1 November 1953: 3. In Folio 45, Box 2072, DCW Collection.
42. Ibid.
43. Ibid.
44. This included teaching himself how to repair and remove part of a descending colon, performed soon after his first appendectomy. Wilson, *Big-Little World*, p. 114.
45. Ibid., p. 115.
46. Pritham recalled for Wilson that the principals of sanitation were 'just taking hold' at the Maine general by the 1890s. Ibid., p. 38.
47. Ibid., p. 116.
48. Wilson, *Twelve Who Cared*, p. 212.
49. Ibid.
50. Publisher Ruth Hardin, in taking stock of overall demand concluded local sales were insufficient. Letter from Ruth Hardin to Dorothy Clark Wilson, 26 August 1974. Folios 37 and 38, Box 2088, DCW Collection. Normally, a minimum of 1000 sales a year was required for a reprint.
51. Wilson, *Twelve Who Cared*, p. 200.
52. 'Maine Doctor Dares Danger of Snow, Water, Bitter Cold', *Oakland Tribune*, 11 January 1929, p. 3. In Folio 45, Box 2072, DCW Collection.
53. See, for instance, D. Brown, *Inventing New England: Regional Tourism in the Nineteenth Century* (Washington, D.C.: Smithsonian Institution Press, 1995).
54. The regional nostalgia for small town mill life is observable by 1870. See D. Brown (ed.), *A Tourist's New England, Travel Fiction 1820–1920* (Hanover, NH and London: University Press of New England, 1999). This nostalgic desire to cling to the small New England village, and to link it to New England's colonial Yankee heritage is also treated, and debunked, in J. S. Wood and M. B. Steinitz, *The New England Village* (Baltimore, MD: Johns Hopkins University Press, 2002).
55. According to Conforti, by the twentieth century the imaginative relocation of 'real' New England to the northernmost reaches of the region, New Hampshire, Vermont and Maine, was complete. And thus, 'the regional periphery was reimagined as the centre of New England identity'. J. Conforti, *Imagining New England: Explorations of Regional Identity from the Pilgrims to the mid-Twentieth Century* (Chapel Hill, NC: University of North Carolina Press, 2001). See especially ch. 6, pp. 263–309.
56. R. W. Sandwell, 'Introduction', in R. W. Sandwell (ed.) *Beyond the City Limits: Rural History in British Columbia* (Vancouver: University of British Columbia Press, 1999), p. 6.
57. See, for instance, R. Kline, *Consumers in the Country: Technology and Social Change in Rural America* (Baltimore, MD: Johns Hopkins University Press, 2000).

4 Smith, 'Putting Hyperactivity in its Place'

1. S. A. Modée, 'Post Sputnik Panic', *English Journal*, 69 (1980), p. 56.
2. For example, in an episode of *The Simpsons* entitled 'Brother's Little Helper' (first broadcast 3 October 1999), Bart is tricked into taking 'Focusin' by his father Homer. Although

Bart quickly becomes a model student, he also develops paranoia and starts behaving even more erratically than normal. By the end of the episode, his parents have switched him onto Ritalin, and the episode ends with Bart singing, to the tune of 'Popeye, the Sailor Man': 'When I can't stops my fiddlin', I just takes me Ritalin, I'm poppin' and sailin' man!' In a 21 February 1999 episode of *The Sopranos*, entitled 'Down Neck', mobster Tony Soprano's son, Anthony, Jr, is diagnosed with ADHD by a school psychologist. Although Tony suspects that ADHD is nothing more than a 'way for these psychologists to line their pockets', and thinks that 'all he [Anthony, Jr] needs is a whack upside the head', his wife Carmella is appalled, demanding, 'You'd hit someone who's sick? You'd hit someone with polio?'.

3.   J. L. Rapoport, I. T. Lott, D. F. Alexander, A. U. Abramson, 'Urinary Noradrenaline and Playroom Behaviour in Hyperactive Children', *Lancet*, 296 (1970), p. 1141; M. A. Stewart, 'Urinary Noradrenaline and Playroom Behaviour in Hyperactive Children', *Lancet*, 297 (1971), p. 140.

4.   Anon., 'Minimal Brain Dysfunction', *Lancet*, 302 (1973), pp. 487–8.

5.   D. N. Livingstone, *Putting Science in its Place* (Chicago, IL: University of Chicago Press, 2003), p. 3.

6.   E. Dyck, 'Prairies, Psychedelics and Place: The Dynamics of Region in Psychiatric Research', *Health and Place*, 15 (2009), p. 890.

7.   M. Jackson, *The Borderland of Imbecility: Medicine, Society and the Fabrication of the Feeble Mind in Late Victorian and Edwardian England* (Manchester: Manchester University Press, 2000).

8.   G. Grob, *The Mad Among Us: A History of the Care of America's Mentally Ill* (New York: The Free Press, 1994), p. 193.

9.   M. T. Brancaccio, 'Educational Hyperactivity: The Historical Emergence of a Concept', *Intercultural Education*, 11 (2000), p. 165; R. Mayes and A. Rafalovich, 'Suffer the Restless Children: The Evolution of ADHD and Paediatric Stimulant Use, 1900–80', *History of Psychiatry*, 18 (2007); S. Sandberg and J. Barton, 'Historical Development', in *Hyperactivity and Attention Disorders of Childhood*, ed. Seija Sandberg (Cambridge: Cambridge University Press, 2002), p. 4; P. H. Wender, *ADHD: Attention-Deficit Hyperactivity Disorder in Children and Adults* (Oxford: Oxford University Press, 2000), p. 3.

10. For example, the often-cited example of Charles Bradley, 'The Behavior of Children Receiving Benzedrine', *American Journal of Psychiatry*, 94 (1937).

11. George F. Still, 'The Goulstonian Lectures on Some Abnormal Psychical Conditions in Children. Lecture II', *Lancet*, 159 (1902), pp. 1079–82.

12. Franklin G. Ebaugh, 'Neuropsychiatric Sequelae of Acute Epidemic Encephalitis in Children', *American Journal of Diseases of Children*, 25 (1923); A. A. Strauss and H. Werner, 'Disorders of Conceptual Thinking in the Brain-Injured Child', *Journal of Nervous and Mental Disease*, 96 (1942); F. T. Thorpe, 'Prefrontal Leucotomy in Treatment for Post-Encephalitic Conduct Disorder', *British Medical Journal*, 1 (1946).

13. What this 'pre-history' of hyperactivity did establish, however, was the notion that deviant childhood behaviour could be caused by neurological dysfunction. This has also been recognised by sociologist Adam Rafalovich. A. Rafalovich, 'The Conceptual History of Attention-Deficit/Hyperactivity Disorder: Idiocy, Imbecility, Encephalitis, and the Child Deviant, 1877–1929', *Deviant Behavior*, 22 (2001), p. 107. See also: M. Smith, 'The Uses and Abuses of the History of Hyperactivity', in L. Graham (ed.) *Deconstructing ADHD: Critical Guidance for Teachers and Teacher Educators* (New York: Peter Lang, 2010).

14. M. W. Laufer and E. Denhoff, 'Hyperkinetic Behavior Syndrome in Children', *Journal of Pediatrics*, 50 (1957); M. W. Laufer, E. Denhoff, and G. Solomons, 'Hyperkinetic Impulse Disorder in Children's Behavior Problems', *Psychosomatic Medicine*, 19 (1957).

15. H. Fischer, '50 Years Ago in the *Journal of Pediatrics*: Hyperkinetic Behavior Syndrome in Children', *Journal of Pediatrics*, 150 (2007).

16. Laufer, Denhoff, and Solomons, 'Hyperkinetic Impulse Disorder in Children's Behavior Problems', p. 41; Mayes and Rafalovich, 'Suffer the Restless Children: The Evolution of ADHD and Paediatric Stimulant Use, 1900–1980', p. 444.

17. Laufer, Denhoff, and Solomons, 'Hyperkinetic Impulse Disorder in Children's Behavior Problems', p. 41.

18. Ibid., p. 44.

19. J. Jacobs Brumberg, *Fasting Girls: The History of Anorexia Nervosa* (Cambridge, MA: Harvard University Press, 1989); A. Young, *The Harmony of Illusions: Inventing Post-traumatic Stress Disorder* (Princeton, NJ: Princeton University Press, 1995).

20. L. Kanner, *Child Psychiatry*, 3rd edn (Springfield, IL: Charles C. Thomas, 1957), p. 528; J. Schrager et al., 'The Hyperkinetic Child: An Overview of the Issues', *Journal of the American Academy of Child Psychiatry*, 5 (1966).

21. I. Bernstein, *Promises Kept: John F. Kennedy's New Frontier* (New York: Oxford University Press, 1991), p. 10.

22. Barbara Ehrenreich and Deirdre English, *For Her Own Good: 150 Years of the Experts' Advice to Women* (Garden City, New York: Anchor Books, 1979), p. 232.

23. H. G. Shane, 'Elementary Schools During the Fabulous Fifties', *Education Digest*, 26 (1961), p. 19.

24. T. Taylor, 'Editorial: Take a Good Look This Year', *Grade Teacher*, 76 (1958–9), p. 5.

25. A. V. Keliher, 'I Wonder as I Wander', *Grade Teacher*, 76 (1958–1959), p. 143.

26. P. Hoyt, 'What Is Ahead for Our Schools', *Grade Teacher*, 76 (1958–9), p. 20.

27. G. L. Gutek, *Education in the United States: An Historical Perspective* (Englewood Cliffs, NJ: Prentice Hall, 1986), pp. 275–9.

28. Capitalization in original. A. S. Knowles, 'For the Space Age: Education as an Instrument of National Policy', *Phi Delta Kappa*, 39 (1958), p. 306.

29. L. Berkner quoted in H. G. Rickover, *American Education – a National Failure: The Problem of Our Schools and What We Can Learn from England* (New York: E. P. Dutton and Co., INC, 1963), p. 57.

30. S. L. Warren, 'Implementation of the President's Program on Mental Retardation', *American Journal of Psychiatry*, 121 (1964/5), pp. 550–1.

31. A. S. Trace., *What Ivan Knows That Johnny Doesn't* (New York: Random House, 1961), p. 3.

32. Rickover, *American Education – a National Failure: The Problem of Our Schools and What We Can Learn from England*, p. 71.

33. J. D. McLeod and Karen Kaiser, 'Childhood Emotional and Behavioral Problems and Educational Attainment', *American Sociological Review*, 69 (2004); K. G. Nadeau, 'Career Choices and Workplace Challenges for Individuals with ADHD', *Journal of Clinical Psychology*, 61 (2005); L. Tarnapol, 'Author's Comment', *Exceptional Children*, 36 (1969–70), p. 368.

34. J. B. Conant, *The American High School Today: A First Report to Interested Citizens* (New York: McGraw-Hill, 1959), pp. 45–50, 55–6.

35. A. Davids and J. Sidmond, 'A Pilot Study – Impulsivity, Time Orientation, and Delayed Gratification in Future Scientists and in Underachieving High School Students', *Exceptional Children*, 29 (1962–3), p. 170.

36. Ibid., p. 174.

37. P. O. Edwards, 'Discipline and the Elementary School', *Grade Teacher*, 74 (1956–7), pp. 127, 129.

38. N. E. Cutts, 'Troublesome or Troubled', *Grade Teacher*, 76 (1958–9), p. 56; A. V. Keliher, 'You, the Psychologist and the Child', *Grade Teacher*, 74 (1956–7), p. 143.

39. G. Rochlin, 'Discussion of David E. Reiser's "Observations of Delinquent Behavior in Very Young Children"', *Journal of the American Academy of Child Psychiatry*, 2 (1963), p. 66.

40. K. Reeves, 'Each in His Own Good Time', *Grade Teacher*, 74 (1956–7), p. 8.

41. These advertisements began in the 1956–7 volume of *Grade Teacher*.

42. Ironically, food allergists long suspected that food sensitivities could manifest themselves in behavioural abnormalities. Moreover, one of the most successful alternative theories regarding the aetiology of hyperactivity has been San Francisco allergist Ben Feingold's claim that food additives cause hyperactivity. B. F. Feingold, *Why Your Child Is Hyperactive* (1974; New York: Random House, 1996); A. Schonwald, 'ADHD and Food Additives Revisited', *AAP Grand Rounds*, 19 (2008); M. Smith, 'Into the Mouths of Babes: Hyperactivity, Food Additives, and the Reception of the Feingold Diet', in M. Jackson (ed.), *Health and the Modern Home* (New York: Routledge, 2007). M. Smith, *An Alternative History of Hyperactivity: Food Additives and the Feingold Diet* (New Brunswick, NJ: Rutgers University Press, 2011)

43. P. Conrad and D. Potter, 'From Hyperactive Children to ADHD Adults: Observations on the Expansion of Medical Categories', *Social Problems*, 47 (2000); S. Gundle, 'Discussion of Masterson, Tucker and Berk's 'Psychopathology in Adolescence, Iv: Clinical and Dynamic Characteristics', *American Journal of Psychiatry*, 120 (1963/4), p. 365; L. Y. Huey et al., 'Adult Minimal Brain Dysfunction and Schizophrenia: A Case Report', *American Journal of Psychiatry*, 134 (1977), p. 1563; J. F. Masterson, Jr, 'The Symptomatic Adolescent Five Years Later: He Didn't Grow out of It', *American Journal of Psychiatry*, 123 (1966/7), pp. 1338, 1345; J. F. Masterson, Jr, K. Tucker, and G. Berk, 'Psychopathology in Adolescence, Iv: Clinical and Dynamic Characteristics', *American Journal of Psychiatry*, 120 (1963/4), p. 363.

44. Masterson, Jr, 'The Symptomatic Adolescent Five Years Later: He Didn't Grow out of It', 1338, 1344.

45. B. Barton and K. D. Pringle, 'Today's Children and Youth: I. As Viewed from the State', *Children*, 7 (1960), p. 55; A. V. Keliher, 'You and the Psychological Experts', *Grade Teacher*, 74 (1956–7), p. 113; E. A. Richards, 'Today's Children and Youth: II. As Seen by National Organizations', *Children*, 7 (1960), p. 60.

46. D. Schreiber, 'The Dropout and the Delinquent: Promising Practices Gleaned from a Year of Study', *Phi Delta Kappa*, 44 (1963), p. 217.

47. Lyndon B. Johnson quoted in D. Schreiber, 'The Low-Down on Dropouts', in E. H. Grant (ed.), *PTA Guide to What's Happening in Education* (New York: Scholastic Book Services, 1965), p. 245.

48. Ibid., p. 246, D. W. Snepp, 'Can We Salvage the Drop-Outs?', *Clearing House*, 31 (1956–1957), p. 49.

49. Hoyt, 'What Is Ahead for Our Schools', p. 20.

50. Rickover, *American Education – a National Failure: The Problem of Our Schools and What We Can Learn from England*, pp. 50–1.

51. J. B. Conant, *Slums and Suburbs* (New York: McGraw-Hill, 1961), p. 145.

52. Ironically, the author of this letter argued that such an 'overwhelming amount of home-work reduced the student's ability to really learn his subjects' and resulted in students becoming 'disenchanted with science and engineering'. M. F. Beall, 'Disenchanted Students', *Science*, 175 (1972), p. 123.

53. D. Barclay, 'A Turn for the Wiser', *Pediatrics*, 23 (1959), p. 760.

54. K. Minde et al., 'The Hyperactive Child in Elementary School: A 5 Year, Controlled, Followup', *Exceptional Children*, 38 (1971–2), pp. 219, 221.

55. Ibid., p. 221.

56. It should be emphasized that Conant himself strongly advocated increasing funding for slums and slum schools in order to improve high school completion rates in such areas. Conant, *Slums and Suburbs*, pp. 2–3.

57. L. M. Dunn, 'Special Education for the Mildly Retarded – Is Much of It Justifiable?', *Exceptional Children*, 35 (1968–9), p. 20; J. J. McCarthy, 'SEIMCs [Special Education Instruction Materials Centers] and the Teacher of Children with Learning Disabilities: A Useful Partnership', *Exceptional Children*, 34 (1967–8), p. 627; E. Siegel, 'Learning Disabilities: Substance or Shadow', *Exceptional Children*, 34 (1967–8), pp. 433, 435.

58. H. S. Adelman, 'The Not So Specific Learning Disability Population', *Exceptional Children*, 37 (1970–1), p. 530.

59. J. B. Conant, 'Recommendations for the Junior-High School', *Education Digest*, 26 (1961), p. 7.

60. Conant, *The American High School Today*, pp. 44–5.

61. S. E. B. Schuck and F. M. Crinella, 'Why Children with ADHD Do Not Have Low IQs', *Journal of Learning Disabilities*, 38:3 (2005).

62. S. A. Rippa, *Education in a Free Society: An American History*, 7th ed (New York: Longman, 1992), pp. 262–3.

63. I. N. Berlin, 'Mental Health Consultation in Schools as a Means of Communicating Mental Health Principles', *Journal of the American Academy of Child Psychiatry*, 1 (1962), pp. 674–5; P. J. Doyle, 'The Organic Hyperkinetic Syndrome', *Journal of School Health*, 32 (1962), pp. 299, 304; P. L. Gardner, 'Guidance: An Orientation for the Classroom Teacher', *Clearing House*, 36 (1961–2); E. H. Grant, 'Forward', in Grant (ed.), *PTA Guide to What's Happening in Education*, p. iii; T. P. Millar, 'Schools Should Not Be Community Health Centers', *American Journal of Psychiatry*, p. 125 (1968/9), p. 119; E. Mumford, 'Teacher Response to School Mental Health Problems', *American Journal of Psychiatry*, 125 (1968/9), pp. 76–8.

64. Keliher, 'You, the Psychologist and the Child', p. 143, W. W. Wattenberg, 'Mental Health and Illness', *Education Digest*, 26 (1961), p. 11.

65. T. C. Lovitt, 'Assessment of Children with Learning Disabilities', *Exceptional Children*, 34 (1967–8), p. 234.

66. Doyle, 'The Organic Hyperkinetic Syndrome', p. 304; B. K. Keogh, 'Hyperactivity and Learning Disorders: Review and Speculation', *Exceptional Children*, 38 (1971–2), p. 101; H. G. Wadsworth, 'A Motivational Approach Towards Remediation of Learning Disabled Boys', *Exceptional Children*, 38 (1971–2), pp. 32–4.

67. J. Peterson, 'The Researcher and the Underacheiver: Never the Twain Shall Meet', *Phi Delta Kappa*, 44 (1963), p. 381.

68. J. W. Gardner, 'No Easy Victories', *American Statistician*, 22 (1968), p. 14.

69. P. Schrag and D. Divoky, *The Myth of the Hyperactive Child: And Other Means of Child Control* (1975; New York: Penguin Books, 1982), pp. 111–15. See, for example, the

increase in advertisements during the 1970s for hyperactivity drugs such as Ritalin and
Cylert in journals such as the *American Journal of Psychiatry*.

70. Association of American Universities, A National Defense Education Act for the 21st
Century Renewing Our Commitment to US Students, Science, Scholarship, and Security (2006), http://www.aau.edu/education/NDEAOP.pdf.

71. Italics in original. H. Hendrick, *Child Welfare: Historical Dimensions, Contemporary
Debate* (Bristol: The Policy Press, 2003), p. 253.

5 Finkel, 'Why Canada Has a Universal Medical Insurance Programme and the United States Does Not'

1. H. Boushey and J. Wright, 'Health Insurance Data Brief #2: Insurance Coverage in the
United States', http://www.cepr.net/publications/health_insurance_2_2004_04.html.
Of course, the number of Americans without coverage throughout the year is considerably higher than the number without coverage at any point during a year. In 2005, the
number without coverage at the time that they were polled by the Census Bureau was
44.8 million. 'US Census Bureau News', 23 March 2007. Among those with coverage
in the early 2000s, only 70 million were covered by public programmes while 170 million had private coverage. J. S. Hacker, *The Divided Welfare State: The Battle Over Public
and Private Social Benefits in the United States* (Cambridge: Cambridge University Press,
2002), p. 6.

2. Lipset has most forcefully made this argument in *American Exceptionalism* (New York:
W.W. Norton, 1996), p. 91. His detailed examination of attitudinal surveys comparing
the two countries is *Continental Divide: The Values and Institutions of the United States
and Canada* (New York: Routledge, 1990). *Continental Divide,* while demonstrating
that Canadians as a whole are more liberal than Americans, demonstrates interestingly
that French Canadians are more liberal than other Canadians. This evidence alone
should cause questioning of any essentialist explanations of popular attitudes. As late
as the 1950s, French Canadians were, on average, more conservative than Americans,
never mind anglophone Canadians. Though the hold of the Catholic Church over the
population was slipping, it virtually evaporated during the so-called 'Quiet Revolution'
of the 1960s when the state took greater control over social services, health and education, traditional areas of Church authority in Quebec. The Church suddenly had to
win individuals' support for spiritual reasons rather than through a demonstration of its
institutional power. While state and institutional power are not the only determinants of
popular attitudes, they play an important role. Lipset's account largely ignores the factors
shaping popular attitudes, and implies that at work in the different attitudes among the
populations he studies is an American essentialism, an anglophone Canadian essentialism, and a francophone Canadian essentialism. On the changes in Quebec society during
the postwar period, see Paul-André Linteau, René Durocher, Jean-Claude Robert, and
François Ricard, *Quebec Since 1930* (Toronto: James Lorimer, 1991), Part 3.

3. A. Maioni, *Parting at the Crossroads: The Emergence of Health Insurance in the United
States and Canada* (Princeton, NJ: Princeton University Press, 1998), p. 31.

4. P. E. Bryden, *Planners and Politicians: Liberal Politics and Social Policy 1957–68* (Montreal and Kingston: McGill-Queen's University Press, 1997).

5. Maioni, *Parting at the Crossroads*, p. 164.

6. C. Lindblom, *Politics and Markets: The World's Political-Economic Systems* (New York: Basic Books, 1997), p. 347.
7. A. C. Cairns, *Reconfigurations: Canadian Citizenship and Constitutional Change* (Toronto: McClelland and Stewart, 1995), p. 34.
8. On workmen's compensation, see J. F. Witt, *The Accidental Republic: Crippled Working-men, Destitute Widows, and the Remaking of American Law* (Cambridge, MA: Harvard University Press, 2004); R. H. Babcock, 'Blood on the Factory Floor: The Workers' Compensation Movement in Canada and the United States', in R. B. Blake and Jeff Keshen (eds), *Social Welfare Policy in Canada: Historical Readings* (Toronto: Copp Clark, 1995).
9. In 1973–4, for example, the federal grant to Newfoundland covered 81.5 per cent of the province's medical bills and 57.6 per cent of its hospital costs while the grant to Ontario paid 44.8 per cent of medical care and 49.4 per cent of hospital costs. Eugene Vayda and Raisa B. Deber, 'The Canadian Health Care System: A Developmental Overview', in Raymond B. Blake and Jeff Keshen, *Social Welfare Policy in Canada: Historical Readings* (Toronto: Copp Clark, 1995), p. 316.
10. Changes to the Unemployment Insurance Act in 1971 raised the percentage of the workforce covered by the legislation from 80 per cent to 96 per cent. Leslie Pal, *State, Class, and Bureaucracy: Canadian Unemployment Insurance and Public Policy* (Montreal, QC: McGill-Queen's University Press, 1988), pp. 43–4. But a series of government assaults on the generosity of the programme, beginning in 1975, resulted in the programme covering no more than 41 per cent of the unemployed in 1997, a figure 1 per cent below the percentage of the work force covered by unemployment insurance in 1940, when the program was introduced. See G. Campeau, *From UI to EI: Waging War on the Welfare State* (Vancouver: UBC Press, 2005).
11. From the beginning, while the federal government shared the costs of unemployment insurance with the states, it was up to the states to determine eligibility for unemployment insurance and the level of benefits in the programme. A. S. Orloff, 'The Political Origins of America's Belated Welfare State', in M. Weir, A. S. Orloff and Theda Skocpol (eds), *The Politics of Social Policy in the United States* (Princeton, NJ: Princeton University Press, 1988), p. 40.
12. Comparisons of the level of support provided by Canadian and American social programmes include J. Myles, *When Markets Fail: Social Welfare in Canada and the United States* (New York: United Nations Research Institute for Social Development, 1995); M. V. Levine, 'Public Policies, Social Institutions, and Earnings Inequality: Canada and the United States, 1970–95', joint issue, *American Review of Canadian Studies* and *Canadian Review of American Studies*, 26:3 (Autumn 1996), pp. 315–9; and M. Baker, 'Eliminating Child Poverty: How Does Canada Compare?', *American Review of Canadian Studies* (Spring 1995), pp. 79–110. The latter also compares programmes in North America with programmes in other industrialized nations. On medical care provision in the two countries, see D. Blumenthal, C. Vogeli, L. Alexander and M. Pittman, *A Five-Nation Hospital Survey: Commonalities, Differences and Discontinuities* (New York: Commonwealth Fund, 2004). The weakness of the welfare states in both Canada and the United States relative to most continental European nations is evident in G. Esping-Anderson, *The Three Worlds of Welfare Capitalism* (Princeton, NJ: Princeton University Press, 1990). A recent article that demonstrates the extent to which the limited social benefits for the destitute in the United States have been weakened in recent years, particularly since the passage of the Personal Responsibility and Work Opportunity Reconciliation

Act, 1996, is Janine Fitzgerald, 'The Disciplinary Apparatus of Welfare Reform', *Monthly Review*, 56:6 (November 2004), pp. 53–62.

13. The degree of equality within countries is measured by the Gini coefficient, a measure that would yield a figure of 1 if all wealth was held by a single individual and 0 if all wealth was equally distributed among all members of the population. By the mid-1990s, according to this measure, there was significantly greater equality in Canada, which had a Gini of .293 in 1997 than in the US, whose Gini the same year was .371. By contrast, the Gini in Sweden in 1995 was .223. But other continental European countries, such as France (Gini of .269) and Germany (Gini of .289) ranked only slightly higher than Canada in equal distribution of income. Lars Osberg, 'How Much Does Employment Matter for Equality in Canada and Elsewhere?' in David A. Green and Jonathan R. Kesselman, eds., *Dimensions of Inequality in Canada* (Vancouver: UBC Press, 2006),169. Osberg's calculations are based on the microdata provided by the Luxemburg Income Study.

14. B. D. Palmer, *Working Class Experience: Rethinking the History of Canadian Labour, 1800–1991*, 2nd edn (Toronto: McClelland and Stewart, 1992), p. 256.

15. On the Canadian Seamen's Union episode, see John Stanton, *Life and Death of a Union: The History of the Canadian Seamen's Union, 1936–49* (Toronto: Steel Rail, 1978); and W. Kaplan, *Everything that Floats: Pat Sullivan, Hal Banks, and the Seamen's Unions of Canada* (Toronto: University of Toronto Press, 1987).

16. I. Abella, *Nationalism, Communism and Canadian Labour: The CIO, The Communist Party of Canada and the Canadian Congress of Labour, 1935–56* (Toronto: University of Toronto Press, 1973).

17. N. Lichtenstein, *Labor's War at Home: The CIO in World War 11* (Cambridge: Cambridge University Press, 1982).

18. M. Davis, *Prisoners of the American Dream: Politics and Economy in the History of the US Working Class* (London: Verso, 1986), ch. 3.

19. On the history of the CCF and NDP, see N. Penner, *From Protest to Power: Social Democracy in Canada 1900–Present* (Toronto: James Lorimer and Company, 1992).

20. P. Starr, *The Social Transformation of American Medicine* (New York: Basic Books, 1982), p. 288.

21. For example, Canadians were asked by the Gallup organization in November 1943: 'Do you think that workers would be better off if all the industries in Canada were owned and run by the Dominion government after the war, or do you think that workers would be better off if these industries were left under private management?' The response: 39 per cent chose government ownership despite the use of 'all the industries in Canada' in the question; 47 per cent chose private ownership and operation, while 14 per cent were undecided. Interestingly, by November 1945, when the Gallup asked the question again, only 21 per cent wanted a primarily government-run economy while 64 per cent now opted for private enterprise and 15 per cent were undecided. The Cold War, though unannounced, had begun and the tremendous anti-communist, and anti-socialist propaganda that people experienced cooled their ardour for a system of public ownership of the major means of production, distribution, and exchange. Library and Archives Canada, National Liberal Federation Papers, MG 28 1V–3, Vol. 961.

22. R. Bothwell, I. Drummond and J. English, *Canada Since 1945: Power, Politics, and Provincialism*, rev. edn (Toronto: University of Toronto Press, 1989), p. 53.

23. I. Bernstein, *A Caring Society: The New Deal, the Worker, and the Great Depression: A History of the American Worker, 1933–41* (Boston, MA: Houghton Mifflin, 1985), pp. 285, 290, 301.

24. Lichtenstein, *Labor's War at Home*, pp. 216–19.

25. A. Finkel, 'Trade Unions and the Welfare State in Canada, 1945–90', in C. Gonick, P. Phillips and J. Vorst, *Labour Gains, Labour Pains: Fifty Years of PC 1003* (Winnipeg: Society for Socialist Studies, 1995), p. 62.

26. G. Makahonuk, 'Masters and Servants: Labour Relations in the Saskatchewan Civil Service, 1905–45', *Prairie Forum*, 12:2 (Autumn 1987), pp. 257–76.

27. D. Morton with T. Copp, *Working People* (Ottawa: Deneau, 1984), pp. 204–5; John Boyko, *Into the Hurricane: Attacking Socialism and the CCF* (Winnipeg: J. Gordon Shillingford Publishing 2006).

28. Penner, *From Protest to Power*, pp. 85–6.

29. Penner, *From Protest to Power*, pp. 91–5; Palmer, *Working-Class Experience*, pp. 304–5.

30. M. M. Poen, *Harry S. Truman Versus the Medical Lobby* (Columbia, MO: University of Missouri Press, 1979); T. R. Marmor, *The Politics of Medicare*, 2nd edn (Chicago, IL: Aldine, 2000); Maioni, *Parting at the Crossroads*.

31. J. Klein, 'The Business of Health Security: Employee Health Benefits, Commercial Insurers, and the Reconstruction of Welfare Capitalism, 1945–60', *International Labour and Working Class History Journal*, 58 (Autumn 2000), pp. 293–313.

32. A. Finkel, *Social Policy and Practice in Canada: A History* (Waterloo: Wilfrid Laurier University Press, 2006), pp. 125–47.

33. R. Radosh, *American Labor and United States Foreign Policy* (New York: Random House, 1969).

34. The gap in thinking on international trade unionism between the Canadian and American trade union movements of the late 50s is evident in A. Carew, 'Charles Millard, A Canadian in the International Labour Movement: A Case Study of the ICFTU 1955–61', *Labour/Le Travail*, 37 (Spring 1996), pp. 121–48.

35. A. Finkel, 'Canadian Immigration Policy and the Cold War, 1945–80', *Journal of Canadian Studies*, 21:3 (Summer 1986), pp. 58–60.

36. S. M. Lipset, *Continental Divide*, p. 154. Lipset notes that in the early eighties 28 per cent of Canadians but only 9 per cent of Americans identified themselves as working class or poor, when asked to indicate to what class they belonged. The pollsters then provided alternative class designations to all respondents who had been unable to identify themselves as members of a particular social class. The gap then closed somewhat between the Canadians and Americans but with 35 per cent of Canadians having identified themselves as working class or poor while only 28 per cent of Americans did so.

37. D. Martin, *Thinking Union: Activism and Education in Canada's Labour Movement* (Toronto: Between the Lines, 1995), p. 6; J. Clemens and A. Karabegovic, 'Union Rates Not a Result of Choice', Fraser Forum, http://www.fraserinstitute.ca/admin/books/chapterfiles/Mar05ffunionrate.

38. On Liberal debates during this period, see Bryden, *Planners and Politicians*.

39. Bryden, *Planners and Politicians*, pp. 8–14. The history of hospital care in Canada before hospitalization insurance is best summarized in D. Gagan and R. Gagan, *For Patients of Moderate Means: A Social History of the Voluntary Public General Hospital in Canada, 1890–1950* (Montreal, QC: McGill-Queen's University Press, 2002).

40. No doubt people felt too intimidated by the power of physicians to go to the public hearings of a Royal Commission to tell all. In the entire body of the Commission's hearings,

I found only one testimony from an individual who was poor and claimed that she had received poorer medical care (in this case, for her asthmatic son) than she would have in a public system. Her doctor's public refutation of her story would have served as a warning to others who might have been thinking of telling their individual stories. Library and Archives Canada, RG 33, Series 78, Royal Commission on Health Services. The testimony of the one individual complainer and her doctor are: Vol. 22, File 355, Brief of Mrs. Marguerite Miles, Toronto, n.d; File 375, Dr. C. Collins-Williams, Toronto, n.d.

41. A. Finkel, 'Trade Unions and the Welfare State in Canada', pp. 67–9; M. G. Taylor, *Health Insurance and Canadian Public Policy: The Seven Decisions That Created the Canadian Health Insurance System*, rev. edn (Montreal, QC: McGill-Queen's, 1987), p. 166.

42. M. Poen, *Harry S. Truman Versus the Medical Lobby*, p. 66.

43. M. G. Taylor, *Health Insurance and Canadian Public Policy*, p. 166, indicates that 80 per cent of Canadians supported a federal health insurance scheme when polled in 1944 and again in 1949. In Britain, in December 1942, 70 per cent of respondents in a Gallup Poll favoured a government insurance scheme 'even if it would mean ... paying more insurance than you are paying now'. Lawrence R. Jacobs, *The Health of Nations: Public Opinion and the Making of American and British Health Policy* (Ithaca, NY: Cornell University Press, 1993), p. 69.

44. Starr, *The Social Transformation of American Medicine*, p. 278.

45. E. Berkowitz and K. McQuaid, *Creating the Welfare State: The Political Economy of Twentieth Century Reform* (New York: Praeger, 1980), p. 137.

46. Poen, *Harry S. Truman Versus the Medical Lobby*, pp. 88–90.

47. Judging, for example, by the relative restraint of Canadian Medical Association briefs to the Royal Commission on Health Services. Library and Archives Canada, Royal Commission on Health Services, RG 33, Series 78, Vol. 6, Report No. 67, 16 October 1962; and Vol. 19, File 278, April 1962.

48. Maioni, *Parting at the Crossroads*, 113.

49. Hacker, *The Divided Welfare State*, p. 232. See also Klein, 'The Business of Health Security'.

50. S. I. David, *With Dignity: The Search for Medicare and Medicaid* (Westport, Connecticut: Greenwood Press, 1985), pp. 146–7.

51. D. A. Fraser, then vice president of the UAW and director of the Chrysler Department, told a conference on health care in 1976 that the cost of prepurchased private insurance for workers in the automobile industry in the US was six weeks wages per year. Douglas A. Fraser address in J. Alex Murray (ed), *Health Care Delivery Systems in North America: The Changing Concepts*, Canadian-American Seminar, University of Windsor, November 11–12, 1976 (n.p.:n.p, 1977), pp. 101–8.

52. C. Gordon, 'Dead on Arrival: Health Care Reform in the United States'. *Studies in Political Economy*, 39 (Autumn 1992), p. 148.

53. J. Hacker, *The Divided Welfare State*, 261.

54. M. Fisk, 'US Health Care Reform and Corporate Structure', *Capital and Class*, 52 (Spring 1994), pp. 19–20.

55. C. Gordon, 'Dead on Arrival', p. 152. Gordon offers the best outline of the economic interests that have opposed universal public medical insurance throughout American history in C. Gordon, *Dead on Arrival: The Politics of Health Care in Twentieth Century America* (Princeton, NJ: Princeton University Press, 2004).

56. M. Watkins, 'Ontario: Discrediting Social Democracy', *Studies in Political Economy*, 43 (Spring 1994), pp. 139–48; M. G. Cohen, 'British Columbia: Playing Safe is a Dan-

gerous Game', *Studies in Political Economy*, 43 (Spring 1994), pp. 149–60; P. Hansen, 'Saskatchewan: The Failure of Political Imagination', *Studies in Political Economy*, 43 (Spring 1994), pp. 161–7.

57. On Quebec unions and politics see Ralph Guntzel, '"Rapprocher les lieux de pouvoir": the Quebec Labour Movement and Quebec Sovereigntism', *Labour/Le Travail*, 46 (Autumn 2000), pp. 369–95; C. Lipsig-Mummé, 'The Web of Dependence: Quebec Unions in Politics Before 1976', in A. G. Gagnon (ed.), *Quebec: State and Society* (Toronto: Methuen, 1984); C. Lipsig-Mummé, 'Future Conditional: Wars of Position in the Quebec Labour Movement', *Studies in Political Economy*, 36 (Autumn 1991), pp. 73–107.

58. T. Skocpol, *Protecting Soldiers and Mothers: The Political Origins of Social Policy in the United States* (Cambridge, MA: Belknap Press of Harvard University Press, 1992), p. 2.

59. A. Klaus, *Every Child a Lion: The Origins of Maternal and Infant Health Policy in the United States and France, 1890–1920* (Ithaca, NY: Cornell University Press, 1993), p. 289; B. Cass and C. V. Baldock (eds), *Women, Social Welfare and the State in Australia* (Sydney 1983), p. 19.

60. K. K. Sklar, 'The Historical Foundations of Women's Power in the Creation of the American Welfare State, 1830–1930', in S. Koven and S. Michel (eds), *Mothers of a New World: Maternalist Politics and the Origin of Welfare States* (New York: Routledge, 1993), p. 44.

61. L. Gordon, 'Social Insurance and Public Assistance: The Influence of Gender in Welfare Thought in the United States', *American Historical Review*, 97:1 (February 1992), p. 49.

62. Skocpol, *Protecting Soldiers and Mothers*, pp. 534–5; F. Davis, *Moving the Mountain: The Women's Movement in America Since 1960* (New York: Simon and Schuster, 1991), p. 31.

63. An important exception was Women Strike for Peace, whose explicit purpose was to fight Cold War thinking. Amy Swerdlow, 'Ladies' Day at the Capitol: Women Strike for Peace Versus HUAC', *Feminist Studies*, 8:3 (Autumn 1982), pp. 493–520.

64. J. Vickers, P. Rankin and C. Appelle, *Politics As If Women Mattered: A Political Analysis of the National Action Committee on the Status of Women* (Toronto: University of Toronto Press, 1993), p. 44.

65. S. A.Hewlett, *A Lesser Life: The Myth of Women's Liberation in America* (New York: Morrow, 1986); F. Davis, *Moving the Mountain*, pp. 280–4, 352.

66. R. J. Simon and G. Danziger, *Women's Movements in America: Their Successes, Disappointments, and Aspirations* (New York: Praeger, 1991), p. 62.

67. C. Backhouse, 'The Contemporary Women's Movement in Canada and the United States: An Introduction', in C. Backhouse and D. H. Flaherty (eds), *Challenging Times: The Women's Movement in Canada and the United States* (Montreal, QC: McGill-Queen's, 1992), pp. 12–13.

68. W. Brown, 'Finding the Man in the State', *Feminist Studies*, 18:1 (Spring 1992), pp. 11–12.

69. Jane Jenson argues that feminists' hostility to the state in France and Britain has weakened their ability to struggle against welfare-state cuts that hit women hardest. In both countries, the feminist discourse of difference has been subverted by conservative politicians and used against women. J. Jenson, 'Both Friend and Foe: Women and State Welfare', in R. Bridenthal, C. Koonz and S. Stuard (eds), *Becoming Visible: Women in European History*, 2nd edn (Boston, MA: Houghton Miflin, 1987), pp. 535–66.

70. L. Gordon, 'The Welfare State: Towards a Socialist-Feminist Perspective', in R. Miliband and L. Panitch (eds), *Socialist Register, 1990* (London: Merlin, 1990), pp. 171–200; F.

F. Piven, 'Ideology and the State: Women, Power, and the Welfare State', in L. Gordon (ed.), *Women, the State and Welfare* (Madison: University of Wisconsin Press, 1990), pp. 250–64.

71. S. Michel, *Children's Interests/Mothers' Rights: The Shaping of America's Child Care Policy* (New Haven, CT: Yale University Press 1999), p. 238.

72. Ibid., p. 279.

73. On the NCWC, see N. E. S. Griffiths, *The Splendid Vision: Centennial History of the National Council of Women of Canada 1893–1993* (Ottawa: Carleton University Press, 1993); and V. Strong-Boag, *The Parliament of Women: The National Council of Women of Canada 1893–1929* (Ottawa: National Museums of Canada, 1976).

74. Alison Prentice *et al.*, *Canadian Women: A History*, Second Edition (Toronto: Harcourt Brace, 1996), p. 230.

75. J. Vickers, 'The Intellectual Origins of the Women's Movement in Canada', in C. Backhouse and D. H. Flaherty (eds), *Challenging Times: The Women's Movement in Canada and the United States* (Montreal, QC: McGill-Queen's, 1992), pp. 39–60.

76. Michel, *Children's Interests/Mothers' Rights*, p. 296.

77. On women and the movement for social welfare in Canada, see C. Andrew, 'Women and the Welfare State', *Canadian Journal of Political Science*, 17:4 (December 1984), pp. 667–83; and T. McCormick, *Politics and the Hidden Injuries of Gender: Feminism and the Making of the Welfare State* (Ottawa: CRIAW, 1991).

78. Finkel, *Social Policy and Practice in Canada*, pp. 180–1.

79. Prentice *et al.*, *Canadian Women: A History*, pp. 446–8.

80. Vickers, 'The Intellectual Origins of the Women's Movement in Canada', p. 45.

81. Ibid., p. 40.

82. See, for example, the essays in C. Baines, P. Evans and S. Neysmith (eds), *Women's Caring: Feminist Perspectives on Social Welfare* (Toronto: McClelland and Stewart, 1991) as well as A. Bullock, 'Community Care: Ideology and Lived Experience', in R. Ng, G. Walker and J. Muller (eds), *Community Organizations and the Canadian State* (Toronto: Garamond, 1990), pp. 65–82.

83. Vickers *et al.*, *Politics As If Women Mattered*, pp. 4, 12–14, 183.

84. A majority of Canadians voted for parties that opposed the Canadian–American Free Trade Agreement, but their votes were split between the Liberals and the NDP, allowing the Conservatives, who supported the agreement, to be re-elected and to sign the agreement. On women's struggles against the agreement, see Vickers *et al.*, *Politics As If Women Mattered*, pp. 272–3; and M. G. Cohen, 'The Canadian Women's Movement and Its Efforts to Influence the Canadian Economy', C. Backhouse and D. H. Flaherty, *Challenging Times: The Women's Movement in Canada and the United States* (Montreal, QC: McGill-Queen's, 1992), pp. 215–24.

85. Prentice *et al.*, *Canadian Women: A History*, pp. 448, 457.

86. P.-A. Linteau, R. Durocher, J.-C. Robert and F. Rivard, *Quebec Since 1930* (Toronto: James Lorimer, 1991), p. 449; Alison Prentice *et al.*, *Canadian Women: A History*, pp. 414–15, 447. On the Quebec women's movement more generally, see Clio Collective, *Quebec Women: A History* (Toronto: Women's Press, 1987).

87. N. Fraser and L. Gordon, 'Contract vs. Charity: Why is there no Social Citizenship in the US?', *Socialist Review*, 22:3 (July/September 1992), pp. 45–67.

88. In 1988, 95 per cent of Canadians indicated that they preferred Canada's public medical care system to the American system. But 61 per cent of Americans also preferred the Canadian system when it was described to them. About 10 per cent of Americans in

1976 and 12 per cent in 1981 believed some form of socialism would be good for the United States. S. M. Lipset, *Continental Divide: The Values and Institutions of the United States and Canada* (New York: Routledge, 1990), pp. 138, 166.

6 Smith and Mawdsley, 'Alberta Advantage'

1. The term 'Alberta Advantage' was a product of Premier Ralph Klein's government in the 1990s and early 2000s. See the Province of Alberta government website, http://www.alberta.ca/home/43.cfm, accessed 1 June 2008.
2. See, for example, G. Feldberg, M. Ladd-Taylor, A. Li, and K. McPherson (eds), *Women, Health and Nation: Canada and the United States Since 1945* (Montreal: McGill-Queens University Press, 2003).
3. See, for example, Tim Cook, *Clio's Warriors: Canadian Historians and the Writing of World Wars* (Vancouver: UBC Press, 2006); and J. Colgrove, *State of Immunity: The Politics of Vaccination in Twentieth-Century America* (Berkeley, CA: University of California Press, and N.Y.: Milbank Memorial Fund, 2006).
4. J. H. Thompson and S. J. Randall, *Canada and the United States: Ambivalent Allies, 3rd Edition* (Athens, GA: University of Georgia Press, 2002), pp. 2, 7, 156–7, 166.
5. Mustard gas is sometimes cited as dichlorethyl sulphide. The military testing programs used sulfur mustard, nitrogen mustard, and lewisite. C. Pechura and D. P. Rall, eds. *Veterans at Risk: The Health Effects of Mustard Gas and Lewisite* (Washington, DC: National Academy Press, 1993), p. v. Mustard gas, or sulfur mustard, was developed in the early nineteenth century. It is a colourless, oily liquid at normal air temperatures. Its name is derived from the smell, sometimes like mustard, horseradish or even garlic, and its yellow-brown colour when mixed with other chemicals. Its vapour is a powerful irritant. It is also a persistent gas, meaning it remains within a given environment for a long time after its introduction. 'Toxicological Profile for Sulfur Mustard', Agency for Toxic Substances and Disease Registry (ATSDR), Public Health Services, Atlanta, Georgia: US Department of Health and Human Services, 2003, www.atsdr.cdc.gov/tfacts49.html, accessed 26 January 2006, courtesy of Donald Macnab.
6. J. Bryden, *Deadly Allies: Canada's Secret War, 1937–47* (Toronto: McClelland & Stewart, 1989), p. 173; K. Freeman, 'The Unfought Chemical War', *Bulletin of Atomic Scientists*, 47:10 (December 1991), pp. 30–9; C. Pechura and D. P. Rall (eds), *Veterans at Risk: The Health Effects of Mustard Gas and Lewisite* (Washington, DC: National Academy Press, 1993), p. v; B. Goodwin, *Keen as Mustard: Britain's Horrific Chemic Warfare Experiments in Australia* (Queensland, Australia: University of Queensland Press, 1998); D. Avery, *The Science of War: Canadian Scientists and Allied Military Technology During the Second World War* (Toronto: University of Toronto Press, 1998), pp. 10–12, 122–50.
7. U. Trumpener, 'The Road to Ypres: The Beginnings of Gas Warfare in World War I', *Journal of Modern History*, 47: 3 (1975), pp. 460–80. The Germans first used chlorine gas, and in 1917 they used mustard gas or sulfur mustard. See also Freeman, 'The Unfought Chemical War', pp. 2, 30–9. During World War 2, the Allied governments conducted mostly animal experiments, of which humans were just a small part. There were also dozens of other gases investigated during the war, as indicated in the material contained in Record Group 175 – Records of the Chemical Warfare Service and Record Group 227 – Records of the Office of Scientific Research and Development, National Archives II, College Park, Maryland.

8. According to Donald Avery, 'the June 1925 Geneva Protocal, held under the auspices of the League of Nations, ... banned the offensive, or first, use of chemical and biological weapons, and was signed by thirty-eight countries including ... Canada. 'The U.S. signed the treaty but the Senate did not ratify it. Avery, *The Science of War*, quote p. 16, and see p. 122. See also, J. E. van Courtland Moon, 'Project SPHINX: The Question of the Use of Gas in the Planned Invasion of Japan', *Journal of Strategic Studies*, 12 (1989), pp. 303–23, especially p. 317.

9. There was a mustard gas accident in December 1943 when the Germans bombed seventeen Allied ships off the coast of Italy at Bari Harbor. The gas, which had been carried aboard one US ship, was released into the air and water, affecting hundreds of allied soldiers and a thousand Italian civilians, many of whom died. R. Evans, *Gassed: A History of British Chemical Warfare Experiments on Humans* (London: House of Stratus, 2000), p. 322.

10. The Suffield tests, and those in Australia, helped the Allies develop a classification system: Class A (man cannot remain on the field of battle), Class B (injured and should be evacuated), Class C (injured but can keep fighting). The goal was to produce Class A enemy soldiers who are incapacitated and can no longer fight. Freeman, 'The Unfought Chemical War', p. 38.

11. Pechura and Rall (eds), *Veterans at Risk*, p. v; Avery, *The Science of War*, p. 128.

12. Thompson and Randall, *Canada and the United States*, pp. 6–7, 156–7, 166; J. A. Keshen, *Saints, Sinners, and Soldiers: Canada's Second World War* (Vancouver: UBC Press, 2004), pp. 4, 13.

13. L. P. Brophy, W. O. Miles and R. C. Cochrane, *U.S. Army in World War II, the Technical Services, volume on The Chemical Warfare Service: From Laboratory to Field* (Washington, DC: Office of the Chief of Military History, Department of the Army, 1959), p. 45; Avery, *The Science of War*, pp. 128–42, 150; Moon, 'Project SPHINX', pp. 303–23, especially p. 307.

14. M. Harrison, 'The Medicalization of War – The Militarisation of Medicine', *Social History of Medicine*, 9:2 (August 1996), pp. 267–76.

15. D. J. Rothman, *Strangers at the Bedside: A History of How Law and Bioethics Transformed Medical Decision Making* (New York: Basic Books, 1991), p. 30; Pechura and Rall (eds), *Veterans at Risk; S. Lederer, Subjected to Science: Human Experimentation in America before the Second World War* (Baltimore, MD: Johns Hopkins University Press, 1995); G. Baader, S. E. Lederer, M. Low, F. Schmaltz and A. V. Schwerin, 'Pathways to Human Experimentation, 1933–45: Germany, Japan, and the United States', OSIRIS, 20:1 (2005), pp. 205–31, especially pp. 224, 229.

16. Rothman, Strangers as the Bedside, p. 30.

17. Bryden, *Deadly Allies*; Freeman, 'The Unfought Chemical War', pp. 30–9; Goodwin, *Keen as Mustard*; Evans, *Gassed*; and the documentary films *Secret War: Oddyssey of Suffield Volunteers* (Insight Film and Video Productions, Canada, 2001); and *Keen as Mustard: The Story of Top Secret Chemical Warfare Experiments* (Yarra Bank Films, Australia, 1989).

18. J. Moreno, *Undue Risk: Secret State Experiments on Humans* (New York: Routledge, 2001); Avery, *The Science of War; Pechura and Rall* (eds), Veterans at Risk.

19. Freeman, 'The Unfought Chemical War'; Pechura and Rall (eds), *Veterans at Risk*, pp. 1, 10, 36; Evans, Gassed, pp. 54, 365.

20. There were 60,000 personnel exposed to mustard agents in the Navy alone. There were 1000 servicemen in the Army exposed at Edgewood, one of five testing locations, plus

there were about 90,000 military and civilan munitions workers. The Army has not made most of its records available and thus these figures are still incomplete. Freeman, 'The Unfought Chemical War'; Pechura and Rall (eds), Veterans at Risk, pp. 1, 10, 36; K. Freeman, 'The VA's Sorry, The Army's Silent', Bulletin of the Atomic Scientists, 49:2 (1 March 1993), pp. 39–43.

21. Bryden, *Deadly Allies*, p. 168; Lederer, *Subjected to Science*, p. 140; Rothman, *Strangers at the Bedside*, p. 30; Pechura and Rall (eds), *Veterans at Risk*.

22. Britain was eager for a large testing site because it no longer had access to French-controlled land in Algeria after Germany occupied France. Bryden, *Deadly Allies*, pp. 61–2; Avery, *The Science of War*, pp. 3–13, 130–1; Environment Canada, 'Suffield: History and Status: Land Expropriation for Military Research,' last updated 15 February 2005, http://www.mb.ec.gc.ca/nature/whp/nwa/suffield/dd02s02.en.html#use, accessed 11 November 2006.

23. B. Y. Card, 'Suffield Experimental Station (1941–5) – Strategic Centre in 'Canada's Secret War', unpublished four-page essay written for Remembrance Day for the Lethbridge Herald, 15 October 2004, author's possession, courtesy of Brigham Young Card via Robert Lampard.

24. J. T. Hugill, 'Trials of High Altitude Mustard Spray on Human Observers', Suffield Experimental Station, 20 December 1942, Defence Research Reports, Defence Research and Development Canada, http://pubs.drdc-rddc.gc.ca, accessed 16 May 2008.

25. D. Chown, 'Suffield, Chemical, Biological Warfare, and Canadian/U.S. Relations', *Peace Magazine* (February/March 1989), pp. 12–14, accession number 94.230, box 1, Provincial Archives of Alberta, Edmonton; Bryden, *Deadly Allies*, pp. 61, 168; Avery, *The Science of War*, pp. 130–1; Keshen, *Saints, Sinners, and Soldiers*, p. 48.

26. Bryden, *Deadly Allies*, pp. 168, 169, 171, 174. The 1947 Nuremberg Code established international ethical standards for research on humans, although the extent to which researchers implemented it in the following years remains the subject of much scholarly investigation. Moreno, *Undue Risk*, pp. 53–85.

27. Bryden, *Deadly Allies*, p. 174.

28. 'The Casualty Producing Power of Mustard Spray', Suffield Experimental Station, 4 January 1943, Defence Research Reports, Defence Research and Development Canada, http://pubs.drdc-rddc.gc.ca, accessed 16 May 2008.

29. W. Somerville, 'Comparison of the Protection Against Liquid Mustard Offered by 1 and 2 Layers of U.S. (CCR) Impregnated Clothing', Suffield Experimental Station, 20 September 1943, Defence Research Reports, Defence Research and Development Canada, http://pubs.drdc-rddc.gc.ca, accessed 16 May 2008.

30. Pechura and Rall (eds), Veterans at Risk, pp. 4–5, 64–6, 388; unpublished telephone notes and written testimony from veterans, National Academy of Sciences Archives, Washington, DC; and documentary films *Secret War*; and *Keen as Mustard*.

31. 'The Casualty Producing Power of Mustard Spray', Suffield Experimental Station, 4 January 1943; and B. A. Griffith and A. W. Birnie, 'Vapour Danger from Gross Mustard Contamination', Suffield Experimental Station, 8 October 1943, both at Defence Research Reports, Defence Research and Development Canada, http://pubs.drdc-rddc.gc.ca, accessed 16 May 2008.

32. Pechura and Rall (eds), *Veterans at Risk*, pp. 4–5, 64–6, 388; unpublished telephone notes and written testimony from US veterans, National Academy of Sciences Archives, Washington, DC; and documentary films Secret War; and Keen as Mustard.

33. Norman Amundson and John Dickson, quoted, in Brian Hauk, 'In WWII, Canadian Army Used Soldiers as Guinea Pigs for Chemical Weapons', *Vancouver Sun*, 19 November 2002. See also, 'Physiological Effect of Mustard Vapour at Low Temperatures', Suffield Experimental Station, 31 March 1944; and W. Somerville, 'The Protection Against Mustard Gas Vapour in the Chamber Afforded By A. V. Impregnated Khaki Drill Shirts and Trousers', 8 June 1944, Suffield Experimental Station, both in Defence Research Reports, Defence Research and Development Canada, http://pubs.drdc-rddc.gc.ca, accessed 16 May 2008.

34. 'Casualty Producing Power of Unthickened Mustard Sprayed from Low Altitudes Under Temperate Conditions', Suffield Experimental Station, 16 May 1944, Defence Research Reports, Defence Research and Development Canada, http://pubs.drdc-rddc.gc.ca, accessed 16 May 2008.

35. John Dickson, quoted in Hauk, 'In WWII, Canadian Army Used Soldiers as Guinea Pigs for Chemical Weapons'. See also, Bryden, *Deadly Allies*, pp. 166, 173.

36. See, for instance, Keshen, *Saints, Sinners, and Soldiers*, p. 280; and F. Milano, 'Gulf War Syndrome: The "Agent Orange" of the Nineties', *International Social Science Review*, 75:1–2 (2000), pp. 16–25.

37. Peter Neary, Chair, Veterans Affairs Canada – Canadian Forces Advisory Council, 'The Origins and Evolution of Veterans Benefits in Canada, 1914–2004', 15 March 2004, www.vac-acc.gc.ca/clients/sub.cfm?source=forces/nvc/reference#17, accessed 25 May 2008; 'When Service Affects Health,' Veterans Affairs Canada, 19 February 2004, www.vac-acc.gc.ca/general/sub.cfm?source=department/press/chemical_back, accessed 25 May 2008; Marnie Ko, 'Exposing Sufferville', *National Post*, 11 November 2004, www.marnieko.com/mustardgas.html, accessed 25 May 2008; 'Ex-soldiers File Suit Over Chemical Testing', *Edmonton Journal*, 8 November 2006, p. A9.

38. Freeman, 'The VA's Sorry, The Army's Silent', pp. 39–43; J. B. Perlin, Acting Under Secretary for Health, Department of Veterans Affairs, 'Under Secretary for Health's Information Letter: Health Effects Among Veterans Exposed to Mustard Gas and Lewisite Chemical Warfare Agents', 14 March 2005, www1.va.gov/vhapublications/ViewPublication.asp?pub_ID=1257, accessed 25 May 2008. For information on the Australian government response, see Goodwin, Keen as Mustard, and on the British government response, see Evans, Gassed.

39. The Axis scientists conducted mustard gas research to benefit the military and the medical community, but these human experiments were often deadly and conducted on people who were treated as dehumanized, racial 'others'. Japan conducted human experiments in Manchuria and used chemical and biological weapons against the Chinese during World War 2. The Germans conducted mustard gas experiments during World War 1 and on German cadets and concentration camp prisoners during World War 2. Baader, et al, 'Pathways to Human Experimentation, 1933–45', pp. 205–31, quote on p. 230. See also V. Spitz, *Doctors from Hell: The Horrific Account of Nazi Experiments on Humans* (Boulder, Co: Sentient Publications, 2005), ch. 9.

40. H. S. Fischgrund, 'Mustard Gas Claims', 13 August 1991, copy sent to Dr. Constance Pechura by Fischgrund 18 February 1992, National Academy of Sciences archives.

41. 'The Protection Afforded Against Mustard Gas Vapour by CCR Impregnated (Aqueous Method) Khaki Drill Trousers', Suffield Experimental Station, 22 June 1944, Defence Research Reports, Defence Research and Development Canada, http://pubs.drdc-rddc.gc.ca, accessed 16 May 2008.

42. Lederer, *Subjected to Science*.

43. Bryden, *Deadly Allies*, p. 176.
44. Bryden, *Deadly Allies*, p. 168.
45. US Office of Scientific Research and Development, Committee on Medical Research, *Advances in Military Medicine*, vol. 2 (Boston, MA: Little, Brown and Co. 1948), Part V: Chemical-Warfare Agents, pp. 532–620.
46. Pechura and Rall (eds), Veterans at Risk, p. 2.
47. On the controversial career of Rhoads, see S. E. Lederer, '"Porto Ricochet": Joking about Germs, Cancer, and Race Extermination in the 1930s', *American Literary History*, 14:4 (Winter 2002), pp. 720–46.
48. Brophy, Miles, and Cochrane, *The Chemical Warfare Service: From Laboratory to Field*, p. 100.
49. Joe Clark to Joyce Sorochan, 22 August 1988, Accession number 94.230, box 1, Provincial Archives of Alberta, Edmonton.
50. Defence R. and D. Canada Suffield, 'Chemical/Biological (CB Plus) Exposure Chamber Facility', 21 February 2005, http://www.suffield.drdc-rddc.gc.ca/Facilities/CB/FS2004_01_CBPLUS/index_e.html, accessed 12 November 2006.
51. For example, in 2006, the CounterACT Research Center of Excellence at the University of Medicine and Dentistry of New Jersey [UMDNJ] at Rutgers University received $19 million to design therapies to counteract chemical terrorism, include mustard gas. www.ninds.nih.gov/funding/research/counterterrorism/counterACT_home.htm, and www.counteract.rutgers.edu, both accessed 23 April 2008.
52. At Suffield, scientists are helping to test a product to alleviate exposure to nerve gas agents. Researchers have developed a drug, known as Protexia®, from a protein produced in the milk of transgenic goats. 'PharmAthene Awarded $1.7 Million NIH Grant for Protexia®', 18 October 2006, www.prnewswire.com/cgi-bin/stories.pl?ACCT=104&STORY=/www/story/10–18–2006. The term 'transgenic' refers to an animal or plant with genes from a different species.
53. Moon, 'Project SPHINX', p. 318.
54. V. Cohn, *Four Billion Dimes* (Minneapolis, MN: Minneapolis Star and Tribune, 1955), p. 55.
55. D. M. Oshinsky, *Polio: An American Story* (New York: Oxford University Press, 2005), pp. 92–128.
56. See A. M. Brandt, 'Polio, Politics, Publicity, and Duplicity: Ethical Aspects in the Development of the Salk Vaccine', *International Journal of Health Services*, 8:2 (1978), p. 264. See also Oshinsky, *Polio*, p. 200. For Dr Julius S. Youngner, see ibid., pp. 175, 205–6.
57. Christopher J. Rutty, 'Do Something! ... Do Anything!: Poliomyelitis in Canada, 1927–62' (PhD thesis, University of Toronto, 1995), p. 333. For information on the role of Connaught Laboratories, see Ibid., pp. 314–7.
58. Rutty, 'Do Something!', p. 332.
59. Constitution Act of 1867, <http://laws.justice.gc.ca/en/const/c1867_e.html> (last accessed: 20 May 2008); Cameron to McGinnis, May 20, 1954, Series 1: Country Files, 'Canada', Box 1, Gov. Rel. (For.) Records, March of Dimes Archives, White Plains, New York (henceforth denoted as MDA).
60. 'City Children to Share Test On Polio Vaccine', Edmonton Journal, 19 May 1954, p. 1; '20,000 Alberta Children Slated For Polio Tests', Edmonton Journal, 26 May 1954, p. 17. Halifax, Nova Scotia, also accepted on 21 May with 5,559 children, followed by Winnipeg on June 3 with 11,081 children. Other provinces declined to participate because

they were not prepared or because 'the amount [of vaccine] was not large enough to make a thorough test of vaccine effectiveness.' See Rutty, 'Do Something!', p. 333.

61. 'Changes At "Royal Alex" Add To Operating Costs', Edmonton Journal, 29 May 1954, p. 5.

62. 'Polio Vaccinations to Start in City Week of 14 June' Edmonton Journal, 2 June 1954, p. 17. Dublin to Van Riper, 20 May 1954, Series 1: Country Files, 'Canada', Box 1, Gov. Rel. (For.) Records, MDA.

63. Smith to Dublin, 20 May1954, Series 1: Country Files, 'Canada', Box 1, Gov. Rel. (For.) Records, MDA.

64. Dublin to Smith, 25 May 1954, Series 1: Country Files, 'Canada', Box 1, Gov. Rel. (For.) Records, MDA, p. 2.

65. Smith to Dublin, 28 May 1954, Series 1: Country Files, 'Canada', Box 1, Gov. Rel. (For.) Records, MDA.

66. Dublin to Press, 28 May 1954, Series 1: Country Files, 'Canada', Box 1, Gov. Rel. (For.) Records, MDA.

67. Huckell to Van Riper, 25 May 1954, Series 1: Country Files, 'Canada', Box 1, Gov. Rel. (For.) Records, MDA; Dublin to Smith, 25 May 1954, Series 1: Country Files, 'Canada', Box 1, Gov. Rel. (For.) Records, MDA, p. 2; Smith to Dublin, 28 May 1954, Series 1: Country Files, 'Canada', Box 1, Gov. Rel. (For.) Records, MDA; Dublin to Press, 28 May 1954, Series 1: Country Files, 'Canada', Box 1, Gov. Rel. (For.) Records, MDA.

68. 'U.S. Doctor Checks Polio Vaccination', Edmonton Journal, 18 June 1954, p. 25.

69. Smith to Dublin, 21 June 1954, Series 1: Country Files, 'Canada', Box 1, Gov. Rel. (For.) Records, MDA.

70. Rutty, 'Do Something!', p. 249.

71. Russell Frederick Taylor, Polio 53 (Edmonton: University of Alberta Press, 1990), p. 16.

72. Donald F. Smith, 'Polio Globulin Still In Short Supply', Drumheller Mail, 5 August 1953, p. 13; 'Poliomyelitis Vaccine Trial Schedule', Drumheller Mail, 7 July 1954, p. 13.

73. 'Parents of 3,515 Children Give Polio Test Permission,' Edmonton Journal, 7 June 1954, p. 17.

74. Rutty, 'Do Something!', p. 130.

75. Rutty, 'Do Something!', p. 130. It should also be noted that the Alberta government as early as 1927 showed concern for polio patients. In 1927, provincial authorities built the 'Provincial Special Hospital for Infantile Paralysis' in Edmonton with treatment given 'at cost.' See Ibid., p. 82.

76. Rutty, 'Do Something!', p. 83.

77. Ibid., p. 254.

78. Ibid., p. 333.

79. R. E. Curran, Canada's Food and Drug Laws (Chicago, IL: Commerce Clearing House, Inc., 1954), p. 193.

80. McGinnis to Cameron, May 24, 1954, Series 1: Country Files, 'Canada', Box 1, Gov. Rel. (For.) Records, MDA.

81. Rutty, 'Do Something!', p. 341.

82. Oshinsky, Polio, pp. 168, 198, 199.

83. Rutty, 'Do Something!', p. 322.

84. Ibid., p. 330.

85. Cameron to McGinnis, May 20, 1954, Series 1: Country Files, 'Canada', Box 1, Gov. Rel. (For.) Records, MDA.

86. Rutty, 'Do Something!, ' pp. 327–8, 332.

87. Oshinsky, *Polio*, pp. 192, 193.
88. Rutty, 'Do Something!, ' pp. 331–2.
89. Oshinsky, *Polio*, p. 195.
90. Oshinsky, *Polio*, p. 196; Rutty, 'Do Something!', p. 329.
91. Oshinsky, *Polio*, p. 197.
92. Dublin to Van Riper, May 20, 1954, Series 1: Country Files, 'Canada', Box 1, Gov. Rel. (For.) Records, MDA.
93. Taylor, *Polio* 53, pp. 13–22.
94. Rutty, 'Do Something!', p. 254; Josephson to Kingsbury, March 3, 1948, Series 1: Country Files, 'Canada', Box 1, Gov. Rel. (For.) Records, MDA.
95. Dublin to Van Riper, May 20, 1954, Series 1: Country Files, 'Canada', Box 1, Gov. Rel. (For.) Records, MDA.
96. Oshinsky, *Polio*, p. 177.
97. D. S. Burke, 'Lessons learned from the 1954 Field Trial of Poliomyelitis Vaccine, Clinical Trials 1 (2004), p. 4; Marcia Lynn Meldrum, 'Departures from the Design: The Randomized Clinical Trial in Historical Context, 1946–70' (PhD thesis, State University of New York, 1994), p. 154.
98. Oshinsky, *Polio*, p. 185.
99. A. K. Brownlee, 'Statistics of the 1954 Polio Vaccine Trials', *Journal of the American Statistical Association*, 50 (1955), p. 1007.
100. Dublin to Van Riper, 20 May 1954, Series 1: Country Files, 'Canada', Box 1, Gov. Rel. (For.) Records, MDA.
101. Osborne to Regional Reps., 25 May1954, Series 1: Country Files, 'Canada', Box 1, Gov. Rel. (For.) Records, MDA.
102. Rutty, 'Do Something!', p. 54.
103. Rutty, 'Do Something!', pp. 236, 328.
104. Smith to Dublin, 27 July 1954, Series 1: Country Files, 'Canada', Box 1, Gov. Rel. (For.) Records, MDA.
105. Dublin to Van Riper, 20 May 1954, Series 1: Country Files, 'Canada', Box 1, Gov. Rel. (For.) Records, MDA.
106. Francis to Amies, 25 May 1954, Series 1: Country Files, 'Canada', Box 1, Gov. Rel. (For.) Records, MDA.
107. 'Polio Test Report Set For April 12', *New York Times*, 23 March 1955, p. 33; William L. Laurence, 'Salk Polio Vaccine Proves Success; Millions Will Be Immunized Soon; City Schools Begin Shots April 25', *New York Times*, 13 April 1955, p. 1; J. Kluger, *Splendid Solution: Jonas Salk and the Conquest of Polio* (New York: G. P. Putnam's Sons, 2004), p. 294; J. R. Paul, *A History of Poliomyelitis* (New Haven, CT: Yale University Press, 1971), p. 432.
108. D. Bookchin and J. Schumacher, *The Virus and the Vaccine* (New York: St. Martin's Press, 2004), pp. 33–6; P. A Offit, *The Cutter Incident: How America's First Polio Vaccine Led to the Growing Vaccine Crisis* (New Haven, CT: Yale University Press, 2005), pp. 113–18.
109. Kluger, *Splendid Solution*, p. 251; J. S. Smith, *Patenting the Sun: Polio and the Salk Vaccine* (New York: William Morrow & Company, Inc., 1990), p. 237.
110. Kluger, *Splendid Solution*, p. 250.
111. Meldrum, 'Departures from the Design,' p. 128; Oshinsky, *Polio*, p. 190.
112. Offit, *Cutter Incident*, p. 89.
113. Edward Shorter, *The Health Century* (New York: Doubleday, 1987), pp. 196, 197, 199, 201, 203; Bookchin, *The Virus and the Vaccine*, pp. 60–70.

114. S. Shah, 'Testing Drugs on Prisoners: The Easy Out', *Boston Globe*, 17 August 2006; 'Study Finds a Widespread Risk Of Reactions to Some Medicines', *New York Times*, 18 October 2006, p. A15.

115. G. Harris, 'Halt Is Urged for Trials of Antibiotic in Children', *New York Times*, June 8, 2006, p. A16.

116. P. Marck, 'Altachem Cleared to Test Pre-Cancer Therapy', *Edmonton Journal*, 2 September 2005, p. E1.

117. 'Capital Health and University of Alberta launch Alberta's first Phase 1 clinical trials facility', *Canada NewsWire*, Ottawa, 26 June 2007, p. 1.

118. P. Galison and B. Hevly (eds), *Big Science: The Growth of Large-Scale Research* (Stanford, CA: Stanford University Press, 1992).

7 De Burgos, 'Placing Illness in its Cultural Territory in Veracruz, Nicaragua'

1. D. Banerji, 'The Political Economy of Western Medicine in Third World Countries', in J. B. McKinlay (ed.), Issues on the Political Economy of Health Care (New York: Tavistock, 1984), pp. 257–82; B. J. Good, Medicine, Rationality, and Experience: An anthropological Perspective (Cambridge: Cambridge University Press, 1994); A. Kleinman, Writing at the Margin: Discourse between Anthropology and Medicine (Berkeley, CA: University of California Press, 1995); E. Martin, The Woman in the Body: A Cultural Analysis of Reproduction (Boston, MA: Beacon Press 1987); S. Sontag, Illness as Metaphor (New York: Farrar, Straus and Giroux, 1978); N. Schepper-Hughes, Death without Weeping: The Violence of Everyday Life in Brazil (Berkeley, CA: University of California Press (1992); N. Schepper-Hughes and M. M. Lock, 'The Mindful Body: A Prolegomenon to Future Work in Medical Anthropology', Medical anthropology Quarterly, 1:1 (1987), pp. 6–41; A. Young, 'Internalizing and Externalizing Medical Belief Systems: an Ethiopian Example', *Social Science & Medicine, 10:3–4 (1976), pp. 147–56.*

2. Good, Medicine, Rationality, and Experience: An Anthropological Perspective; Kleinman, Writing at the Margin: Discourse between Anthropology and Medicine; Martin, The Woman in the Body: A Cultural Analysis of Reproduction; Sontag, Illness as Metaphor; Schepper-Hughes, Death without Weeping; Schepper-Hughes and Lock, 'The Mindful Body: A Prolegomenon to Future Work in Medical Anthropology'.

3. Good, *Medicine, Rationality, and Experience: An Anthropological Perspective*, pp. 53, 43.

4. H. De Burgos, *Suchitoto: ciudad y memoria* (San Salvador: Dirección Nacional de Publicaciones, 1999); W. R. Fowler, The Cultural Evolution of Ancient Nahua Civilizations: The Pipil-Nicarao of Central America (Norman and London: University of Oklahoma Press, 1989); Veracruceños abhor the term 'Indios', Spanish for Indian, and call themselves 'Indígenas', Spanish for Indigenous. They find the term 'Indios' pejorative, and think it is sad anachronistic misnomer that anthropologist in particular should avoid using. Thus, throughout this article I use the term 'Indigenous' with a capital 'I', to refer to Veracruceños and other Indigenous people for the following reasons. First, instead of using the lowercase 'I' for Indigenous, I use the capital 'I' to make a distinction between 'indigenous', meaning 'local' or 'home-grown', and Indigenous peoples in general. Stephen Greymorning makes a similar argument against the erroneously over-used term 'Indian' to designate Indigenous or Native people and uses uppercase 'I' in Indigenous when referring to Natives peoples, see Stephen Greymorning. A Will to Survive: Indig-

enous Essays on the Politics of Culture, Language, and Identity: Indigenous Essays on the Politics of Culture, Language and Identity (Boston, MA: McGraw-Hill, 2004). Since the 1970's, many Indigenous communities in Nicaragua, as well as in other parts of the world, gradually started to adopt the term 'Indigenous' as a self-designation used when presenting their claims in international forums such as the United Nations. Since the 1970's, many Indigenous communities in Nicaragua, as well as in other parts of the world, gradually started to adopt the term 'Indigenous' as a self-designation used when presenting their claims in international forums such as the United Nations. Currently, the term 'Indigenous', as argued by Niezen, 'is not only a legal category and an analytical concept but also an expression of identity, a badge worn with pride, revealing something significant and personal about its wearer's collective attachments', Currently, the term 'Indigenous', as argued by Niezen, 'is not only a legal category and an analytical concept but also an expression of identity, a badge worn with pride, revealing something significant and personal about its wearer's collective attachments'. See R. Niezen, The Origins of Indigenism: Human Rights and the Politics of Identity (Berkeley, CA: University of California Press, 2003), p. 3. Migrations of Nahua groups from Mexico to Central America are perhaps some of the best-known examples of large-scale population movements of 'New World' cultural history (Fowler, The Cultural Evolution of Ancient Nahua Civilizations).

5. P. F. Healy, *Archaeology of the Rivas Region, Nicaragua* (Waterloo, Ontario: Wilfrid Laurier University Press, 1980); S. R. Urtecho, Cultura e Historia Prehispánica del Istmo de Rivas (León, Nicaragua: Editorial Hospicio-León, 1960), p. 87.

6. Urtecho, *Cultura e HistoriaPrehispánica del Istmo de Rivas*, pp. 87–9.

7. H. De Burgos, 'Indigenous Medicine and Identity in Nicaragua' (PhD dissertation, University of Alberta, Edmonton, Canada, 2006).

8. Good, *Medicine, Rationality, and Experience: An Anthropological Perspective*; Kleinman, *Writing at the Margin: Discourse between Anthropology and Medicine*.

9. G. Lakoff and M. Johnson, *Metaphors We Live By* (Chicago, IL: The University of Chicago Press, 1980).

10. G. Gordillo, *Landscapes of Devils: Tensions of Place and Memory in the Argentinean Chaco* (Durham: Duke University Press, 2004), p. 3.

11. H. Baer, M. Singer and I. Susser, *Medical Anthropology and the World System* (Westport, CT: Praeger, 2003), p. 8.

12. R. Handler, *Nationalism and the Politics of Culture in Quebec* (Wisconsin: University of Wisconsin Press, 1988).

13. L. Garro, 'Cultural Configurations of the self', *Transcultural Psychiatry*, 40:1 (March 2003), pp. 91–108.

14. Central to my analysis is a particular category of people encountered at the fieldwork site. Given their unconcealed political militancy, and their roll in preserving and vitalizing their community's 'Indigenous culture', I refer to these people as Culturally Conservative Leaders. Around ten men and two women constitute the core of this group. They promote marital endogamy, local cultural values, rituals, historical awareness, and traditions as a way of resisting what they call 'an engulfing mestizo culture'. Most CCL are well-versed in national and international politics, Indigenous rights, and issues of globalization. In the past, some of them have served as leaders in important national and international Indigenous organizations. Nowadays, they continue to be active in the Nicaraguan Indigenous movements and the Parlamento Indígena de América. Although

all CCL are part of the monéxico (Nahua for council of elders), not all members of the monéxico are part of the CCL group. In many ways CCLs are an elite group.

15. Cultural consultant and CCL Esban Gonzáles interviewed by the author in Veracruz during the research.

16. C. Geertz, 'The integrative revolution: primordial sentiments and civil politics in the new states', in C. Geertz (ed.), Old Societies and New States (New York: Free Press, 1963); F. J. Gil-White, 'How thick is blood? The plot thickens ...: If ethnic actors are primordialists, what remains of the circumstantialist/primordialist controversy?', Ethnic and Racial Studies, 22:5 (1999), pp. 789–820; E. Shils, 'Primordial, Personal, Sacred, and Civil Ties', British Journal of Psychology, 8 (1957), pp. 130–45.

17. B. Anderson, Imagined Communities: Reflections on the Origin and Spread of Nationalism (London; New York: Verso, 2006).

18. M. Sahlins, Historical Metaphors and Mythical Realities: Structure in the Early History of the Sandwich Islands (ASAO Special Publication, Ann Arbor, MI: University of Michigan Press, 1995), p. 7.

19. G. Gordillo, Landscapes of Devils: Tensions of Place and Memory in the Argentinean Chaco; M. Taussig, Mimesis and Alterity: A Particular History of the Senses (London: Routledge, 1993).

20. C. Esteva-Fabrigat, Mestizaje in Ibero-America (Tucson, AZ: University of Arizona Press, 1995).

21. L. Field, 'Post-Sandinista Ethnic Identities in Western Nicaragua', American Anthropologist, 100:2 (1998), p. 435.

22. A. Knight, 'Racism, Revolution, and Indigenism: Mexico, 1910–40', in Graham (ed.), The Idea of Race in Latin America, 1870–1940 (Austin, TX: University of Texas, 1990), p. 73.

23. Field, 'Post-Sandinista Ethnic Identities in Western Nicaragua', p. 438.

24. M. Rizo Zeledón, 'Etnicidad, legalidad y demandas de las comunidades indígenas del norte, centro y del Pacífico de Nicaragua', in G. Romero (ed.), Persistencia indígena en Nicaragua (Managua: CIDCA, 1992), p. 88.

25. Similar to the colonial shilling, pesos duros (Spanish currency during the colony) were intended to serve as universal money, as opposed to local currency, which was considered pesos sencillos or simple; see W. G. Sumner, 'The Spanish Dollar and the Colonial Shilling', American Historical Review, 3 (July 1898, 2002), pp. 607–19.

26. De Burgos, 'Indigenous Medicine and Identity in Nicaragua'.

27. Hoyt, The Many Faces of Sandinista Democracy. Monographs in International Studies. Latin American Series, Number 27 Athens (Ohio: Ohio University for International Studies. 1997). p. 85.

28. G. V. Romero, Persistencia Indígena en Nicaragua (Managua: CIDCA-UCA, 1992).

29. In the 1960s, Juan Salinas, an individual with no relation to the community and under the protection of the Somoza dictatorship, fraudulently claimed ownership of over one-sixth of the Veracruz territory. During the Sandinista agrarian reform, which did not include communally owned lands, the land Salinas had illegally claimed were confiscated and allocated to a cooperative comprized of people from Veracruz.

30. Cultural consultant and CCL Arturón Morales interviewed by the author in Veracruz during the research.

31. P. Gow, 'Land, People, and Paper in Western Amazona', in Eric Hirsch and Michael O'Hanlon (eds.), The Anthropology of Landscape: Perspectives on Place and Space (Oxford: Oxford University Press, 1995), p. 59.

32. G. Gordillo, 'The Crucible of Citizenship: ID-Paper Fetishism in the Argentinean Chaco', *American Ethnologist*, 33:2 (2006), pp.162–76.

33. F. Barth, *Ethnic Groups and Boundaries: The Social Organization of Difference* (Boston, MA: Little, Brown and Company, 1969).

34. G. W. White, *Nationalism and Territory: Constructing Group Identity in Southeastern Europe* (Lanham, MD: Rowman & Littlefield Pub Inc., 2000).

35. M. Saltman, *Land and Territoriality* (Oxford; New York: Berg, 2002).

36. J. Friedman, *Cultural Identity and Global Process* (London: Sage, 1994), p. 117.

37. Sahlins, *Historical Metaphors and Mythical Realities: Structure in the early History of the Sandwich Islands*, p. 5.

38. R. Borofsky, *Making History: Pukapukan and Anthropological Constructions of Knowledge* (Cambridge: Cambridge University Press, 1989).

39. B. Anderson, *Imagined Communities: Reflections on the Origin and Spread of Nationalism; The Invention of Tradition* (Cambridge: Cambridge University Press, 1992).

40. Borofsky, *Making History*.

41. Ibid., p. 144.

42. Barth, *Ethnic Groups and Boundaries*.

43. P. Bourdieu, *Language & Symbolic Power* (Cambridge: Polity Press, 1991).

44. Cultural consultant and CCL Conchita Gonzáles intervied by the author in Veracruz during the research.

45. Cultural consultant and CCL Alfredo López interviewed by the author in Veracruz during the research.

46. M. Bloch, 'People into Places: Zafimaniry Concepts of Clarity', in E. Hirsch and Michael O'Hanlon (eds), *The Anthropology of Landscape: Perspectives on Place and Space* (Oxford: Oxford University Press, 1995).

47. Cultural consultant and CCL Pedro Gonzáles interviewed by the author during the research. Gonzáles also claims that since the Sandinista agrarian reform was not to handle communally owned lands, Indigenous communal lands were to be formally demarcated as Indigenous territory in order to exempt them from the agrarian amendment. Once Indigenous lands had been properly demarcated, adjacent lands were confiscated and used as state farms and cooperatives during the Sandinista revolution.

48. Cultural consultant and CCL Alfredo López interviewed by the author during the research.

49. Cultural consultant and CCL Pedro Gonzáles interviewed by the author during the research CCL.

50. R. Keesing, Kwaio Religion: The Living and the Dead in a Solomon Island Society (New York: Columbia University Press, 1982), p. 76.

51. Taussig, Mimesis and Alterity: A Particular History of the Senses.

52. Gordillo, Landscapes of Devils: Tensions of Place and Memory in the Argentinean Chaco, p. 5.

53. Cultural consultant and CCL Alfredo López interviewed by the author during the research.

54. Cultural consultant, healer and CCL Felipe Urrútia interviewed by the author during the research.

55. Cultural consultant and healer Agustina Pavón interviewed by the author during the research.

56. Cultural consultant and CCL Alfredo López interviewed by the author during the research.

57. Cultural consultant and CCL Alfredo López interviewed by the author during the research.

58. Cultural consultant and healer Cipriano M. interviewed by the author during the research.

59. A. Dávila Bolaños, Medicina Pre-colombina de Nicaragua (Estelí, Nicaragua: Editorial Imprenta, 1974), p. 38; I am here artificially separating the natural from the supernatural based on a Western model, since in Veracruz the supernatural is only another level of reality from the natural world; Evans-Pritchard, similarly argued that to suggest that 'for the Azande people supernatural agency is regarded as the cause of illness, hardly reflects their view of the matter, because from their point of view nothing can be more natural than witchcraft', see E. E. Evans-Pritchard, Witchcraft, Oracles, and Magic among the Azande (Oxford: Clarendon, 1937), pp. 80–3.

60. G. Foster, 'Hippocrates' Latin American Legacy: "Hot" and "Cold" in Contemporary Folk Medicine', in R. K. Wetherington (ed.), Colloquia in Anthropology, 2 (Dallas, TX: Southern Methodist University and Fort Burgwin Research Center, 1968), pp. 3–19.

61. For a similar discussion in the Peruvian Amazon see P. Gow, 'Land, People, and Paper in Western Amazona'in Eric Hirsch and Michael O'Hanlon (ed.), The Anthropology of Landscape: Perspectives on Place and Space (Oxford: Oxford University Press, 1995).

62. L. Garro, 'Cultural Configurations of the self', Transcultural Psychiatry.

63. D. Bolaños, Medicina Pre-colombina de Nicaragua, p. 38.

64. Ibid., p. 58.

65. See M. Taussig, Mimesis and Alterity: A Particular History of the Senses; June Nash, We Eat the Mines and the Mines Eat Us: Dependency and Exploitation in Bolivian Tin Mines (New York: Columbia University Press, 1993), for a discussion of similar beliefs.

66. Regrettably, ten people passed on in the community during the period of my fieldwork; a young man was killed accidentally by one of his own sibling during a fight at a party; another had a dreadful bicycle crash that broke his neck; a young teenager was killed by neurocysticercosis caused by eating contaminated pork; two other youths died of mysterious causes while in Costa Rica; and the rest, mainly children and elders, died from infectious and chronic illnesses, particularly diabetes and moto (tetanus).

67. Cultural consultant and CCL Alex Morales interviewed by the author during the research.

68. Snake powder is prepared by drying its flesh and grinding it until a fine powder is obtained.

69. Cultural consultant and healer Cipriano M. interviewed by the author during the research.

70. This same tree is also regarded as sacred in the Afro-Cuban religion of Santeria, see L. Cabrera, El Monte (Miami: Ediciones Universal, 1995).

71. Cultural consultant and healer Agustina Pavón interviewed by the author during the research.

72. Cultural consultant, CCL and healer Felipe Urrutia interviewed by the author during the research.

73. Cultural consultant and healer Cipriano M. interviewed by the author during the research.

74. S. Hall, 'Cultural Identity and Diaspora', in J. Rutherford (ed.), Identity, Community, Culture Difference (London: Lawrence and Wishart, 1990).

75. Cultural consultant and CCL Alfredo López interviewed by the author during the research.

76. De Burgos, 'Indigenous Medicine and Identity in Nicaragua'.
77. Ibid.
78. Taussig, Mimesis and Alterity: A Particular History of the Senses.
79. See Dávila Bolaños, Medicina Pre-colombina de Nicaragua.
80. Bioenergetics is a diagnostic method developed by a Japanese physician, Yoshiaki Omura, in 1978, and introduced to Nicaragua by the Germans who in the 1980s came as internationalist to work with the Sandinistas. The method was initially called 'Bi-Digital' or 'Ring-Test' (Fundación Comunidad del Hospital Natural de Nicaragua, 1993, p. 29). Bioenergetics is based on the applications of an electro-magnetic field between the patient, the medicaments and the healers. Based on this technique, the healer seeks to detect the illness, its possible causes and its treatment.
81. R. Campos Navarro, Nosotros los Curanderos: Experiencias de una curandera tradicional en el México de Hoy (Ciudad de México: Nueva Imagen, 1997); S. Cosminsky, 'The Evil Eye in a Chiché Community', in C. Maloney (ed.), The Evil Eye (New York: Columbia University Press, 1976), pp. 163–74; G. Foster, 'Hippocrates' Latin American Legacy'; A. Rubel, C. O'Nell and R. Collado-Ardon, Susto: A Folk Illness (California: University of California Press, 1984); N. Schepper-Hughes and D. Stewart, 'Curanderismo in Taos country, New Mexico –a Possible Case of Anthropological Romanticism?', Western Journal of Medicine, 139 (1983), pp. 875–84.
82. Bolaños, Medicina Pre-colombina de Nicaragua, p. 52.
83. Cosminsky, 'The Evil Eye in a Chiché Community', p. 164.
84. Kleinman, Writing at the Margin: Discourse between Anthropology and Medicine, p. 23.
85. S. Pigg, 'Acronyms and Effacements: Traditional Medical Practitioners (TMP) in International Health Development', Social and Medicine, 41:1 (1995).
86. C. O. Sauer, 'The Fourth Dimension of Geography', in C. O. Sauer (ed.), Selected Essays, 1963–75 (Berkeley, CA: Turtle Island Foundation, 1974); C. M. Fletcher, 'Equivocal Illness and Cultural Landscape in Nova Scotia' (Ph.D. Dissertation, Université de Montréal, Canada, 2002), p. 28.
87. A. R. Damasio, Descartes' Error: Emotion, Reason, and the Human Brain (New York: G. P. Putnam, 1994).

8 Piper, 'Chronic Disease in the Yukon River Basin, 1890–1960'

1. W. H. Fry to Bishop Stringer, 25 November 1919, COR 251 file 16, Yukon Archives [hereafter YA].
2. W. A. Geddes to A. Coldrick, 25 January 1934, COR 260 file 17, YA; News from Bishop Stringer, 31 May 1921, COR 251 file 20, YA.
3. Humans, in turn and in keeping with prevailing interpretations in environmental history, are considered as part of, not separate from, the rest of nature.
4. A. W. Crosby, 'Virgin Soil Epidemics as a Factor in the Depopulation of the Americas', The William and Mary Quarterly, 33 (April 1976), pp. 289–99; A. W. Crosby, Ecological Imperialism: The Biological Expansion of Europe, 900–1900 (Cambridge; New York: Cambridge University Press, 1986); L. Piper and J. Sandlos, 'A Broken Frontier: Ecological Imperialism in the Canadian North', Environmental History, 12:4 (2007), pp. 759–95.
5. Current research on northern tuberculosis includes most importantly R. Fortuine, Must we all Die? Alaska's Enduring Struggle with Tuberculosis (Fairbanks, AL: University of

Alaska Press, 2005); M. E. Kelm, *Colonizing Bodies: Aboriginal health and healing in British Columbia 1900–50* (Vancouver: UBC Press, 1998); P. S. Grygier, *A Long Way from Home: The Tuberculosis Epidemic among the Inuit* (Montreal & Kingston: McGill-Queen's University Press, 1994); ch. 1 and 2 in F. J. Tester and P. Kulchyski, *Tammarniit (Mistakes): Inuit relocation in the Eastern Arctic* (Vancouver: UBC Press, 1994). For an invaluable study from southern Canada see M. Lux, *Medicine that Walks: Disease, Medicine, and Canadian Plains Native Peoples, 1880–1940* (Toronto: University of Toronto Press, 2001).

6.   See, for example, the register of Baptisms, Burials and Marriages, 1887–1902, for Buxton Mission, COR O/S 001b, file 2, and the Confirmation, Marriage, and Burial Records for Aklavik, COR 261, file 5, YA. For discussion of missionary medical knowledge see Walter J. Vanast, 'Arctic bodies, frontier souls: missionaries and medical care in the Canadian North, 1896–1926', (PhD dissertation: University of Wisconsin – Madison, 1996); See also M. McCarthy, *From the Great River to the Ends of the Earth: Oblate Missions to the Dene, 1847–1921* (Edmonton: University of Alberta Press and Western Canadian Publishers, 1995). Evidence drawn from this database is hereafter referenced as Cause of Death Database with specific year(s) or reference number(s) indicated.

7.   J. Cruikshank's, *Do Glaciers Listen? Local Knowledge, Colonial Encounters, and Social Imagination* (Vancouver: University of British Columbia Press, 2005) is focused upon from the St. Elias range.

8.   The health history of Alaska has received much more sustained study than that of the Yukon. This paper will draw upon secondary references to the health history of Alaska, as appropriate. See in particular Fortuine, *Must we all Die?*; R. Fortuine, *Chills and Fever: Health and Disease in the Early History of Alaska* (Fairbanks, AL: University of Alaska Press, 1989).

9.   See for examples, The Elders of Tsiigehtshik with Michael Heine, Alestine Andre, Ingrid Kirtsch and Alma Cardinal, *Gwichya Gwich'in Googwandak. The History and Stories of the Gwichya Gwich'in, As Told by the Elders of Tsiigehtshik* (Tsiigehtchik: Gwich'in Social and Cultural Institute, 2007). *Gwichya Gwich'in Googwandak* which although focused on the Gwich'in in the Mackenzie delta region, makes reference to a larger area including the northern Yukon; Heritage Branch, Yukon, Fort Selkirk Elders Oral History Project, 2 vols (recorded 21 July 1985, transcribed February–March 1987); C. McClellan, *My Old People Say: An Ethnographic Survey of Southern Yukon Territory*, parts 1 and 2 (Ottawa: National Museum of Man; available from National Museums of Canada, 1975).

10. K. S. Coates, *Best Left as Indians: Native-White Relations in the Yukon Territory, 1840–1973* (Montreal-Kingston: McGill-Queen's University Press, 1991); K. S. Coates and W. R. Morrison, *Land of the Midnight Sun: a History of the Yukon*, 2 edn (Montreal-Kingston: McGill-Queen's University Press, 2005).

11. K. Morse, *The Nature of Gold: An Environmental History of the Klondike Gold Rush* (Seattle, WA: University of Washington Press, 2003), pp. 48–58.

12. For environmental toxins and health see J. A. Roberts and N. Langston, 'Toxic Bodies/ Toxic Environments: An Interdisciplinary Forum', *Environmental History* 13:4 (2008), pp. 629–703. One of the better known northern issues linking environmental toxins and ill-health is the concern about the role of concentrated Persistent Organic Pollutants (POPs) in Arctic environments, see D. Leonard Downie and Terry Fenge (eds), *Northern lights against POPs: combatting toxic threats in the Arctic* (Montreal, QC: Published for the Inuit Circumpolar Conference Canada by McGill-Queen's University Press, 2003).

13. R. J. Bowerman, 'Alaska Native Cancer Epidemiology in the Arctic', *Public Health*, 112:1 (1998), pp. 7–13; N. M. Edwards, 'Cancer in Point Hope, Alaska: Science, Language,

and Knowledge', (PhD dissertation: Arizona State University, 2000). See also S. Kirsch, *Proving Grounds: Project Plowshare and the Unrealized Dream of Nuclear Earthmoving* (New Brunswick, NJ: Rutgers University Press, 2005).

14. For some instances of post-1950s developments see P. R. Mulvihill, D. C. Baker, W. R. Morrison, 'A Conceptual Framework for Environmental History in Canada's North', *Environmental History*, 9:4 (2001), pp. 611–26.

15. V. Stefansson, *Cancer: Disease of Civilization? An Anthropological and Historical Study* (New York: Hill and Wang, 1960).

16. Fortuine, *Chills and Fever*, p. 85.

17. For discussion of difficulties in discerning cancer in the historical record see B. Clow, *Negotiating Disease: Power and Cancer Care, 1900–1950* (Montreal and Kingston: McGill-Queen's University Press, 2001), pp. 20–5.

18. Robert McDonald diary, 11 July 1872, YA. Robert McDonald fonds, 86/97, MSS 195. Archives of the Ecclesiastical Province of Rupert's Land, Winnipeg.

19. Fortuine, *Chills and Fever*, p. 276.

20. Clow, *Negotiating Disease*, pp. 16–17 for survival from different kinds of cancers.

21. Figures from Coates, *Best Left as Indians*, Table 8 'Sex Ratios, Yukon Population, 1901–51' data from Canada Census.

22. Ibid, Table 7.

23. Cause of Death Database, 1905, 1925, 1929, 1931 for examples.

24. M. K. Lux, 'Disease and Growth of Dawson City: The Seamy Underside of a Legend,' *The Northern Review*, 3:4 (1989), pp. 96–117.

25. Morse, *Nature of Gold*, n. 128.

26. A. Duncan, *Medicine, Madams and Mounties: Stories of a Yukon Doctor, 1933–47* (Vancouver: Raincoast Books, 1989), p. 80.

27. Duncan, *Medicine, Madams and Mounties*, p. 81.

28. F. Wilson and D. Hawkins, 'Arsenic in Streams, Stream Sediments, and Ground Water, Fairbanks Area, Alaska,' *Environmental Geology*, 2:4 (July 1978), pp. 195–202.

29. P. T. Rowe, 'The Yukon Country', *The Chautauquan* (Jan. 1899). Abstract of a lecture delivered at Sitka, Alaska.

30. See the Native American Ethnobotany Database (University of Michigan) http://herb.umd.umich.edu/ for details on how each of these plants were used in indigenous cancer treatments.

31. See Cause of Death Database, ID 1819.

32. There is little evidence of preventative measures or even much effort at early detection being taken with regards to cancer before the 1950s. In 1949, pamphlets advising people to see their doctor if they had suspicious pain were distributed to Yukon residents, see 'Health newsletter, ' September 1949, in GOV 1886, file 36496, part 2, YA. For the importance of early detection from the late 1920s see Clow, *Negotiating Disease*, p. 50. For the history of radiation therapy in Canada see C. Hayter, *An Element of Hope: Radium and the Response to Cancer in Canada, 1900–40* (Montreal: McGill-Queen's University Press, 2005). After 1953 the Yukon territorial government was funding, in cooperation with the federal government, a 'Cancer Control Grant Detection and Treatment Project,' see GOV 2286, file 10, YA.

33. Duncan, *Medicine, Madams and Mounties*, p. 27.

34. For just two examples of women who chose to leave the Yukon for health reasons see K. Coates and B. Morrison, *The Sinking of the Princess Sophia: Taking the North Down with Her* (Fairbanks, AL: University of Alaska Press, 1991), pp. 17–19.

35. C. K. LeCapelain, Memorandum 'Treatment of Tubercular Patients from the NWT and Yukon', 10 July 1950, GOV 2206, file 1, YA.

36. Charles Camsell History Committee, *The Camsell Mosaic: the Charles Camsell Hospital, 1945–85* (Edmonton: Charles Camsell History Committee, 1985), p. 47.

37. *The Camsell Mosaic*, p. 16.

38. B. G. Sivertz to P. E. Moore, 16 January 1957, See also B. G. Sivertz to W. L. Falconer, 29 August 1957 both in RG 85, vol. 2075, file 554/600, part 3, Library and Archives Canada [hereafter LAC].

39. R. T. Boyd, *The Coming of the Spirit of Pestilence: Introduced Infectious Diseases and Population Decline among Northwest Coast Indians, 1774–1874* (Vancouver and Toronto: University of British Columbia Press, 1999), pp. 9–15, 61–3 and part I of Fortuine, *Chills and Fever* for discussions of the earliest evidence of tuberculosis.

40. Fortuine, *Must we all Die?*, p. 10.

41. Their arrival also led to outbreaks of measles, influenza, diphtheria, typhoid, and dysentery. See Morse, *Nature of Gold*, p. 163.

42. P. R. Donald and J. F. Schoeman, 'Tuberculous Meningitis', *New England Journal of Medicine*, 351:17 (2004), pp. 1719–20.

43. D. B. Shimkin, 'The Economy of a Trapping Center: The Case of Fort Yukon, Alaska', *Economic Development and Cultural Change*, 3:3 (1955), pp. 225.

44. Cause of Death Database, ID 1166, 1476, 1403, 1494, 1477 for some examples.

45. Coates, *Best Left as Indians*, Table 7.

46. Major epidemics in the Yukon basin included a combined measles and influenza epidemic known as the 'Great Sickness' that originated in Alaska in 1900 and spread along the Yukon River, reaching Fort Selkirk and later the Mackenzie district. The Spanish flu in 1918–19 principally affected the southernmost part of the Yukon basin. Robert J. Wolfe, 'Alaska's Great Sickness, 1900: An Epidemic of Measles and Influenza in a Virgin Soil Population', *Proceedings of the American Philosophical Society*, 126 (April 1982), pp. 91–121; Fortuine, *Chills and Fever*, 215–26. For Spanish flu see various correspondence in spring of 1919 related to Skagway and Champagne Landing in particular in RG 18, series A–1, vol. 567, file G6, LAC. Also interview with Johnnie Johns, in Skookum Jim Oral History Project fonds, COR 1096 (88/58 R), YA.

47. See Cause of Death Database.

48. M. Docherty to W. L. Falconer, 16 April 1955, RG 29, vol. 2970, file 851–4–096, part 1, LAC.

49. G. Mitman, 'In Search of Health: Landscape and Disease in American Environmental History', *Environmental History*, 10:2 (2005), pp. 184–210; K. Thompson, 'Wilderness and Health in the Nineteenth Century', *Journal of Historical Geography*, 2:2 (1976), pp. 145–61; .

50. R. Campbell, *In Darkest Alaska: Travel and Empire Along the Inside Passage* (Philadelphia, PA: University of Pennsylvania Press, 2007).

51. E. B. Osborn, *Greater Canada the Past, Present and Future of the Canadian North-West* (London: Chatto & Windus, 1900), pp. 1–2.

52. For another example see G. Bryce, *The Remarkable History of the Hudson's Bay Company including that of the French Traders of North-Western Canada and of the North-West, XY, and Astor Fur Companies* (Toronto: W. Briggs, 1900), p. 477 and for discussion of historical perceptions of the Canadian North see Janice Cavell, 'The Second Frontier: The North in English-Canadian Historical Writing', *Canadian Historical Review*, 83:3 (2002) and S. Grant, 'Arctic Wilderness – And Other Mythologies', *Journal of Canadian Studies*, 32:2 (1998).

53. Bryce, *Remarkable History*, p. 395, for discussion see Bill Waiser, 'Bill Waiser', A Very Long Journey: Distance and Northern History', in *Northern Visions: New Perspectives on the North in Canadian History* (Peterborough, Ontario: Broadview Press, 2001), pp. 37–44.

54. I. S. Shepherd, *The Cruise of the U.S. Steamer 'Rush' in Behring Sea Summer of 1889* (San Francisco, CA: Bancroft, 1889), p. 119.

55. Bryce, *Remarkable History*, p. 3.

56. See [name ommitted], RG 85, vol. 973, file 14246, LAC.

57. A. C. Duncan to J. Gibben, 26 May 1944, GOV 2206, file 7, YA.

58. William C. Stewart to The Commissioner, Yukon Territory, 17 December 1949, RG 91, series 2, vol. 65, file 813, LAC.

59. J. E. Gibben to H.L. Keenleyside, 4 September 1947, RG 91, series 2, vol. 65, file 813, LAC.

60. E. J. Young, Colonel, Acting General Director Medical Services to Command Medical Officer, Edmonton, 16 September 1947, RG 91, series 2, vol. 65, file 813, LAC.

61. J. E. Gibben to H. Melzter, March 10, 1949, RG 91, series 2, vol. 65, file 813, LAC.

62. Ibid.

63. J. Locke, 'Report on a Tuberculosis Survey in the Yukon Territory', [1949] RG 91, series 2, vol. 65, file 813, LAC.

64. J.E. Gibben to R. A. Gibson, 31 July 1950, GOV 2206, file 1, YA.

65. B. P. Duncan to Dr. Stone, Regional Director, Indian Health Services, Charles Camsell Hospital, 7 February 1950, RG 85, vol. 742, file 554/201, LAC; See also C. K. LeCapelain, Memorandum for the Commissioner, 25 November 1950, RG 85, vol. 178, file 552–1–1, part 2, LAC.

66. See Grygier, *A Long Way from Home*, p. 73. The US government also sent Alaska Natives south to a sanatorium established in Washington state for treatment. See Fortuine, *Must we all Die?*, pp. 123–6.

67. R. A. Gibson to P. E. Moore, 21 June 1945, GOV 2206, file 1, YA; LeCapelain, Memorandum, 25 November 1950. See also C. K. LeCapelain, Memorandum 'Treatment of Tubercular Patients from the NWT and Yukon', 10 July 1950, GOV 2206, file 1, YA.

68. For details on early epidemics and state response to them see F. Montizambert, MD Director General of Public Health, Ottawa, 4 July 1901; F. Montizambert to A. E. Porter, 1900; the Semi-annual report on the Sanitary condition of the Dawson Health District (with vital and other statistics) for the half year ending Dec 31 1900; all in RG 29, vol. 2, file 937013, part 2, LAC; also Ronald L. Lautaret, 'Alaska's Greatest Disaster: The 1918 Spanish Influenza Epidemic', *Alaska Journal* 16 (1986).

69. Fortuine, *Must we all Die?*, pp. 21–3; *Chills and Fever*, ch. 8.

70. Gold Commissioner to Major R. E. Tucker, Officer Commanding 'B' Division RCMPolice Dawson, 29 November 1920, GOV 1843, file 251, parts 1 and 2, YA.

71. Fortuine, *Chills and Fever*, p. 185.

72. Bishop Stringer to C. F. Johnson, 20 June 1921, COR 252, file 11 A, YA.

73. Coates, *Best Left as Indians*, p. 97.

74. As well, of course, the federal government paid the health expenses of Native peoples as wards of the state.

75. G.I MacLean to O.S. Finnie, Director, NWT and Yukon Branch, 18 August 1928, GOV 1929, file 403–2, parts 1–5, YA. See also Coates, *Best Left as Indians*, p. 95.

76. H. A. Proctor to Dr. Moore, 14 March 1949, RG 85, vol. 742, file 554/201, LAC.

77. 'Report on Teslin Mission, June–Sept 1931', COR 258, file 6, YA.

78. This is in contrast to Coates suggestion that this system was dispensed with in 1905, *Best Left as Indians*, p. 174.
79. McClellan, *My Old People Say*, part 1, p. 224.
80. McClellan, *My Old People Say*, part 2, pp. 343–99 for life-cycle including birth practices; See also J. Cruikshank in collaboration with A. Sidney, K. Smith and A. Ned, *Life Lived Like a Story: Life Stories of Three Yukon Native Elders* (Vancouver: University of British Columbia Press, 1990), p. 246; Cause of Death Database records twelve of thirty-three women or children who died in childbirth whose race/ethnicity was known before 1939 as Native or Metis. Shimkin, in 'Economy of a Trapping Center', p. 225 also describes low mortality in childbirth among the residents of Fort Yukon, noting that surviving birth was less difficult than surviving childhood and in particular childhood tuberculosis.
81. A. Andre and A. Fehr, *Gwich'in Ethnobotany: Plants used by the Gwich'in for Food, Medicine, Shelter and Tools* (Gwich'in Social and Cultural Institute and Aurora Research Institute, 2002) including references to cure for respiratory problems. See also McDonald diaries, 15 April 1879, McDonald notes that his wife 'Julia went to gather liquorice roots'.
82. Cause of Death Database, ID 4384.
83. *Fort Selkirk Elders Oral History Project*, pp. 3, 28.
84. Archie Linklater diaries, MSS O/S 6 (95/30), YA.
85. Frank Foster diaries, MSS 62 (82/415), YA.
86. Controller of Yukon Territory, 4 March 1938 in RG 85, vol. 742, file 554/201, LAC.
87. J. Cruikshank, 'The Gravel Magnet: Some Social Impacts of the Alaska Highway on Yukon Indians', in K. Coates (ed.), *The Alaska Highway: Papers of the 40th Anniversary Symposium* (Vancouver: University of British Columbia Press, 1985), p. 183.
88. P. E. Moore to Regional Superintendent, Foothills Region, 24 May 1957, GOV 2319, file 1, YA.
89. R. A. Gibson, Director to G. A. Jeckell, Controller, 16 May 1944, GOV 2206, file 7, YA.
90. G. A. Jeckell to R. A. Gibson, 31 May 1944, GOV 2206, file 7, YA – decided not to because too expensive and would require significant modification to be made into a permanent facility.
91. Copy of letter from J. L. Coudert, OMI to T. A. Crerar, 10 October 1944, GOV 2206, file 7, YA.
92. Memorandum for the Advisory Committee on Northern Development: Northern Health Services, 29 March 1954, RG 85, vol. 1335, file 554/119, part 5, LAC – technically ten years after Coubert's letter to Crerar, but the sentiment in place since 1920s with Aklavik.
93. For a recent contribution to this extensive literature see S. Tillotson, *Contributing Citizens: Modern Charitable Fundraising and the Making of the Welfare State, 1920–66* (Vancouver: UBC Press, 2008).
94. See for example, A.H. Gibson wire to Ivan Schultz, 23 October 1950, GOV 2206, file 1, YA.
95. For discussion of the construction plans see H. W. Firth to Paul Martin, 30 July 1949, J. E. Gibben to R. A. Gibson, 9 September 1949, H. W. Firth to R.A. Gibson, plus attachments, 11 October 1949 all in RG 85, vol. 742, file 554/201, LAC.
96. H. A. Proctor to Dr Moore, 14 March 1949, RG 85, vol. 742, file 554/201, LAC.

97. Ibid.
98. Copy of letter from the Sisters of St Ann, per Sister Mary Mark, Supr. to Hon Colin Gibson, 9 September 1949, RG 85, vol. 742, file 554/201, LAC.
99. Commissioner J. E. Gibben to R. A. Gibson, Director, Northern Administration Branch, 7 February 1950, RG 85, vol. 742, file 554/201, LAC.
100. William C. Stewart to A. H. Gibson, 2 October 1950, RG 85, vol. 459, file 554 / 200, part 2, LAC.
101. A. H. Gibson to William C. Stewart, 27 October 1950, GOV 2206, file 1, YA.
102. See 'Progress Notes' dated 13 May 1954, 8 August 1958, 29 May 1959, 5 May 1960, 12 May 1960, 7 November 1960, 8 March 1963, 17 March 1964, 14 September 1964, 4 January 1965, 20 August 1965, 24 November 1965, 13 May 1966, 10 August 1966, 25 October 1966, 25 November 1966 in GOV 2206, file 1, YA.
103. Report 15 May 1958 Re: [name omitted], GOV 2319, file 1, YA.
104. D. R. Kinloch, Superintendent, Yukon Health Service to Commissioner of Yukon Territory, 1 April 1965 and Outline of Conditions Respecting 'Transportation Assistance (Medical)' – Government of the Yukon Territory, both in GOV 2319, file 3, YA.
105. Also hired a chief medical officer, J. M. Michael *From Sissons to Meyer: the Administrative Development of the Yukon Government, 1948–79* (Whitehorse: Yukon Archives, 1987).
106. John S. Willis, Yukon Territory Health Program, Northern Health Service, 17 November 1956, GOV 2319, file 3, YA.
107. Report of Public Health Nurse to Commissioner of Yukon Territory, 22 March 1954, GOV 2286, file 9, YA.
108. Jeckell to Gibson, 31 May 1944; for pre-war segregation see above and Coates, *Best Left as Indians*, pp. 95–6.
109. B. P. Duncan to William C. Stewart, 13 November 1950, GOV 2206, file 1, YA.
110. Granted, this description was used by Moore to justify not paying more for Native patients in the Yukon. H. A. Young to W. G. Brown, 4 June 1953, RG 85, vol. 459, file 554 / 200, part 2, LAC.
111. Duncan to Stewart, 13 November 1950.
112. Gibson to Stewart, 27 October 1950.
113. Gwich'in Social and Cultural Institute [hereafter GSCI], Elders' Biographies Project 1999–2001, interview with Lydia Elias, 19 & 21 July 2001, Tapes 35, 36.
114. Cruikshank, 'Gravel Magnet', p. 183; See also Grygier, *A Long Way from Home* for more extensive discussion from the Eastern Arctic.
115. GSCI, Arctic Red River Oral History Project 1989, interview with Annie Norbert, March 1990, Tape 1.

9 Lux, 'An Ideal Home for the Consumptive'

1. A. J. Ray, *Indians in the Fur Trade* (Toronto: University of Toronto Press, 1974), p. 46.
2. Chief John Snow, *These Mountains are Our Sacred Places* (Toronto: Samuel Stevens, 1977), p. 2.
3. I rely here on I. McKay, 'A Note on Region in Writing the History of Atlantic Canada', *Acadiensis* 29:2 (2000), p. 91; I. McKay, 'The Liberal Order Framework: A Prospectus for a Reconnaissance of Canadian History', *Canadian Historical Review*, 81:4 (December 2000), p. 625.
4. S. Razack, 'When Place Becomes Race, in S. Razack (ed.), *Race, Space, and the Law: Unmapping a White Settler Society* (Toronto: Between the Lines, 2002), p. 1; A. Bash-

ford, *Imperial Hygiene; A Critical History of Colonialism, Nationalism and Public Health* (New York: Palgrave Macmillan, 2004), p. 13.

5. M. J. Davies, 'Mapping "Region" in Canadian Medical History: The Case of British Columbia ' *Canadian Bulletin of Medical History*, 17:1–2 (2000), p. 78; see also 'Written on the Landscape: Health and Regionalism in Canada', special volume *Journal of Canadian Studies*, 41:3 (Autumn 2007).

6. C. Jones and R. Porter (eds), *Reassessing Foucault: Power, Medicine and the Body* (London: Routledge, 1994), pp. 1–2 .

7. R. McGowen, 'Power and Humanity, or Foucault among the Historians ' in Jones and Porter (eds) *Reassessing Foucault*, p. 108.

8. K. Ott, *Fevered Lives: Tuberculosis in American Culture since 1870* (Cambridge, MA: Harvard University Press, 1996), p. 1.

9. Understanding the cause did not necessarily imply a cure, at least until after 1944 when Albert Schatz and Selman Waksman discovered the antibiotic streptomycin, the first biomedical treatment for tuberculosis.

10. W. D. Johnston, 'Tuberculosis', in K. Kiple (ed.), *The Cambridge World History of Human Diseases* (Cambridge: Cambridge University Press, 1993), pp. 1059–61.

11. The physicians, N. J. Lindsay, E. H. Rouleau, R. D. Sanson, H. G. Mackid, A. E. Willis, R. G. Brett, J. D. Lafferty, A. E. Porter, G. Macdonald, and G. Arthur Inges practised in Calgary, Banff, and High River, Alberta.

12. The Aboriginal people of southern Alberta, were signatories to Treaty Six (1876) and Treaty Seven (1877).

13. A. Morris, *Treaties of Canada with the Indians of Manitoba and the North-West Territories* (1880; Saskatoon: Fifth House, 1991), p. 369.

14. Ibid.

15. Treaty Seven Elders and Tribal Council, *The True Spirit and Original Intent of Treaty Seven* with Walter Hildebrandt, Sarah Carter, and Dorothy First Rider (Montreal, QC: McGill-Queen's University Press, 1996), pp. 111–2; Snow, *These Mountains are Our Sacred Places*, p. 29.

16. Snow, *These Mountains are Our Sacred Places*, p. 39.

17. J. L. Tobias, 'Protection, Civilization, Assimilation: An Outline History of Canada's Indian Policy ' *Western Canadian Journal of Anthropology*, 6:2 (1976), pp. 13–30.

18. McKay, 'The Liberal Order Framework', p. 625.

19. The Stoney never abandoned their efforts to increase their land base despite the establishment of the Bighorn reserve in 1947–8, Snow, *These Mountains are Our Sacred Places*, p. 103.

20. C. Harris, *Making Native Space: Colonialism, Resistance, and Reserves in British Columbia* (Vancouver: University of British Columbia Press, 2002), p. xviii.

21. Scholars from a number of disciplines have studied the continuities between different institutions of isolation acknowledging Foucault's famous 'carceral archipelag' A. Bashford and C. Strange (eds.), *Isolation: Places and Practices of Exclusion* (London: Routledge, 2003), p. 2; M. Foucault, *Discipline and Punish: The Birth of the Prison*, trans. A. Sheridan, 2 edn (New York: Vintage, 1975); *Madness and Civilization: A History of Insanity in the Age of Reason* (New York: Vintage, 1984) .

22. The concept of internal frontier is addressed by Ann Laura Stoler, 'European Identities and the Cultural Politics of Exclusion in Colonial Southeast Asia', in F. Cooper and A. L. Stoler (eds), *Tensions of Empire: Colonial Cultures in a Bourgeois World* (Berkeley, CA: University of California Press, 1997), p. 199.

23. Gerald Friesen, *The Canadian Prairies: A History* (Toronto: University of Toronto Press, 1987), pp. 149–50.

24. T. Binnema and M. Niemi, 'Let the Line be Drawn Now: Wilderness, Conservation, and the Exclusion of Aboriginal People from Banff National Park in Canada', *Environmental History*, 11:4 (2006), p. 727.

25. D. Breen, *The Canadian Prairie West and the Ranching Frontier* (Toronto: University of Toronto Press, 1983), p. 11.

26. Friesen, *The Canadian Prairies*, p. 237; J. Jennings, 'Policemen and Poachers: Indian Relations on the Ranching Frontier', in A. Rasporich and H. Klassen (eds), *Frontier Calgary: Town, City, and Region, 1875–1914* (Calgary: McClelland and Stewart West, 1975), p. 93.

27. see M. K. Lux, *Medicine that Walks: Disease, Medicine, and Canadian Plains Native People, 1880–1940* (Toronto: University of Toronto Press, 2001), pp. 20–70.

28. Canada. House of Commons Debates, 27 April 1882, p. 1186.

29. Binnema and Niemi, 'Let the Line be Drawn Now', p. 727.

30. Snow, *These Mountains are Our Sacred Places*, p. 13.

31. Binnema and Niemi, 'Let the Line be Drawn Now', p. 727.

32. Ibid., p. 728.

33. Ibid., p. 725.

34. Snow, These Mountains are Our Sacred Places, p. 6.

35. 'Sanitarium' is an older form that often referred to spa-like health resorts, while 'sanatorium' came to be associated with the treatment of tuberculosis, *Valley Echo*, 36 (1955), pp. 3, 5.

36. R. Lampard, 'Robert George Brett', *Alberta History* (Spring 2003), p. 15.

37. G. McDougall and F. Harris, *Medical Clinics and Physicians of Southern Alberta* (Calgary: University of Calgary Press, 1991), p. 184.

38. Lampard, 'Robert George Brett', p. 15.

39. 'Banff Sanitarium' advertisement reprinted in McDougall and Harris, *Medical Clinics and Physicians of Southern Alberta*, p. 180.

40. McDougall and Harris, *Medical Clinics and Physicians of Southern Alberta*, p. 185; Brett's medical enterprise eventually included two drugstores and another hospital at Canmore, D. J. Hall, 'Brett, Robert George', in *Dictionary of Canadian Biography Online*, vol. 15.

41. Sarah Carter, *Lost Harvests: Prairie Indian Reserve Farmers and Government Policy* (Montreal, QC: McGill-Queen's University Press, 1990), pp. 161–2.

42. E. Churchill, 'Tsuu T'ina: A History of a First Nations Community, 1890–1940' (PhD diss. University of Calgary, 2000), p. 173.

43. Snow, *These Mountains are Our Sacred Places*, pp. 46, 50.

44. Quoted in Churchill, 'Tsuu T'ina', p. 82.

45. Ibid., p. 245.

46. On the Blackfoot reserve east of Calgary crude death rates exceeded birth rates in seven of ten years after 1884, Lux, *Medicine that Walks*, pp. 61, 63 (Tables 1.9 and 1.11).

47. The population dropped from 384 in 1885 to 329 in 1890, Churchill, 'Tsuu T'ina', p. 553.

48. Dr Neville Lindsay to assistant Indian Commissioner Forget, 31 May 1895, Records of the department of Indian Affairs, RG 10, vol. 3949, file 126,345, Library and Archives Canada (hereafter LAC); 'scrofula' refers to tuberculosis with abscess of the cervical lymph glands; 'phthisis' refers to pulmonary tuberculosis.

49. Lux, *Medicine that Walks*, p. 63 (Table 1.11).

50. Lindsay to Forget, 31 May 1895, RG10, vol. 3949, file 126,345, LAC.
51. Gage quoted in *Calgary the Denver of Canada: Its adaptability as a Health Resort and as a Site for the Dominion Sanatorium* (Calgary: Calgary Herald, 1895), p. 2.
52. *Calgary the Denver of Canada*, p. 3.
53. Ibid., p. 5.
54. Ibid., pp. 8, 9.
55. Ibid., pp. 11–15.
56. Ott, *Fevered Lines*, p. 40; see also E. Abel, *Tuberculosis and the Politics of Exclusion: A History of Public Health and Migration to Los Angeles* (New Jersey; Rutgers University Press, 2007).
57. 'J. D. Lafferty', Heber C. Jamieson papers, 25/1 Box 1, file 8, University of Alberta Archives.
58. McDougall and Harris, *Medical Clinics and Physicians of Southern Alberta*, pp. 21, 91, 159.
59. Wherrett, *The Miracle of the Empty Beds* (Toronto: University of Toronto Press, 1977), p. 39.
60. Ott, *Fevered Lines*, p. 28 .
61. G. D. Stanley, 'Early Days at the Muskoka San', *Calgary Historical Bulletin*, 18:1 (May 1953), p. 18.
62. Ibid., p. 19.
63. Ott, *Fevered Lines*, p. 1.
64. Wherrett, *The Miracle of the Empty Beds*, p. 182.
65. Ott, *Fevered Lives*, p. 7; Georgina Feldberg explains this era as the consolidation of the middle-class state in *Disease and Class: Tuberculosis and the Shaping of Modern North American Society* (New Brunswick, New Jersey: Rutgers University Press, 1995), p. 6.
66. McKay, 'The Liberal Order Framework', p. 637.
67. P. H. Bryce, *Report on the Indian Schools of Manitoba and the North-West Territories* (Ottawa: Government Printing Bureau, 1907), p. 18, RG 10, vol. 4037, file 317,021, LAC.
68. On residential schools generally see J. R. Miller, *Shingwauk's Vision* (Toronto: University of Toronto Press, 1996); J. Milloy, *A National Crime: the Canadian Government and the Residential School System, 1879 to 1986* (Winnipeg: University of Manitoba Press, 1999).
69. Lafferty to McLean, Dec. 1908, RG 10, vol. 3957, file 140,754–1 LAC.
70. Bryce to Pedley, 5 Nov. 1909, RG 10, vol. 3957, file 140,754–1 LAC; Linda Bryder, *Below the Magic Mountain: A Social History of Tuberculosis in Twentieth-Century Britain* (Oxford: Clarendon Press, 1988), p. 65.
71. D. C. Scott to Deputy Superintendent General Indian Affairs, 28 Mar. 1911, RG 10, vol. 3957, file 140,754–1 LAC.
72. Canada, House of Commons *Sessional Papers*, vol. 12, no.27, 1907, Annual Report of the Chief Medical Officer, p. 274.
73. Ibid, p. 276.
74. The reasons for tuberculosis decline in the Western world are not altogether clear, but it is apparent that improved sanitation, higher levels of prosperity, and cleaner workplaces had an impact, L. Bryder, *Below the Magic Mountain* (Oxford: Clarendon Press, 1988), p. 2; F. B. Smith, *The Retreat of Tuberculosis, 1850–1950* (London Croom Helm, 1988), p. 1; T. McKeown, *The Modern Rise of Population* (London: Edward Arnold, 1976), p.

92; R. Dubos and J. Dubos, *The White Plague: Tuberculosis, Man And Society* (Boston, MA: Little, Brown, 1952), p. 185.

75. Wherrett, *The Miracle of the Empty Beds*, pp. 174–96.
76. Quoted in C. Stuart Houston, *R. G. Ferguson: Crusader Against Tuberculosis* (Toronto: Dundurn, Associated Medical Services, 1991), p. 51.
77. Bashford, *Imperial Hygiene*, p. 64.
78. In 1924 forty beds at Saskatchewan's Fort Qu'Appelle sanatorium were allocated for Aboriginal patients in order to pay debts to the federal government. These beds were the extent of sanatorium treatment for Aboriginal people in the Canadian west, *R.G. Ferguson*, p. 92.
79. Stewart to Bracken, 14 November 1934, RG29 (Records of the department of National Health and Welfare) vol. 1225, file 311–T7–16, LAC.
80. Dr Wodehouse, executive secretary CTA to Dr Carmichael, 4 September 1924, RG 10 vol. 3958, file 140,754–3, LAC.
81. In Alberta there were hospitals on the Blood, Blackfoot, Stoney, and Hobbema reserves.
82. Churchill, 'Tsuu T'ina', p. 394.
83. Lafferty to McLean Dec 1908, RG10, vol. 3957, file 140,754–, LAC.
84. F. A. Corbett to Graham, 7 Dec 1920, RG10, vol. 4092, file 546898, LAC.
85. quoted in Churchill, 'Tsuu T'ina', p. 396.
86. Churchill, 'Tsuu T'ina', p. 393.
87. McGill Papers, M742, box 4, file 36 'Correspondence, 1928–41' Glenbow Archives Institute (GAI).
88. Baker Memorial Sanatorium, 1917–37, file 73.315/37, box 2, Public Archives of Alberta (PAA); *Calgary the Denver of Canada*, p. 5 .
89. quoted in Churchill, 'Tsuu T'ina', p. 413 .
90. P. H. Bryce, *The Story of a National Crime: Being an Appeal for Justice to the Indians of Canada* (Ottawa: James Hope and Sons, 1922).
91. Wherrett, *Miracle of the Empty Beds*, p. 110.
92. On these transformations in Canada see, for example, Gagan and Gagan, *For Patients of Moderate Means*; in the United States see Charles Rosenberg, *The Care of Strangers: The Rise of America's Hospital System* (New York: Basic Books, 1987); R. Stevens, *In Sickness and Wealth: American Hospitals in the Twentieth Century* (New York: Basic Books, 1989); D. Rosner, *A Once Charitable Enterprise: Hospitals and Health Care in Brooklyn and New York, 1885–1915* (New York: Cambridge University Press, 1982); J. D. Thompson and G. Goldin, *The Hospital: A Social and Architectural History* (New Haven, CT: Yale University Press, 1975).
93. J. Wishart, 'Class Difference and the Reformation of Ontario Public Hospitals, 1900–35', *Labour Le Travail*, 48 (2001), pp. 27–61; M. Cortiula, 'Social Class and Health Care in a Community Institution: The Case of Hamilton City Hospital', *Canadian Bulletin of Medical History*, 6 (1989), pp. 133–45; Gagan and Gagan, *For Patients of Moderate Means*, pp. 39–40.
94. M.-E. Kelm, *Colonizing Bodies: Aboriginal Health and Healing in British Columbia, 1900–50* (Vancouver: University of British Columbia Press, 1998), pp. 136–7; for the north see K. Coates, *Best Left as Indians; Native-White Relations in the Yukon Territory, 1840–1973* (Montreal and Kingston: McGill-Queen's University Press, 1991), p. 95; in Manitoba the St Boniface sanatorium operated by the Grey Nuns had a separate 'Indian Building', J. D. Adamson to J. McEachern, 15 July 1939, RG29, vol. 2590, file 800–1–D297, part 1, LAC.

95. Wherrett, *The Miracle of the Empty Beds*, p. 117.
96. J. W. Fry to Ian McKenzie, minister of Veterans Affairs, 4 Oct. 1945, RG29, vol. 2592, file 800–1–D479, part 1, LAC.
97. Edmonton *Bulletin*, 2 November 1945.
98. Officers Alberta Provincial Command of the Canadian Legion to Prime Minister, 13 Oct 1945, RG29, vol. 2592, file 800–1–D479, part 1, LAC.
99. J. Allison Glen to Mr. Mayor, RG29, vol. 2592, file 800–1–D479, part 1 LAC.
100. Edmonton *Bulletin*, 14 November 1945, 'Protest Indian Hospital Here'.
101. H. Darling, Superintendent RCMP, Edmonton, 26 Nov 1945, 'Confidential and Urgent' RG29, vol. 2592, file 800–1–D479, part 1 LAC.
102. Minister of National Health and Welfare to W.H Hobbins, 27 November 1945, RG 29, vol. 2592, file 800–1–D479, part 1 LAC.
103. Charles Camsell was born in the north. As a geologist, commissioner of the Northwest Territories, and deputy minister of Mines and Resources he took a direct role in much of the mining development in the north. His life spanned the era of technological and economic change that was captured in the term 'opening the north'. Charles Camsell, *Son of the North* (Toronto: Ryerson, 1954).
104. P. E. Moore to Max Freedman, 4 Dec 1945, RG 29, vol. 2592, file 800–1–D479, part 1 LAC.
105. C. Gray, 'Profile: Percy Moore', *Canadian Medical Association Journal*, 126 (February 1982), p. 416; Institutional expansion continued and by the 1960s there were twenty-two Indian hospitals in Canada, most of them in similarly borrowed military buildings, T. Kue Young, *Health Care and Cultural Change* (Toronto: University of Toronto Press, 1988), p. 88.

10 Živković, 'Places of Power and Memory in Post-Milošević Serbia'

1. C. A. Meier, 'The Dream in Ancient Greece and its use in Temple Cures', in G. E. von Grunebaum and R. Caillois (eds), *The Dream and Human Societies* (Berkeley, CA: University of California Press, 1966), p. 318.
2. See for instance N. Munn, 'Symbolism in a Ritual Context: Aspects of Symbolic Action', in J. J. Honigmann (ed.), *Handbook of Social and Cultural Anthropology* (Chicago, IL: Rand McNally, 1973); J. Dow, 'Universal Aspects of Symbolic Healing: A Theoretical Synthesis', *American Anthropologist*, 88:1 (1986); L. J. Kirmayer, 'The Cultural Diversity of Healing: Meaning, Metaphor and Mechanism', British Medical Bulletin, 69 (2004).
3. M. Douglas, *Purity and Danger* (1966; London and New York, Routledge, 2002); M. Douglas, *Natural Symbols: Explorations in Cosmology* (New York: Pantheon Books, 1982).
4. M. Taussig, *The Devil and Commodity Fetishism in South America* (Chapel Hill, NC: University of North Carolina Press, 1980).
5. Interview with the author.
6. D. Pjević, *Kremansko proročanstvo: Izvor novih inspiracija (u svetlu novih dogadjaja)* (Kremna: Turistička agencija Kremnaturist, 2005).
7. Pjević, *Kremansko proročanstvo*, p. 15.
8. N. R. Kazimirović *Čaranje, gatanje, vrčanje i proricanje u našem narodu: prilog ispitivanju tajanstvenih duhovnih pojava* (Biblioteka reprint izdanja. Beograd: Knjižarnica Milorada P. Milanovića, 1941).

9. See S. Pavlović '"Mirror, Mirror on the Wall...": Prophecies, Horoscopes, and the Politics of the Paranormal in Serbia', *Spaces of Identity*, 1:1 (1992–2000).
10. Pjević, *Kremansko proročanstvo*, p. 89–90)
11. V. Antonić, *Kremansko neproročanstvo: studije jedne obmane* (Beograd: Voja Antonić, 2002).
12. Pjević, *Kremansko proročanstvo*, p. 15.
13. Ibid., p. 85.
14. Ibid., p. 86.
15. See Y. Bilu, 'Oneirobiography and Oneirocommunity in Saint Worship in Israel: A Two-Tier Model for Dream-Inspired Religious Revivals', *Dreaming*, 10:2 (2000).
16. P. Bokun *Poreklo kremanskih proročanstava* (Beograd: Draganić, 2002), p.27.
17. i.e. J. Marić, *Kakvi smo mi Srbi? Prilozi za karakterologiju Srba*, 3rd edn (Beograd: J. Marić, 1998).
18. i.e. D. Kecmanović, *Ethnic Times: Exploring Ethnonationalism in the Former Yugoslavia* (Westport, CT: Praeger Publishers, 2001)
19. M. Živković, 'Inverted Perspective and Serbian Peasants: Antiquities and the Byzantine Revival in Serbia', in A. C. Gow (ed.), *Hyphenated Histories: Central European Bildung and Slavic Studies in the Contemporary Academy* (Leiden: Brill, 2007).
20. Živković, 'We are Gypsy People Cursed by Fate: Dealing with Balkan Stigma in Serbia and Croatia', paper read at the Second Conference of the Association for Balkan Anthropology (ABA), 4–7 September 1997, at Bucharest, Romania; Živković, 'Jelly, Slush and Red Mists: Poetics of Amorphous Substances in Serbian Jeremiads of the 1990s', *Anthropology and Humanism*, 25:2; D. Iordanova, *Cinema of Flames: Balkan Film, Culture and the Media* (London: British Film Institute, 2001)
21. M. Ivy, *Discourses of the Vanishing: Modernity, Phantasm, Japan* (Chicago, IL and London: The University of Chicago Press, 1995), and L. Greenfeld, *Nationalism: Five Roads to Modernity* (Cambridge, MA and London: Harvard University Press, 1992).
22. V. Ćorović, *Sveti Sava u narodnom predanju* (Biblioteka Nasledje; kolo 1, knj. 1. Beograd: Narodno delo; Zadruga pravoslavnog sveštenstva SFRJ, 1990), V. Čajkanović, *Mit i religija u Srba: izabrane studije*, ed. V. Djurić (Beograd: Srpska književna zadruga, 1973), and *O magiji i religiji*. ed. S. Velmar-Janković (Biblioteka Baština; 8. Beograd: Prosveta, 1985)
23. M. Bećković, 'Srpska geografija je opredmećena biografija Svetog Save', in M. M. Radivojević and S. M. Stanišić (eds), *Živi zlatokrug: Pesme i zapisi o Svetom Savi* (Loznica: Samostalna izdavačka radnja Dragan Djordjević, 1990), pp. 84, 86, emphasis added.
24. See for instance N. Munn, 'The Transformation of Subjects into Objects in Walbiri and Pitjantjara Myth', in R. M. Berndt (ed.), *Australian Aboriginal Anthropology: Modern Studies in the Social Anthropology of the Australian Aborigines* (Nedlands: University of Western Australia Press, 1970).
25. K. Basso, *Wisdom Sits in Places: Landscape and Language among the Western Apache* (Albuquerque, NM: University of New Mexico Press, 1996).
26. Munn, 'Symbolism in a Ritual Context', p. 597.
27. Glas javnosti Internet edition, Sunday, 12 October 2003 www.glas-javnosti.co.yu accessed 27 October 2007.

INDEX